T0227150

Anesthesia, Sedation, and Pain Control

Editors

SHANNON E.G. HAMRICK
CALEB ING

CLINICS IN
PERINATOLOGY

www.perinatology.theclinics.com

Consulting Editor
LUCKY JAIN

December 2019 • Volume 46 • Number 4

ELSEVIER

1600 John F. Kennedy Boulevard • Suite 1800 • Philadelphia, Pennsylvania, 19103-2899

http://www.theclinics.com

CLINICS IN PERINATOLOGY Volume 46, Number 4
December 2019 ISSN 0095-5108, ISBN-13: 978-0-323-75550-4

Editor: Kerry Holland
Developmental Editor: Casey Potter

© **2019 Elsevier Inc. All rights reserved.**

This periodical and the individual contributions contained in it are protected under copyright by Elsevier, and the following terms and conditions apply to their use:

Photocopying
Single photocopies of single articles may be made for personal use as allowed by national copyright laws. Permission of the Publisher and payment of a fee is required for all other photocopying, including multiple or systematic copying, copying for advertising or promotional purposes, resale, and all forms of document delivery. Special rates are available for educational institutions that wish to make photocopies for non-profit educational classroom use. For information on how to seek permission visit www.elsevier.com/permissions or call: (+44) 1865 843830 (UK)/(+1) 215 239 3804 (USA).

Derivative Works
Subscribers may reproduce tables of contents or prepare lists of articles including abstracts for internal circulation within their institutions. Permission of the Publisher is required for resale or distribution outside the institution. Permission of the Publisher is required for all other derivative works, including compilations and translations (please consult www.elsevier.com/permissions).

Electronic Storage or Usage
Permission of the Publisher is required to store or use electronically any material contained in this periodical, including any article or part of an article (please consult www.elsevier.com/permissions). Except as outlined above, no part of this publication may be reproduced, stored in a retrieval system or transmitted in any form or by any means, electronic, mechanical, photocopying, recording or otherwise, without prior written permission of the Publisher.

Notice
No responsibility is assumed by the Publisher for any injury and/or damage to persons or property as a matter of products liability, negligence or otherwise, or from any use or operation of any methods, products, instructions or ideas contained in the material herein. Because of rapid advances in the medical sciences, in particular, independent verification of diagnoses and drug dosages should be made. Although all advertising material is expected to conform to ethical (medical) standards, inclusion in this publication does not constitute a guarantee or endorsement of the quality or value of such product or of the claims made of it by its manufacturer.

Clinics in Perinatology (ISSN 0095-5108) is published quarterly by Elsevier Inc., 360 Park Avenue South, New York, NY 10010-1710. Months of issue are March, June, September, and December. Business and Editorial Offices: 1600 John F. Kennedy Blvd., Ste. 1800, Philadelphia, PA 19103-2899. Customer Service Office: 3251 Riverport Lane, Maryland Heights, MO 63043. Periodicals postage paid at New York, NY and additional mailing offices. Subscription prices are $309.00 per year (US individuals), $578.00 per year (US institutions), $365.00 per year (Canadian individuals), $708.00 per year (Canadian institutions), $435.00 per year (international individuals), $708.00 per year (international institutions), $100.00 per year (US students), and $195.00 per year (Canadian and international students). International air speed delivery is included in all Clinics subscription prices. All prices are subject to change without notice. **POSTMASTER:** Send address changes to *Clinics in Perinatology*, Elsevier Health Sciences Division, Subscription Customer Service, 3251 Riverport Lane, Maryland Heights, MO 63043. **Customer Service: Telephone: 1-800-654-2452** (U.S. and Canada); **1-314-447-8871** (outside U.S. and Canada). **Fax: 1-314-447-8029. E-mail: journalscustomerservice-usa@elsevier.com** (for print support); **journalsonlinesupport-usa@elsevier.com** (for online support).

Reprints. For copies of 100 or more, of articles in this publication, please contact the Commercial Reprints Department, Elsevier Inc., 360 Park Avenue South, New York, NY 10010-1710. Tel. 212-633-3874; Fax: 212-633-3820; E-mail: reprints@elsevier.com.

Clinics in Perinatology is also pubished in Spanish by McGraw-Hill Interamericana Editores S.A., P.O. Box 5-237, 06500 Mexico D.F., Mexico.

Clinics in Perinatology is covered in *MEDLINE/PubMed (Index Medicus) Current Contents, Excepta Medica, BIOSIS and ISI/BIOMED.*

Contributors

CONSULTING EDITOR

LUCKY JAIN, MD, MBA
George W. Brumley Jr Professor and Chair, Emory University School of Medicine, Department of Pediatrics, Chief Academic Officer, Children's Healthcare of Atlanta, Executive Director, Emory and Children's Pediatric Institute, Atlanta, Georgia, USA

EDITORS

SHANNON E.G. HAMRICK, MD
Associate Professor of Pediatrics, Divisions of Neonatology and Cardiology, Emory University and Children's Healthcare of Atlanta, Emory Children's Center, Atlanta, Georgia, USA

CALEB ING, MD, MS
Associate Professor of Anesthesiology (in Epidemiology), Division of Pediatric Anesthesia, Columbia University Irving Medical Center, New York, New York, USA

AUTHORS

DEAN B. ANDROPOULOS, MD, MHCM
Department of Anesthesiology, Perioperative and Pain Medicine, Anesthesiologist-in-Chief, Texas Children's Hospital, Professor, Anesthesiology and Pediatrics, Vice Chair for Clinical Affairs, Department of Anesthesiology, Baylor College of Medicine, Houston, Texas, USA

KEN BRADY, MD
Division Head, Cardiac Anesthesia, Lurie Children's Hospital of Chicago, Professor, Anesthesiology and Pediatrics, Northwestern University Feinberg School of Medicine, Chicago, Illinois, USA

NICOLA GROES CLAUSEN, MD, PhD
Department of Anesthesiology and Intensive Care, Odense University Hospital, Odense, Denmark

NICOLA DISMA, MD
Department of Anesthesia, IRCCS Istituto Giannina Gaslini, Genoa, Italy

JAMESIA DONATO, MD
Neonatal-Perinatal Medicine Fellow, Division of Neonatology, Children's Mercy Hospital, Kansas City, Missouri, USA

ROBERT A. DYER, MBChB, FCA (SA), PhD
Emeritus Professor, Department of Anaesthesia and Perioperative Medicine, University of Cape Town, Groote Schuur Hospital, Cape Town, South Africa

RONALD BLAINE EASLEY, MD
Department of Anesthesiology, Perioperative and Pain Medicine, Associate
Anesthesiologist-in-Chief for Academic Affairs, Texas Children's Hospital,
Professor, Anesthesiology and Pediatrics, Baylor College of Medicine, Houston, Texas,
USA

NICOLE L. FERNANDES, MBChB, DA (SA), FCA (SA)
Doctor, Department of Anaesthesia and Perioperative Medicine, University of Cape Town,
Groote Schuur Hospital, Cape Town, South Africa

MARÍA V. FRAGA, MD
Associate Professor of Clinical Pediatrics, Perelman School of Medicine, University of
Pennsylvania, Attending Neonatologist, The Children's Hospital of Philadelphia,
Philadelphia, Pennsylvania

YEHUDA GINOSAR, BSc, MBBS
Director, Mother and Child Anesthesia Unit, Associate Professor, Department of
Anesthesiology, Critical Care, and Pain Medicine, Hebrew University – Hadassah School
of Medicine, Director, Anesthesia Research Institute, Faculty, The Wohl Institute for
Translational Medicine, Hadassah Hebrew University Medical Center, Ein Karem
Campus, Jerusalem, Israel; Professor of Anesthesiology, Obstetrics and Gynecology,
Division of Obstetric Anesthesiology, Washington University School of Medicine, Barnes
Jewish Hospital, St Louis, Missouri, USA

ERIN A. GOTTLIEB, MD
Chief of Pediatric Cardiac Anesthesiology, Dell Children's Medical Center, Associate
Professor of Surgery and Perioperative Care, The University of Texas at Austin Dell
Medical School, Austin, Texas, USA

TOM G. HANSEN, MD, PhD
Department of Anesthesiology & Intensive Care – Pediatrics, Odense University Hospital,
Department of Clinical Research – Anesthesiology, University of Southern Denmark,
Odense, Denmark

CELESTE JOHNSTON, RN, DEd, FCAHS
Professor Emeritus, Ingram School of Nursing, McGill University, Montreal, Canada;
Scientist, IWK Health Centre, Halifax, Canada

PETE G. KOVATSIS, MD, FAAP
Assistant Professor, Department of Anesthesiology, Critical Care and Pain Medicine,
Boston Children's Hospital, Harvard Medical School, Boston, Massachusetts, USA

ELIZABETH E. KRANS, MD, MSc
Assistant Professor, Department of Obstetrics, Gynecology and Reproductive Sciences,
University of Pittsburgh, Magee-Womens Research Institute, Pittsburgh, Pennsylvania,
USA

ALLISON LEE, MD, MS
Associate Professor, Department of Anesthesiology, Columbia University Medical Center,
Columbia University, New York, New York, USA

TAMORAH LEWIS, MD, PhD
Assistant Professor, Department of Pediatrics, Divisions of Neonatology and Pediatric
Clinical Pharmacology, UMKC School of Medicine, Children's Mercy Hospital, Kansas
City, Missouri, USA

KATHRYN DEE LIZCANO MacMILLAN, MD, MPH
Clinical Associate, Divisions of Neonatology and Newborn Medicine, and Pediatric Hospital Medicine, Massachusetts General Hospital for Children, Good Samaritan Medical Center, Boston, Massachusetts, USA

CARRIE P. MALAVOLTA, MSN, MBE, PNP
Pediatric Neurology Nurse Practitioner, The Children's Hospital of Philadelphia, Philadelphia, Pennsylvania, USA

CAITLIN E. MARTIN, MD, MPH
Assistant Professor, Department of Obstetrics and Gynecology, Virginia Commonwealth University, Richmond, Virginia, USA

LYNNE G. MAXWELL, MD, FAAP
Emeritus Professor, Anesthesiology and Critical Care, Perelman School of Medicine at the University of Pennsylvania, Senior Anesthesiologist, The Children's Hospital of Philadelphia, Philadelphia, Pennsylvania, USA

CAROL McNAIR, RN(EC), MN, PhD(c), NP-Pediatrics, NNP-BC
Neonatal Nurse Practitioner, Nursing and Child Health Evaluative Sciences, The Hospital for Sick Children, Toronto, Canada

WARWICK NGAN KEE, BHB, MBChB, MD, FANZCA, FHKCA, FHKAM (Anaesthesiology)
Chair, Professor, Department of Anesthesiology, Sidra Medicine, Weill Cornell Medicine–Qatar, Doha, Qatar

JAMES D. O'LEARY, MBBCh, MM, MD, FCARCSI
Associate Professor, Department of Anesthesia, University of Toronto, Toronto, Ontario, Canada

RAYMOND S. PARK, MD
Instructor, Department of Anesthesiology, Critical Care and Pain Medicine, Boston Children's Hospital, Harvard Medical School, Boston, Massachusetts, USA

JAMES M. PEYTON, MBChB, MRCP, FRCA
Assistant Professor, Department of Anesthesiology, Critical Care and Pain Medicine, Boston Children's Hospital, Harvard Medical School, Boston, Massachusetts, USA

KARISHMA RAO, MD
Neonatal-Perinatal Medicine Fellow, Division of Neonatology, Children's Mercy Hospital, Kansas City, Missouri, USA

LAURENCE E. RING, MD
Assistant Professor of Anesthesiology, Director of Fetal Anesthesia, Columbia University Medical Center, New York, New York, USA

ANNA TADDIO, BScPhm, MSc, PhD
Professor, Clinical, Social and Administrative Pharmacy, Leslie Dan Faculty of Pharmacy, University of Toronto, Senior Associate Scientist, Child Health Evaluative Sciences, The Hospital for Sick Children, Toronto, Ontario, Canada

MISHKA TERPLAN, MD, MPH
Senior Researcher, Friends Research Institute, Baltimore, Maryland, USA

EMMETT E. WHITAKER, MD
Assistant Professor of Anesthesiology and Neurological Sciences, University of Vermont Larner College of Medicine, University of Vermont Medical Center, Burlington, Vermont, USA

ROBERT K. WILLIAMS, MD
Chris Abajian, MD & Margret Abajian Professor of Pediatric Anesthesia, University of Vermont Larner College of Medicine, University of Vermont Medical Center, Burlington, Vermont, USA

MARSHA CAMPBELL YEO, RN, PhD NNP-BC
Clinician Scientist, Department of Pediatrics, IWK Health Centre, Associate Professor, School of Nursing, Faculty of Health Professions, Dalhousie University, Halifax, Nova Scotia, Canada

Contents

In 2017, the US Food and Drug Administration warned that exposure to anesthetic medicines for lengthy periods of time or over multiple surgeries may affect brain development in children aged less than 3 years. Since then, the clinical literature continues to find mixed evidence of pediatric anesthesia-related neurotoxicity. However, several new human studies provide strong evidence that a single short exposure to general anesthesia in young children does not cause detectable neurocognitive injury by neuropsychological testing. These newer findings are reassuring, but cannot be extrapolated to children who are deemed to be at highest risk of neurologic injury after anesthesia.

Diagnostic and invasive procedures in premature infants may require general anesthesia. General anesthetics interfere with the development of the immature animal brain. Accelerated apoptosis, disturbed synaptogenesis, and cytoarchitecture are among the mechanisms suspected to underlie this phenomenon. The implications for humans are unknown. This article presents current suspected mechanisms of anesthesia-induced neurotoxicity and elaborates on the difficulties in translating results from animal research to human. Ethical considerations limit the conduct of such experiments in human neonates, but the use of animal models is still considered feasible. Vulnerable periods in brain development need further identification as do neurotoxic and neuroprotective interventions.

Neurodevelopmental outcomes after neonatal congenital heart surgery are significantly influenced by brain injury detectable by MRI imaging techniques. This brain injury can occur in the prenatal and postnatal periods even before cardiac surgery. Given the significant incidence of new MRI brain injury after cardiac surgery, much work is yet to be done on strategies to detect, prevent, and treat brain injury in the neonatal period in order to optimize longer-term neurodevelopmental outcomes.

This article reviews the benefits, risks, and applications of neuraxial anesthesia in neonates.

Raymond S. Park, James M. Peyton, and Pete G. Kovatsis

Safe and effective airway management of neonates requires unique knowledge and clinical skills. Practitioners should have an understanding of neonatal airway anatomy and respiratory physiology and their clinical implications related to airway management. It is vital to recognize the potential sequelae of prematurity. Clinicians should be familiar with the skills and techniques available for managing normal neonatal airways. This review provides stepwise considerations for managing the neonatal airway: specific considerations for neonatal airway management, assessment and preparation, induction and premedication, and techniques and strategies for airway management in patients with normal anatomy and in patients who are difficult to intubate.

Allison Lee and Warwick Ngan Kee

Maternal hemodynamics, positioning, and anesthesia technique for cesarean delivery influence neonatal acid–base balance; direct effects from drugs that cross the placenta also have an influence. Spinal anesthesia limits fetal exposure to depressant drugs and avoids maternal airway instrumentation, but is associated with hypotension. Hypotension may be prevented/treated with vasopressors and intravenous fluids. Current evidence supports phenylephrine as the first-line vasopressor. Fifteen degrees of lateral tilt during cesarean delivery has been advocated to relieve vena caval obstruction, but routine use may be unnecessary in healthy nonobese women having elective cesarean delivery if maternal blood pressure is maintained near baseline.

Nicole L. Fernandes and Robert A. Dyer

Cesarean section (CS) is a common surgical procedure worldwide. The anesthesiologist is responsible, together with obstetrician and neonatologist, for safe perioperative management. A continuum of risk exists for urgent CS. The decision-to-delivery interval is an important audit tool, to ensure international standards are upheld and good outcomes for mother and neonate are achieved. Urgent CS may be performed under either GA or RA, with benefits and risks attributable to each. Specific clinical scenarios require an individualized approach to anesthesia, including hemorrhage, hypertensive disorders, cardiac disease, the difficult airway and fetal compromise. Ongoing training is integral to the provision of safe anesthesia.

Laurence E. Ring and Yehuda Ginosar

Advances in imaging and technique have pushed the boundaries of the types of surgical interventions available to fetuses with congenital and

developmental abnormalities. This review focuses on fundamental aspects of fetal anesthesia, including the physiologic changes of pregnancy,
uteroplacental perfusion, and fetal physiology. We discuss the types of
fetal surgeries and procedures currently being performed and discuss
the specific anesthetic approaches to different categories of fetal surgeries. We also discuss ethical aspects of fetal surgery and anesthesia.

The incidence of neonatal abstinence syndrome owing to prenatal opioid
exposure has grown rapidly in recent decades and it disproportionately affects rural, non-white, and public insurance–dependent populations.
Treatment consists of pharmacologic and nonpharmacologic interventions with wide variability in approaches across the United States. Standardizing clinical assessment, minimizing unnecessary interruptions, and
prioritizing nonpharmacologic and family-centered care seems to improve
hospital outcomes. Neonatal abstinence syndrome may have long-term
developmental and biological effects, but understanding is limited owing
in part confounding biosocial factors. Early intervention and longitudinal
support of the infant and family promote better outcomes.

Women are being disproportionately affected by the opioid crisis,
including during pregnancy. Pain and other vulnerabilities to addiction
differ between men and women. Management of opioid use disorder
should be gender informed and accessible across the lifespan. During
pregnancy, care teams should be multidisciplinary to include obstetrics,
addiction, social work, anesthesia, pediatrics, and behavioral health.
Pain management for women with opioid use disorder requires tailored approaches, including integration of trauma-informed care and addressing
psychosocial needs. Thus, coordinated continued care by obstetric and
addiction providers through pregnancy into postpartum is key to supporting women in recovery.

PROGRAM OBJECTIVE

The goal of *Clinics in Perinatology* is to keep practicing perinatologists, neonatologists, obstetricians, practicing physicians and residents up to date with current clinical practice in perinatology by providing timely articles reviewing the state of the art in patient care.

TARGET AUDIENCE

Perinatologists, neonatologists, obstetricians, practicing physicians, residents and healthcare professionals who provide patient care utilizing findings from *Clinics in Perinatology*.

LEARNING OBJECTIVES

Upon completion of this activity, participants will be able to:
1. Review best practices for assessing pain, safely controlling pain, and sedation in the newborn patient.
2. Discuss current evidence on epidemiology and predictive factors, evolving assessment and treatment models, and current understanding of post-discharge considerations and long-term outcomes for infants with Neonatal Abstinence Syndrome (NAS).
3. Recognize the impact of both giving and not giving anesthetic and sedative agents to care for pediatric patients in the perinatal and neonatal period.

ACCREDITATION

The Elsevier Office of Continuing Medical Education (EOCME) is accredited by the Accreditation Council for Continuing Medical Education (ACCME) to provide continuing medical education for physicians.

The EOCME designates this journal-based CME activity for a maximum of 13 *AMA PRA Category 1 Credit(s)*™. Physicians should claim only the credit commensurate with the extent of their participation in the activity.

All other health care professionals requesting continuing education credit for this enduring material will be issued a certificate of participation.

DISCLOSURE OF CONFLICTS OF INTEREST

The EOCME assesses conflict of interest with its instructors, faculty, planners, and other individuals who are in a position to control the content of CME activities. All relevant conflicts of interest that are identified are thoroughly vetted by EOCME for fair balance, scientific objectivity, and patient care recommendations. EOCME is committed to providing its learners with CME activities that promote improvements or quality in healthcare and not a specific proprietary business or a commercial interest.

The planning committee, staff, authors and editors listed below have identified no financial relationships or relationships to products or devices they or their spouse/life partner have with commercial interest related to the content of this CME activity:
Dean B. Andropoulos, MD, MHCM; Ken Brady, MD; Nicola Groes Clausen, MD, PhD; Nicola Disma, MD; Jamesia Donato, MD; Robert A. Dyer, MBChB, FCA (SA), PhD; R. Blaine Easley, MD; Nicole L. Fernandes, MBChB, DA (SA), FCA (SA); María V. Fraga, MD; Yehuda Ginosar, BSc, MBBS; Erin A. Gottlieb, MD; Shannon E.G. Hamrick, MD; Tom G. Hansen, MD, PhD; Kerry Holland; Caleb H. Ing, MD, MS; Lucky Jain; Celeste Johnston, RN, DEd, FCAHS; Warwick Ngan Kee, BHB, MBChB, MD, FANZCA, FHKCA, FHKAM(Anaesthesiology); Alison Kemp; Elizabeth E. Krans, MD, MSc; Allison Lee, MD; Tamorah Lewis, MD, PhD; Kathryn Dee Lizcano MacMillan, MD, MPH; Carrie P. Malavolta, MSN, CRNP; Caitlin E. Martin, MD, MPH; Lynne G. Maxwell, MD, FAAP; Carol McNair, RN(EC), MN, PhD(c), NP-Pediatrics, NNP-BC; James D. O'Leary, MBBCh, MM, MD, FCARCSI; Raymond S. Park, MD; James M. Peyton, MBChB, MRCP, FRCA; Karishma Rao, MD; Laurence E. Ring, MD; Anna Taddio, BScPhm, MSc, PhD; Mishka Terplan, MD, MPH; Swaminathan Nagarajan; Emmett E. Whitaker, MD; Robert K. Williams, MD; Marsha Campbell Yeo, RN, PhD NNP-BC.

The planning committee, staff, authors and editors listed below have identified financial relationships or relationships to products or devices they or their spouse/life partner have with commercial interest related to the content of this CME activity:
Pete. G. Kovatsis, MD, FAAP: consultant/advisor for Verathon Inc.

UNAPPROVED/OFF-LABEL USE DISCLOSURE

The EOCME requires CME faculty to disclose to the participants:
1. When products or procedures being discussed are off-label, unlabelled, experimental, and/or investigational (not US Food and Drug Administration [FDA] approved); and

2. Any limitations on the information presented, such as data that are preliminary or that represent ongoing research, interim analyses, and/or unsupported opinions. Faculty may discuss information about pharmaceutical agents that is outside of FDA-approved labelling. This information is intended solely for CME and is not intended to promote off-label use of these medications. If you have any questions, contact the medical affairs department of the manufacturer for the most recent prescribing information.

TO ENROLL

To enroll in the *Clinics in Perinatology* Continuing Medical Education program, call customer service at 1-800-654-2452 or sign up online at http://www.theclinics.com/home/cme. The CME program is available to subscribers for an additional annual fee of 244.40 USD.

METHOD OF PARTICIPATION

In order to claim credit, participants must complete the following:
1. Complete enrolment as indicated above.
2. Read the activity.
3. Complete the CME Test and Evaluation. Participants must achieve a score of 70% on the test. All CME Tests and Evaluations must be completed online.

CME INQUIRIES/SPECIAL NEEDS

For all CME inquiries or special needs, please contact elsevierCME@elsevier.com.

CLINICS IN PERINATOLOGY

SERIES OF RELATED INTEREST

Pediatric Clinics
https://www.pediatric.theclinics.com/

THE CLINICS ARE AVAILABLE ONLINE!
Access your subscription at:
www.theclinics.com

Foreword

First, Do No Harm

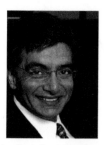

Lucky Jain, MD, MBA
Consulting Editor

One of the foundational principles in medicine that has been passed from generation to generation is rooted in the Latin phrase "primum non nocere": *first do no harm*. The Hippocratic Oath emphasizes it, and we all began our medical careers firmly believing in the principle of nonmaleficence. When confronted with a problem or condition that we are planning to treat, we must give due consideration to any potential harm, particularly when the risk of harm outweighs potential gains. Yet, medicine is replete with practices for which the balance is tilted in the wrong direction. The recently recognized opioid crisis in the United States is an example of how safeguards around potentially harmful therapies can erode over time. It is estimated that more than 700,000 people died from drug overdose from 1999 to 2017 with a majority of deaths in recent years implicating opioids (68% in 2017).[1] On average, a staggering 130 Americans die from opioid overdose every day.[1]

Pregnant women and their newborns have not been spared in this epidemic, which can be described as having occurred in 3 distinct waves (**Fig. 1**).[1] The initial period began with a sharp rise in opioid prescriptions in the 1990s. During this period, the medical profession witnessed a rise in the use of natural and semisynthetic opioids in the 1990s. In phase 2, the culprit was heroin, with a rise in overdose deaths starting in 2010. The third phase (starting in 2013) saw a sharp rise in overuse of fentanyl and other synthetic opioids.

Why is this discussion important to the current issue of the *Clinics in Perinatology* on Anesthesia, Sedation, and Pain Control? For one, neonatologists have struggled with a similar conundrum of pain management in sick newborns, and the impact excessive opioid use may have had on short- and long-term outcomes.[2,3] I often wonder about babies I took care of decades ago who received morphine or fentanyl drips for weeks before being put on methadone regimens to soften their withdrawal.

As is the case with many things in our environment, the pendulum often swings from one extreme to another. Safe delivery of anesthesia, sedation, and pain medicines is of

Clin Perinatol 46 (2019) xv–xvi
https://doi.org/10.1016/j.clp.2019.09.001
0095-5108/19/© 2019 Published by Elsevier Inc.

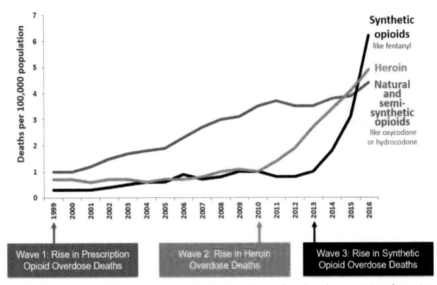

Fig. 1. Three waves of the increasing opioid crisis. (Reproduced with permission from Centers for Disease Control and Prevention. Opioid overdose. Understanding the epidemic. 2017. Available at: http://www.cdc.gov/drugoverdose/epidemic/index.html. Accessed August 25, 2019.)

critical importance to us all, just as it is to minimize unintended harm.[4] These issues have been covered in great depth in this issue of the *Clinics in Perinatology* edited by Drs Ing and Hamrick. As always, I am grateful to the publishing staff at Elsevier, including Kerry Holland and Casey Potter, for their support in covering this important topic for you.

Lucky Jain, MD, MBA
Emory University School of Medicine, and Children's Healthcare of Atlanta
1760 Haygood Drive NE
Atlanta, GA 30322, USA

E-mail address:
ljain@emory.edu

REFERENCES

1. Centers for Disease Control and Prevention. Opioid overdose. Understanding the epidemic. 2017. Available at: http://www.cdc.gov/drugoverdose/epidemic/index.html. Accessed August 25, 2019.
2. Rummans TA, Burton C, Dawson NL. How good intentions contributed to bad outcomes: the opioid crisis. Mayo Clin Proc 2018;93:344–50.
3. Price HR, Collier AC, Wright TE. Screening pregnant women and their neonates for illicit drug use: consideration of the integrated technical, medical, ethical, legal, and social issues. Front Pharmacol 2018;9:961. https://doi.org/10.3389/phar.2018.00961.
4. Walker SM. Long-term effects of neonatal pain. Semin Fetal Neonatal Med 2019;5:101005. https://doi.org/10.1016/j.siny.2019.04.005.

Preface

Anesthesia, Sedation, and Pain Control

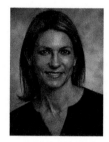 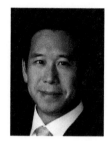

Shannon E.G. Hamrick, MD   Caleb Ing, MD, MS
Editors

In this issue of *Clinics in Perinatology* on Anesthesia, Sedation, and Pain Control, we present articles that describe the delivery of anesthesia care to children in the perinatal and neonatal period and also discuss the impact of giving, as well as not giving, anesthetic and sedative agents to these children. Among these topics, the potential neurotoxic effect of anesthetics, analgesics, and sedatives on the immature brain has generated great interest and concern over the past 2 decades. This phenomenon was initially discovered in animals where there is convincing evidence that anesthetics interfere with neurodevelopment. Translating these studies to humans however has been challenging, as exposure to anesthetic and sedative agents in children is inexorably tied to their need for surgery or treatment of medical conditions. In this issue, the clinical and preclinical investigations into anesthetic exposure and subsequent neurodevelopmental impairment are discussed in addition to neurologic outcomes in children requiring major cardiac surgery. Although there is concern regarding the long-term effects of anesthetics, analgesics, and sedatives, it is unreasonable to forgo use of these agents. Aside from the ethics, there are detrimental effects of repetitive pain on the developing brain, with exposure to pain during rapid brain development leading to altered microstructure and reduced cortical thickness. Thus, subsequent articles discuss the best practices for assessing pain, how to safely control pain and sedation in the newborn (including nonpharmacologic approaches, pharmacologic choices, and epidurals/spinals in operative patients). The delivery of safe anesthetic care in the neonatal and perinatal period is also discussed, with descriptions of airway management in children, as well anesthetic management for the obstetric patient and the impact on the fetus. Finally, the opioid crisis in the United States is addressed, with articles on maternal management and neonatal abstinence syndrome. We hope that,

Clin Perinatol 46 (2019) xvii–xviii
https://doi.org/10.1016/j.clp.2019.09.002
0095-5108/19/© 2019 Elsevier Inc. All rights reserved.
perinatology.theclinics.com

whether you are in the field of obstetrics or perinatology, family practice, pediatrics, neonatology, pediatric surgery, or anesthesiology, you will find this issue a useful reference into these interesting and evolving topics.

Shannon E.G. Hamrick, MD
Divisions of Neonatology and Cardiology
Emory University and
Children's Healthcare of Atlanta
Emory Children's Center
316 F 3rd floor
Atlanta, GA 30322, USA

Caleb Ing, MD, MS
Division of Pediatric Anesthesia
Columbia University Irving Medical Center
622 West 168th Street BHN 4-440
New York, NY 10032, USA

E-mail addresses:
sehamri@emory.edu (S.E.G. Hamrick)
ci2119@cumc.columbia.edu (C. Ing)

Human Studies of Anesthesia-Related Neurotoxicity in Children

A Narrative Review of Recent Additions to the Clinical Literature

James D. O'Leary, MBBCh, MM, MD, FCARCSI

KEYWORDS

- Neonate • Infant • Child • Anesthesia • Toxicity

KEY POINTS

- The US Food and Drug Administration issued a Drug Safety Communication in 2017 on the safety of general anesthetic and sedation drugs in young children stating that exposure to anesthesia medicines for lengthy periods of time or over multiple surgeries may affect brain development in children younger than 3 years.
- Most recent additions to the literature continue to find mixed clinical evidence for adverse neurodevelopmental effects of general anesthesia in young children.
- There is increasing high-quality evidence in humans, consistent with preclinical data, that a single short exposure to general anesthesia in young children does not cause detectable long-term neurocognitive injury.

INTRODUCTION

General anesthesia is frequently required to facilitate medical and surgical procedures in young children.[1,2] In addition to transiently disrupting normal neural activity, there are ongoing concerns that anesthetic drugs can cause long-term neurologic injury in the developing human brain.[3] There is overwhelming preclinical evidence that most commonly used anesthetic drugs can cause neurologic injury in animals,[4] including nonhuman primates.[5] Preclinical studies repeatedly find evidence of brain injury in young animals after lengthy or multiple exposures to general anesthetics. These studies have found that anesthetic drugs can cause a range of acute deleterious structural changes in the developing brain, including altered synaptogenesis,[6]

Financial Disclosures: None.
Department of Anesthesia, University of Toronto, 12th Floor, 123 Edward Street, Toronto, Ontario M5G 1E2, Canada
E-mail address: james.oleary@utoronto.ca

0095-5108/19/© 2019 Elsevier Inc. All rights reserved.

neurogenesis,[7] and neuronal cell death.[8] Long-term adverse changes in behavior, cognition, and learning have also been observed in animal models, including nonhuman primates, after exposure to general anesthetic drugs.[9,10] The evidence supporting anesthesia-related neurotoxicity in humans is, however, less consistent.[11] If preclinical findings translate to humans, pediatric anesthesia-related neurotoxicity may represent a major public health issue. This narrative review aims to provide a summary of clinical research reports investigating pediatric anesthesia-related neuro- toxicity in humans in the time period since the US Food and Drug Administration (FDA) issued a Drug Safety Communication (in 2017) on the use of general anesthetic and sedative medicines in young children.[12]

US FOOD AND DRUG ADMINISTRATION DRUG SAFETY COMMUNICATION

In response to both preclinical and human evidence, the US FDA issued a statement in April 2017 on the safety of general anesthetic and sedation drugs in young children. Anesthetic and sedative drug labels are now required to have warnings that exposure to anesthesia medicines for lengthy periods of time or over multiple surgeries may affect brain development in children younger than 3 years. These label changes were applied to some of the most commonly used anesthetic and sedative drugs (ie, desflurane, etomidate, halothane, isoflurane, ketamine, lorazepam injection, methohexital, midazolam, pentobarbital, propofol, and sevoflurane).[12] Approximately 1 in 7 children in the United States are exposed to general anesthesia drugs before age 3 years, and 1 in 4 of these children are considered to be at highest risk of anesthesia- related neurotoxicity by this FDA warning.[13] Although the FDA Safety Communication does not recommend altering current medical practices and supports that medically necessary procedures in children age less than 3 years should not be delayed, this regulatory change has widespread implications for pregnant women, parents of young children scheduled for surgery, and pediatric health care providers.[14]

CHALLENGES OF STUDYING ANESTHESIA-RELATED NEUROTOXICITY IN HUMANS

Translating preclinical evidence to humans is difficult,[15] and clinical studies of anesthesia-related neurotoxicity — with the capacity to yield high-quality evidence — are inherently challenging to conduct.[16] Despite most preclinical studies supporting that increasing durations of anesthesia exposure can cause long-term neurologic harm, clinical studies are yet to provide consistent high-quality evidence of anesthesia-related neurologic injury in humans.

To date, the majority of studies in humans investigating anesthesia-related neuro- toxicity have relied on retrospective study designs. In addition to the limitations inherent to this study design, such as increased risks of bias and confounding, retro- spective studies of anesthesia-related neurotoxicity tend to have other restrictions. Importantly, despite the nuanced selection of surgical procedures and populations, they typically cannot reliably distinguish between anesthesia-related neurologic injury and other potential health care-related causes of adverse child development during illness or hospitalization (eg, indirect effects of anesthesia, surgical stress response, pain, altered nutrition). Although the widespread cortical injury observed in animal models is commonly hypothesized to manifest as a global decline in cognitive function in humans, there remains potential for a range of neurologic injuries and susceptibility to occur with differential neurodevelopment occurring throughout childhood.[17] Retro- spective studies of anesthesia-related neurotoxicity also tend to rely on repurposed outcome measures (eg, academic performance, clinical diagnoses of behavioral or learning disorders), which may not be able to detect detailed or modest changes in neurodevelopment that can be attributable to anesthesia-related neurologic injury.[18] Further to this, most children typically experience only a single short general anesthetic before age 3 years and there is potential for modest (or no) effect size differences to be associated with the brief exposures experienced by the majority of young children exposed to anesthesia. Prospective studies of anesthesia-related neurotoxicity can have similar inherent difficulties in design and conduct. In addition, a relatively long interval between exposure and measuring outcomes is required due to limitations of assessing detailed neurocognitive development in young children,[19] to differentiate between anesthesia-related neurologic injury and maladaptive behavioral changes that can occur in the postoperative period,[20] and also to better predict achievement in adulthood.[21] This time lag to outcome testing can predispose prospective studies to sample attrition, loss to follow-up, and increased risk of bias from nonrandom missing data.

Despite observational studies (under most conditions) lacking the strength of evidence needed to make causal inference,[22] the previous absence of randomized controlled trials in this field meant that clinical guidelines largely relied on evidence from observational and preclinical studies. However, many of the existing clinical studies are difficult to compare, they have important differences in anesthetic exposures examined (frequency, duration, ages at exposure), outcome measures used, and fidelity of data available.[23] This heterogeneity in study design and methodology has prevented the integration of these (positive and negative) studies for evidence synthesis and, in the absence of higher quality evidence, hindered their interpretation and use for guiding clinical decision making.

Recent research reports of anesthesia-related neurotoxicity have attempted to mitigate for the limitations of previous observational research by using more innovative study designs (eg, sibling comparisons, ambidirectional cohorts, randomized controlled trials) to provide higher quality evidence and also by readdressing some criticisms of early clinical research in this field.

RETROSPECTIVE STUDIES

Overall, retrospective studies have found mixed evidence for an association between exposure to surgery and anesthesia at young ages and long term adverse neurodevelopmental, educational or behavioral outcomes. These studies have been comprehensively summarized in several reviews.[23,24] Of note, the 3 large population-based studies (Ontario, Canada; Manitoba, Canada; Sweden) of educational readiness at primary school entry or later academic achievement have found only modest differences in the outcomes measured,[25–27] and none of these 3 studies found evidence that associations with adverse outcomes are greatest in younger children, who are frequently hypothesized to be at greatest risk for anesthesia-related neurotoxicity.

In recent retrospective studies of anesthesia-related neurotoxicity, there has been a notable increase in the awareness of potential modifying effects of heritable, cultural, and socioeconomic factors on adverse child development associated with anesthesia exposure. To attempt to mitigate for these factors several studies have previously examined differences among siblings. Bartels and colleagues[28] used the Netherlands Twin Registry to measure educational outcomes for 1143 monozygotic twin pairs who were exposed to anesthesia before age 3 years. They found that although exposed children had lower educational achievement scores and more cognitive problems than unexposed children, discordant (exposed vs unexposed) twin pairs did not differ from each other.[28] More recently, O'Leary and colleagues[29] used the Early Development Instrument (a validated population-based measure of child development before primary school entry) data for Ontario, Canada to assemble a cohort of 10,897 biological sibling pairs (ie, children with the same birth mother) who were discordant or concordant for exposure to surgical procedures that require general anesthesia. The Early Development Instrument is a 103-item teacher-completed questionnaire and assesses children's readiness to learn before primary school entry in 5 major domains (physical health and well-being, social knowledge and competence, emotional health and maturity, language and cognitive development, and communication skills and general knowledge).[26] The investigators had previously found small differences in developmental outcomes between children exposed and unexposed to procedures that require general anesthesia in a larger population-based cohort of Ontario, Canada,[26] but when biological siblings were examined they found no differences in odds of early developmental vulnerability or deficits in major developmental domains among siblings exposed or unexposed to surgical procedures that require general anesthesia.[29]

Ing and colleagues[30,31] recently performed a series of secondary analyses of the Western Australia Pregnancy (Raine) cohort. First, they investigated whether increasing duration of exposure to procedures that required general anesthesia was associated with adverse differences in language and cognitive ability. From a cohort of 2868 children, 148 children were exposed to surgical procedures that required general anesthesia and had detailed neuropsychological testing performed at age 10 years. They found that children with exposures of 35 minutes or less (the 50th centile of exposure duration) did not differ from unexposed children, but children with greater than 35 minutes of exposure had increased risks of language deficits (both overall and in receptive language deficits). The investigators caution that the negative findings associated with longer duration exposures may not be attributable to anesthesia exposure alone, but this study does provide additional reassurance that short anesthetic exposures do not seem to cause detectable harm in language or cognitive ability.[31] Second, Ing and colleagues[30] sought to describe a clinical phenotype for neurodevelopmental deficits in children exposed to procedures that required general anesthesia. The investigators used latent class analysis to define 4 exclusive subgroups of neurodevelopmental test outcomes (few or no deficits in any test, language and cognitive deficits, behavioral deficits, or deficits in all domains) in a cohort of 1444 children. Consistent with earlier findings from the Raine cohort,[32] this analysis found that children with language and cognitive deficits were more likely to be exposed to anesthesia and surgery before age 3 years compared with normal children.[30] The investigators support that these findings are likely to be represent specific deficits in higher order brain function and not a widespread neurologic injury, as suggested by the widespread cortical injury seen in many animal studies.

Ing and colleagues[33] also investigated whether age at exposure to anesthesia for commonly performed surgical procedures (ie, circumcision outside the neonatal period, inguinal hernia repair, pyloromyotomy, tonsillectomy) was associated with a modified risk of a subsequent diagnosis of a mental disorder (including developmental delay and attention-deficit hyperactivity disorder [ADHD]). The investigators defined 11 exclusive age at exposure categories (mostly 6-month intervals) in a cohort of 38,493 children aged less than 5 years at exposure assembled from New York and Texas Medicaid databases. After propensity score matching, this study did find that the risk for any mental disorder occurring in childhood was increased after exposure to general anesthesia for commonly performed surgical procedures (hazard ratio; 1.26; 95% confidence interval, 1.22–1.30). However, there was a similar magnitude of increased risk observed for all age at exposure categories evaluated.[33]

A series of studies using a birth cohort (born 1976–1982) from Olmsted County, Minnesota, previously found adverse associations between multiple—but not single—exposures to procedures that require general anesthesia before age 2 to 4 years and subsequent diagnoses of learning disabilities and ADHD.[34,35] However, some clinical practices in this cohort (ie, halothane anesthesia, routine intraoperative monitoring) do not reflect contemporary anesthesia drugs and monitoring standards. Hu and colleagues[36] approached these concerns, by assembling a more recent birth cohort (born 1996–2000) of children born in Olmsted County, Minnesota, who were categorized by exposure to procedures that require general anesthesia before age 3 years. In a propensity matched cohort of 1036 children (463 unexposed, 457 single-exposed, and 116 multiple-exposed), Hu and colleagues[36] found both decreased academic performance in group-administered tests, and increased frequencies of any learning disability (hazard ratio, 2.17; 95% confidence interval, 1.32–3.59) and ADHD (hazard ratio 2.59; 95% confidence interval, 1.59–4.21) for multiply exposed children compared with unexposed children before age 3 years. There were no significant differences between unexposed children and those with single exposures to procedures that require general anesthesia.[36]

AMBIDIRECTIONAL STUDIES

The Pediatric Anesthesia & NeuroDevelopment Assessment (PANDA) study was the first ambidirectional study to report detailed neurodevelopmental testing used to examine the association between anesthesia exposure and adverse neurodevelopmental outcomes. This cohort consisted of 105 discordant sibling pairs, where exposed children had a single anesthetic exposure before age 3 years for inguinal hernia repair and their closest sibling who was unexposed to general anesthesia before age 3 years. Across multiple primary neuropsychological and behavioral outcomes in later childhood (age 8–15 years), Sun and colleagues[37] found no significant differences between young children who had a single anesthetic exposure before age 3 years and their unexposed sibling. The only differences found between groups were higher frequencies of total problems and abnormal internalizing scores for exposed children from the parent-reported Child Behavioral Checklist and adaptive behavior from the Adaptive Behavior Assessment System, Second Edition.[37]

The results of the Mayo Anesthesia Safety in Kids (MASK) study were published in 2018.[38] This ambidirectional observational study investigated whether multiple, but not single, procedures requiring general anesthesia before age 3 years were associated with long-term adverse neurodevelopment outcomes. Warner and colleagues[38] assembled a propensity-guided sample of 997 (411 unexposed, 380 single-exposed, and 206 multiple-exposed) children born in Olmsted County, Minnesota, and performed a comprehensive battery of neuropsychological testing at ages 8 to 12 or 15 to 20 years. The primary outcome was the Wechsler Abbreviated Scale of Intelligence Full-Scale intelligence quotient (FSIQ). There were no significant differences in FSIQ when comparing exposed and unexposed children. There were some select adverse findings in individual domains tested (ie, processing speed and fine motor abilities) for children with multiple, but not single, exposures to procedures that required general anesthesia. There were increased parental reports of problems for both children with single (related to executive function and reading) and multiple (related to executive function, behavior, and reading) exposures compared with unexposed children.

In a secondary analysis of the MASK cohort,[39] Warner and colleagues subsequently investigated whether exposure to procedures that required general anesthesia was associated with differences in Operant Test Battery (OTB) performance. Improving the clinical relevance and translation of animal findings to humans is a priority for directing future clinical research.[40] The OTB may be a valuable outcome measure for comparing relevant outcomes in human and nonhuman primates; child and nonhuman primate completion of the OTB may be indistinguishable, and the OTB is sensitive to a variety of toxicologic injury in both humans and primates. Primates exposed to general anesthesia have demonstrated deficiencies in the OTB, and the aspects of the OTB that are affected by anesthesia exposure in primates have a moderate correlation with IQ in children.[41] In the MASK cohort, Warner and colleagues[39] found no significant differences in any OTB test scores between children exposed or unexposed to surgical procedures that require general anesthesia, suggesting that adverse findings using the OTB in nonhuman primates may not readily translate to children.

RANDOMIZED STUDIES

The General Anesthesia compared to Spinal anesthesia (GAS) Study is the first and, thus far, only randomized controlled trial to investigate whether exposure to general anesthesia in young children adversely effects long term neurodevelopmental outcomes.[42,43] This multicenter equivalence trial by McCann and colleagues[42] compared the effect of awake regional versus sevoflurane anesthesia on neurodevelopmental outcomes for infants who were less than 60 weeks postconceptual age at the time of inguinal hernia repair. The median duration of sevoflurane anesthesia was 54 minutes (interquartile range, 41–70 minutes). The interim (at age 2 years) results were published in 2016,[43] and the final (at age 5 years) results were published in 2019.[42] Both interim and final analyses of the GAS study showed equivalence between awake regional and general anesthesia for infant inguinal hernia repair. Consistent with the prespecified interim findings (using the Bayley Scales of Infant and Toddler Development III), there were no significant differences in the Wechsler Preschool and Primary Scale of Intelligence FSIQ (primary outcome) or a range of other secondary cognitive and behavioral outcomes in the final (5 years) analysis. There was some cross-over between groups (19% of infants in the awake regional group were also exposed to general anesthesia), but the adjusted mean difference in FSIQ between interventions was 0.16 (95% confidence interval, -2.45 to 2.78) with an intention-to-treat analysis and 0.23 (95% confidence interval, -2.59 to 3.06) with as-per-protocol analysis. Intelligence testing at this older age has greater predictive potential for future achievement compared with the interim analysis at age 2 years, and these results provide strong evidence that relatively short exposures to sevoflurane anesthesia do not cause detectable adverse neurodevelopmental outcomes at age 5 years compared with awake regional anesthesia.

SUMMARY

Overall, these recent additions to the clinical literature continue to find mixed evidence of anesthesia-related neurotoxicity in young children. However, neurodevelopment is a function of the interactions between multiple risk and protective factors, including genetic, familial, and environmental influences.[44] For example, persistent poverty is a significant risk factor for impaired cognition in middle childhood[45] that persists into adulthood.[46] Despite advances in study design and methodology used by these more recent additions to the literature, differentiating between potential contributing factors to adverse neurodevelopment remains difficult in clinical studies. As a consequence, the strength of evidence supporting associations between exposure to general anesthesia and learning deficits, mental disorders, or ADHD remains weak.[47]

The recent addition of more high-quality human studies in this field, particularly the GAS Study, provides the strongest evidence to date that, although parents have reported worse outcomes in behavior and executive function in anesthetic-exposed children, a single exposure to general anesthesia in young children does not have detectable risks of long-term neurocognitive injury as measured by neuropsychological testing. These findings are consistent with both previous studies in humans and preclinical studies, which support a dose–response relationship between general anesthesia exposure and adverse cellular outcomes. This finding is reassuring for the majority of young children who experience only a single short exposure to general anesthesia,[13] but these new findings cannot be extrapolated to those children deemed to be at highest risk by the US FDA drug safety communication, that is, those who undergo prolonged or repeated exposures to general anesthesia drugs. The dose threshold for causing anesthesia-related neurologic injury in humans, ages most susceptible to injury, and potential effect modification and confounding from environmental and patient factors, need to be considered in future clinical studies.

REFERENCES

1. Rabbitts JA, Groenewald CB, Moriarty JP, et al. Epidemiology of ambulatory anesthesia for children in the United States: 2006 and 1996. Anesth Analg 2010;111(4):1011–5.
2. Sury MR, Palmer JH, Cook TM, et al. The state of UK dental anaesthesia: results from the NAP5 activity survey. A national survey by the 5th National Audit Project of the Royal College of Anaesthetists and the association of Anaesthetists of Great Britain and Ireland. SAAD Dig 2016;32:34–6.
3. Vutskits L, Xie Z. Lasting impact of general anaesthesia on the brain: mechanisms and relevance. Nat Rev Neurosci 2016;17(11):705–17.
4. Lin EP, Lee JR, Lee CS, et al. Do anesthetics harm the developing human brain? An integrative analysis of animal and human studies. Neurotoxicol Teratol 2017; 60:117–28.
5. Coleman K, Robertson ND, Dissen GA, et al. Isoflurane anesthesia has long-term consequences on motor and behavioral development in infant rhesus macaques. Anesthesiology 2017;126(1):74–84.
6. Briner A, De Roo M, Dayer A, et al. Volatile anesthetics rapidly increase dendritic spine density in the rat medial prefrontal cortex during synaptogenesis. Anesthesiology 2010;112(3):546–56.
7. Stratmann G, Sall JW, May LD, et al. Isoflurane differentially affects neurogenesis and long-term neurocognitive function in 60-day-old and 7-day-old rats. Anesthesiology 2009;110(4):834–48.
8. Jevtovic-Todorovic V, Hartman RE, Izumi Y, et al. Early exposure to common anesthetic agents causes widespread neurodegeneration in the developing rat brain and persistent learning deficits. J Neurosci 2003;23(3):876–82.
9. Paule MG, Li M, Allen RR, et al. Ketamine anesthesia during the first week of life can cause long-lasting cognitive deficits in rhesus monkeys. Neurotoxicol Teratol 2011;33(2):220–30.
10. Raper J, De Biasio JC, Murphy KL, et al. Persistent alteration in behavioural reactivity to a mild social stressor in rhesus monkeys repeatedly exposed to sevoflurane in infancy. Br J Anaesth 2018;120(4):761–7.
11. O'Leary JD, Warner DO. What do recent human studies tell us about the association between anaesthesia in young children and neurodevelopmental outcomes? Br J Anaesth 2017;119(3):458–64.

12. US Food and Drug Administration. Drug Safety Communication: FDA approves label changes for use of general anesthetic and sedation drugs in young children. Available at: https://www.fda.gov/downloads/Drugs/DrugSafety/UCM554644.pdf. Accessed April 17, 2019.

13. Shi Y, Hu D, Rodgers EL, et al. Epidemiology of general anesthesia prior to age 3 in a population-based birth cohort. Paediatr Anaesth 2018;28(6):513–9.

14. Andropoulos DB, Greene MF. Anesthesia and developing brains - Implications of the FDA warning. N Engl J Med 2017;376(10):905–7.

15. Kharasch ED. The challenges of translation. Anesthesiology 2018;128(4):693–6.

16. Walkden GJ, Pickering AE, Gill H. Assessing long-term neurodevelopmental outcome following general anesthesia in early childhood: challenges and opportunities. Anesth Analg 2019;128(4):681–94.

17. Hofacer RD, Deng M, Ward CG, et al. Cell age-specific vulnerability of neurons to anesthetic toxicity. Ann Neurol 2013;73(6):695–704.

18. Clausen NG, Kahler S, Hansen TG. Systematic review of the neurocognitive outcomes used in studies of paediatric anaesthesia neurotoxicity. Br J Anaesth 2018;120(6):1255–73.

19. Beers SR, Rofey DL, McIntyre KA. Neurodevelopmental assessment after anesthesia in childhood: review of the literature and recommendations. Anesth Analg 2014;119(3):661–9.

20. Fortier MA, Del Rosario AM, Rosenbaum A, et al. Beyond pain: predictors of postoperative maladaptive behavior change in children. Paediatr Anaesth 2010;20(5): 445–53.

21. Batty GD, Der G, Macintyre S, et al. Does IQ explain socioeconomic inequalities in health? Evidence from a population based cohort study in the west of Scotland. BMJ 2006;332(7541):580–4.

22. O'Neil M, Berkman N, Hartling L, et al. Observational evidence and strength of evidence domains: case examples. Syst Rev 2014;3:35.

23. Davidson AJ, Sun LS. Clinical evidence for any effect of anesthesia on the developing brain. Anesthesiology 2018;128:840–53.

24. Lei S, Ko R, Sun LS. Neurocognitive impact of anesthesia in children. Adv Anesth 2018;36(1):125–37.

25. Graham MR, Brownell M, Chateau DG, et al. Neurodevelopmental assessment in kindergarten in children exposed to general anesthesia before the age of 4 years: a retrospective matched cohort study. Anesthesiology 2016;125(4):667–77.

26. O'Leary JD, Janus M, Duku E, et al. A population-based study evaluating the association between surgery in early life and child development at primary school entry. Anesthesiology 2016;125(2):272–9.

27. Glatz P, Sandin RH, Pedersen NL, et al. Association of anesthesia and surgery during childhood with long-term academic performance. JAMA Pediatr 2017; 171(1):e163470.

28. Bartels M, Althoff RR, Boomsma DI. Anesthesia and cognitive performance in children: no evidence for a causal relationship. Twin Res Hum Genet 2009; 12(3):246–53.

29. O'Leary JD, Janus M, Duku E, et al. Influence of surgical procedures and general anesthesia on child development before primary school entry among matched sibling pairs. JAMA Pediatr 2019;173(1):29–36.

30. Ing C, Wall MM, DiMaggio CJ, et al. Latent class analysis of neurodevelopmental deficit after exposure to anesthesia in early childhood. J Neurosurg Anesthesiol 2017;29(3):264–73.

31. Ing C, Hegarty MK, Perkins JW, et al. Duration of general anaesthetic exposure in early childhood and long-term language and cognitive ability. Br J Anaesth 2017; 119(3):532–40.
32. Ing C, DiMaggio C, Whitehouse A, et al. Long-term differences in language and cognitive function after childhood exposure to anesthesia. Pediatrics 2012; 130(3):e476–85.
33. Ing C, Sun M, Olfson M, et al. Age at exposure to surgery and anesthesia in children and association with mental disorder diagnosis. Anesth Analg 2017;125(6): 1988–98.
34. Wilder RT, Flick RP, Sprung J, et al. Early exposure to anesthesia and learning disabilities in a population-based birth cohort. Anesthesiology 2009;110(4): 796–804.
35. Sprung J, Flick RP, Katusic SK, et al. Attention-deficit/hyperactivity disorder after early exposure to procedures requiring general anesthesia. Mayo Clin Proc 2012; 87(2):120–9.
36. Hu D, Flick RP, Zaccariello MJ, et al. Association between exposure of young children to procedures requiring general anesthesia and learning and behavioral outcomes in a population-based birth cohort. Anesthesiology 2017;127(2):227–40.
37. Sun LS, Li G, Miller TL, et al. Association between a single general anesthesia exposure before age 36 months and neurocognitive outcomes in later childhood. JAMA 2016;315(21):2312–20.
38. Warner DO, Zaccariello MJ, Katusic SK, et al. Neuropsychological and behavioral outcomes after exposure of young children to procedures requiring general anesthesia: the Mayo Anesthesia Safety in Kids (MASK) Study. Anesthesiology 2018; 129(1):89–105.
39. Warner DO, Chelonis JJ, Paule MG, et al. Performance on the operant test battery in young children exposed to procedures requiring general anaesthesia: the MASK study. Br J Anaesth 2019;122(4):470–9.
40. Disma N, O'Leary JD, Loepke AW, et al. Anesthesia and the developing brain: a way forward for laboratory and clinical research. Paediatr Anaesth 2018;28(9): 758–63.
41. Paule MG, Chelonis JJ, Buffalo EA, et al. Operant test battery performance in children: correlation with IQ. Neurotoxicol Teratol 1999;21(3):223–30.
42. McCann ME, de Graaff JC, Dorris L, et al. Neurodevelopmental outcome at 5 years of age after general anaesthesia or awake-regional anaesthesia in infancy (GAS): an international, multicentre, randomised, controlled equivalence trial. Lancet 2019;393(10172):664–77.
43. Davidson AJ, Disma N, de Graaff JC, et al. Neurodevelopmental outcome at 2 years of age after general anaesthesia and awake-regional anaesthesia in infancy (GAS): an international multicentre, randomised controlled trial. Lancet 2016;387(10015):239–50.
44. McCulloch A. Variation in children's cognitive and behavioural adjustment between different types of place in the British National Child Development Study. Soc Sci Med 2006;62(8):1865–79.
45. Schoon I, Jones E, Cheng H, et al. Family hardship, family instability, and cognitive development. J Epidemiol Community Health 2012;66(8):716–22.
46. Cermakova P, Formanek T, Kagstrom A, et al. Socioeconomic position in childhood and cognitive aging in Europe. Neurology 2018;91(17):e1602–10.
47. Efron D, Vutskits L, Davidson AJ. Can we really suggest that anesthesia might cause attention-deficit/hyperactivity disorder? Anesthesiology 2017;127(2): 209–11.

Anesthesia Neurotoxicity in the Developing Brain

Basic Studies Relevant for Neonatal or Perinatal Medicine

Nicola Groes Clausen, MD, PhD[a], Tom G. Hansen, MD, PhD[b,c],
Nicola Disma, MD[d,*]

KEYWORDS

- General anesthesia • Pediatric anesthesia • Neonatal anesthesia
- Neurocognitive outcome • Neurotoxicity

KEY POINTS

- General anesthetics have been shown to interfere with development of the immature animal brain.
- Anesthesia-induced neurotoxicity has been studied extensively and potential mechanisms identified. Whether this has implications for humans is unknown.
- Owing to animal–human differences in physiology and developmental progress, translation of results is difficult.
- Interventions under general anesthesia might introduce additional factors with the potential to disturb neurodevelopment, particularly in premature infants.

INTRODUCTION

Human brain development is complex and progresses through multiple stages (**Table 1**). General anesthetics have been shown to interfere with development of the immature animal brain by induction of neuronal apoptosis and disturbance of the cerebral cytoarchitecture.[1,2] These findings originated from studies conducted primarily in rodents as well as in nonhuman primates. Human observational studies have both confirmed and rejected associations between exposure to general anesthesia in

[a] Department of Anesthesiology and Intensive Care, Odense University Hospital, J.B. Winsløwsvej 4, Odense C 5000, Denmark; [b] Department of Anesthesiology and Intensive Care – Pediatrics, Odense University Hospital, J.B. Winsløwsvej 4, Odense C 5000, Denmark; [c] Department of Clinical Research – Anesthesiology, University of Southern Denmark, Odense C 5000, Denmark; [d] Department of Anesthesia, IRCCS Istituto Giannina Gaslini, Via G. Gaslini 5, Genoa 16100, Italy
* Corresponding author.
E-mail address: nicoladisma@icloud.com

Clin Perinatol 46 (2019) 647–656
https://doi.org/10.1016/j.clp.2019.08.002
0095-5108/19/© 2019 Elsevier Inc. All rights reserved.

Table 1 Partial steps of normal brain development	
Neurulation	Folding of ectodermal plate around a liquid-filled cavity creating the neural tube; the tube becomes the spinal cord enclosing the spinal canal; the vesicle-filled bulges of ectodermal cells at the anterior end fold up to create the primary brain structures and the ventricle system.
Neurogenesis and gliogenesis	Epithelial progenitor cells lining the early ventricles differentiate into neurons and glia-cells (astrocytes and oligodendrocytes).
Migration	Young neurons migrate toward their destined region of the brain; the signaling and regulation of this process is still poorly understood.
Synaptogenesis	Synapses are areas of physical contact between axons and/or dendrites; one neurone has up to 10,000 of these connections. A signal is transmitted across the synapsis from a sending (presynaptic) site to a receiving (postsynaptic) site. Synapses are maintained and fine-tuned throughout life, which is the basis of *learning*.
Myelination	To optimize signal transmission, each axon and dendrite is covered with myelin provided by oligodendrocytes.

young children and subsequent impaired neurodevelopment.[3–10] However, the compelling evidence from preclinical studies is no longer questioned and should be acknowledged by those who are engaged in the clinical care of neonates.

This narrative review summarizes suspected mechanisms of anesthesia-related neurotoxicity (section I), preclinical studies (section II), and translational difficulties within the field (section III).

SECTION I: SUSPECTED PATHWAYS OF NEUROTOXICITY

In the central nervous system, 2 ligand-gated ion channels, the gamma-aminobutyric acid type A receptor ($GABA_A$-R) and the *N*-methyl-D-aspartic acid receptor, are the main binding sites for anesthetics. Activation of $GABA_A$-R in the immature brain facilitates refinement of neuronal circuits by acting on cell migration, synaptogenesis, DNA synthesis, and cell proliferation. Antagonism of $GABA_A$-R induced by general anesthetics might disturb physiologic neuronal plasticity, especially in the hippocampal dentate gyrus. Moreover, $GABA_A$-R is excitatory during development, rather than inhibitory, and the time at which the receptor shift from excitatory to inhibitor is still not elucidated.[11,12] Of note, both *N*-methyl-D-aspartic acid receptor antagonists and $GABA_A$-R agonists have demonstrated a neurotoxic profile[13,14] in all species studied: nematodes,[15] zebrafish,[16] rodents,[17] pigs,[18] sheep,[19] and nonhuman primates.[20]

Synapse formation is a crucial step in physiologic brain maturation. In rodents and mice, peak synaptogenesis occurs during the first week of life. In rodents exposed to general anesthesia between postnatal day (PND) 5 and 10 the number of synapses was significantly reduced. Contrarily, synapse density on dendritic spines and cortical pyramidal neurons was increased in rodents exposed between PND 15 and 20. Both examples demonstrate the potential of general anesthetics to modify neuronal architecture.[21–24] These modulations have been observed after the administration of clinically relevant doses of anesthetics, and after both prolonged or multiple exposures,[22,25] but the synapse formation disruption might be triggered even by a short anesthesia exposure.

During early brain development, neurons and synapses are generated in excessive numbers. The initial overabundance is followed by DNA-programmed neuronal death (apoptosis). Apoptosis is an integral part of brain development and maintenance, ensuring normal central nervous system morphology and function. As a result, fewer than 50% of neurons survive into adult life. Any interference with this normal apoptotic process may have detrimental effects to the central nervous system.

Apoptosis is induced via 2 main routes involving either mitochondria (intrinsic pathway) or the activation of transmembrane death receptors (extrinsic pathway). Both pathways converge to induce the activation of caspases, the final executioners of cell death. The mitochondrial pathway of apoptosis begins with the permeabilization of the (mitochondrial) outer membrane. Water enters the mitochondrial matrix, which results in swelling of the intermembranal space and rupturing of the outer membrane. Consequently, apoptogenic proteins are released[26,27] comprising cytochrome c,[28] apoptosis-inducing factor,[29] and endonuclease G.[30]

Oscillating calcium concentrations in the cell function represent a signaling pathway and are important for neuronal maturation. Although elevations of calcium are necessary for it to act as a signal, excessive and prolonged increases in the cytoplasm might be lethal for the cell. Exposure of young animals to anesthetics has been shown causing a release of excessive calcium from the endoplasmic reticulum. Although short exposures induce neuroprotection, long exposure can trigger neurotoxicity and the prolonged intracellular calcium elevation could be one of the mechanisms involved. However, the exact mechanism of anesthetic-induced calcium overload is not fully explained, although it does involve the inhibition of mitochondrial function and a significant decrease in the cellular energy with adenosine triphosphate depletion. As a consequence, intracellular calcium and lactate are released, triggering apoptosis. Elevated intracellular calcium was observed even after complete washout of general anesthetics, suggesting a persistent effect. **Fig. 1** illustrates activation of the mitochondrial apoptotic pathway and intracellular calcium release from the endoplasmic reticulum after anesthesia exposure.

Neurotrophins

Neurotrophins play a fundamental role in neuronal survival and differentiation. General anesthetics influence the synthesis of brain-derived neurotrophic factor (BDNF), an important neurotrophin. BDNF promotes neuronal survival through the activation of Trk receptors. Contrarily, neurogenesis is decreased by BDNF activation of p75NTR receptors. Volatile anesthetics facilitate an increase of pro-BDNF with higher affinity to p75NTR than to Trk receptors. The net result is a decrease in neuronal cell survival. Similar to volatile anesthetics, propofol induces neuronal apoptosis via the BDNF pathway.[31,32]

Epigenetic Modifications

Epigenetics is the study of heritable changes in gene expression without changes in the DNA sequence. According to this principle, a phenotype can be changed by external influences (eg, disease, age, and environment) through chromatin remodeling and histone modification without a direct DNA modification. Recent reports suggest general anesthetics to cause cognitive impairments in second-generation offspring of animals exposed to anesthesia while pregnant.[33] It has been hypothesized that intrauterine exposure to anesthetics induces epigenetic changes, which are then embedded in the DNA of the next generation.[34] How this phenomenon translates to humans is unknown, but epigenetic changes might increase the risk of intellectual disability disorders and autism.[35]

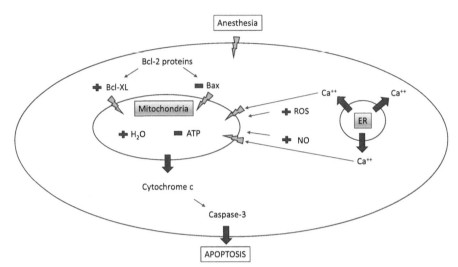

Fig. 1. Bcl-2 family proteins regulate apoptosis by controlling mitochondrial permeability. The antiapoptotic proteins Bcl-2 and Bcl-xL reside in the outer mitochondrial wall and inhibit cytochrome c release. The proapoptotic Bcl-2 proteins (eg, Bax) may reside in the cytosol but translocate to mitochondria following death signaling, where they promote the release of cytochrome c. Anesthesia might be able to regulate levels of Bcl-2 proteins (through upregulations and downregulations) and hence interfere with membrane permeability (H_2O) of mitochondria.[58] Activation of microglia and astrocytes generates an overproduction of free oxygen radicals (ROS)[59] and nitric oxide (NO)[60] causing mitochondrial membrane damage and inducing neuronal death. In fact, the described simultaneous upregulation of Bax and downregulation of Bcl-2 facilitates an accumulation of free oxygen radicals responsible for damage to the cellular membrane (through reduction of both membrane potential and adenosine triphosphate production), which leads to cell death. The ultimate apoptosis activator remains caspase-3.

Further, anesthesia-induced modification of DNA might be responsible for the downregulation of BDNF. In addition to the functions previously explained, BDNF is important for the development of memory. Hence, epigenetic changes might induce memory impairment.[36–38]

SECTION II: ANESTHESIA-RELATED NEUROTOXICITY—OBSERVATIONS FROM PRECLINICAL STUDIES
Studies on Nonhuman Primates

Preclinical studies on nonhuman primates are considered of high relevance owing to the closeness of this species with humans. Experiment performed in rhesus and macaque monkeys showed that general anesthetics induce significant histopathological changes in cerebral tissue. However, vulnerability seemed to differ between cell types. Neurons were affected after exposure from the third trimester through PND 40, whereas oligodendrocytes showed changes continuously. This observation suggests a window of vulnerability, depending on developmental stage and cell type.[39] Of note, the neuronal damage observed was both of apoptotic and necrotic nature.[40]

Minimally invasive methods have recently been introduced to study anesthesia-related neurotoxicity in nonhuman primates. PET targeted at glial activation has been used to monitor the effect of sevoflurane in vivo.[41,42] Activated glia express a translocator protein of 18 kDa used as a PET biomarker for glial activation and neuroinflammation. This method may have an application in humans to monitor the effect of anesthesia.

The toxic effects of several medications have been tested on nonhuman primates. Based on these experiments, the National Center for Toxicologic Research has developed a validated tool for assessment of neurocognition. The Operant Test Battery (OTB) consists of tasks that rely on specific brain functions. These include motivation, color and position discrimination, learning, short-term memory, and time estimation. OTB-findings in nonhuman primates might translate closely to humans.[43] Various experiments on monkeys used the OTB as primary neurocognitive outcome. After 24-hour continuous intravenous ketamine anesthesia, experimental animals completed tasks of learning, color, and position discrimination with less accuracy and with more delay than controls.[44] In monkeys exposed to isoflurane multiple times, motor reflexes were slowed and level of anxiety increased for as long as 12 months after receiving anesthesia.[45]

Recently, the OTB was assessed as a secondary outcome in the Mayo Anesthesia Safety in Kids (MASK) Study.[46] In the MASK study, children exposed to one, multiple, or no anesthesia before the age of 3 years were prospectively assessed with OTB testing at ages 8 to 12 or 15 to 20 years of age. No association between exposure to anesthesia and test scores could be demonstrated. An explanation could be that the effect of anesthesia differs among species. Further, the OTB might not detect neurocognitive impairment in humans as other validated tests could.

SECTION III: TRANSLATIONAL RESEARCH—CHALLENGES AND PITFALLS

Many factors limit the applicability of animal-derived data to humans.[47] The major issues are emphasized here.

Ontogenic Differences Among Species

The human brain has a tremendous potential for neural plasticity and compensation after major cerebral insults, particularly so in early life. It is largely unknown which ontogenic differences in neurodevelopment among humans and animals have an impact on outcome. The morphology and function of the brain is not static, but rather a complex, continuous, and lifelong process.[48,49] What this implies is that a window of vulnerability may extend well into adulthood and beyond. Immediately after birth, the human brain comprises about 25% of its adult size. The relative proportion of specific brain areas varies between species.[50] Additionally, similar brain areas mature at different rates in different species. Even within the same region the various cell layers may mature at different rates. The brainstem and spinal cord of a human newborn are relatively well-developed, whereas the limbic system and cerebral cortex are still immature. Cortical neurons are poorly connected and most synapses are produced after birth. During this peak synaptogenesis period, the rate of cortical synapse formation is estimated to be 2 million new synapses per second. At the age of 2 years, the cerebral cortex comprises more than 100 trillion synapses. The newborn brain contains little myelin, and myelination seems to be virtually an automatic or innate process in that its sequence succession is very predictable and it seems that severe malnutrition is the only single individual environmental factor known to impact myelination. The majority of studies have used rodent pups at PND 7, because this time is optimal to detect increased apoptosis in the most susceptible parts of the brain (eg, stria terminalis, olfactory bulb). This is the right time to provoke apoptosis in this context.[51,52] However, PND 7 corresponds with anesthetic exposure of an extremely premature child and not to the major target population of term babies and young infants.[49] Thus, shifting the time of exposure of experimental animals to PND 10 to 14 may be more appropriate because this timing corresponds with the neonatal period and early infancy. For more details on this please visit: www.translating-time.net.

Anesthetic Techniques and Differences in Vital Parameter Monitoring

In humans, multiparameter monitoring is standard throughout the entire anesthesia procedure. Anesthesiologists are particularly attentive to physiologic parameters (eg, oxygenation, CO_2, blood pressure) and metabolism (eg, hemoglobin, blood glucose, electrolytes, and acid–base balance).[53] Anesthetic protocols used in the majority of animal (rodent) studies differ from those used in normal clinical practice. For example, the use of supraclinical doses and long duration of exposure to anesthetic drugs has in some studies resulted in high mortality (25%–30%).[54] Additionally, the use of multiparameter monitoring and control of airway and respiration are difficult (or even impossible) owing to the small size of the neonatal animals. Small circulating blood volumes preclude repeated blood gas and glucose measurements. As an example, Wu and colleagues[55] studied the effects of mechanical ventilation versus spontaneous breathing on outcome of 14-day-old rats exposed to isoflurane and sevoflurane. Compared with mechanically ventilated rats, spontaneously breathing rats had significantly higher mortality, increased neuroapoptosis, and impaired neurocognitive outcome. Other rodent studies have focused on "an enriched environment." Immature Cynomolgus monkeys exposed to anesthesia were allowed access to mothers and toys in their cages, instead of being placed in an environment of sensory deprivation. As a consequence, it was no longer possible to reproduce any negative long-term cognitive effects.[56]

What this shows is that many factors other than anesthetic drugs themselves can impact neurocognitive outcomes. In an attempt to increase perianesthetic safety of infants and toddlers, the Safetots Initiative promotes and encourages maintenance of normalized metabolism and an environment free of anxiety and discomfort (www.Safetots.org).

In 2014, Pound and Bracken[57] emphasized overall limitations in animal research and emphasized those of animal neuroscience. To improve research quality, preclinical studies should follow detailed research protocols. Hereby, the reproducibility of results between laboratories is attenuated. The *Animal Research: Reporting of in Vivo Experiments* guidelines illustrate responsible conductance and reporting of studies should be performed, the results interpreted and reported (www.nc3rs.org.uk/arrive-guidelines).

SUMMARY

General anesthetics have been shown to interfere with development of the immature animal brain. Anesthesia-induced neurotoxicity has been studied extensively and potential mechanisms identified. Whether this has implications for humans is unknown. Owing to animal–human differences in physiology and developmental progress, the translation of results is difficult. Interventions under general anesthesia might introduce additional factors with the potential to disturb neurodevelopment, particularly in premature infants.

Obvious ethical considerations limit the conductance of experiments in human neonates. The use of animal models is still considered feasible. To identify reasonable neurocognitive outcomes, vulnerable periods in brain development need further identification, as do neurotoxic and neuroprotective interventions.

Best Practices

What is the current evidence for the risk of anesthetic neurotoxicity in the developing brain?

Best practice, guideline, and care path objectives
- General anesthetics have been shown to interfere with development of the immature animal brain.
- Based on the evidence from laboratory studies, the US Food and Drug Administration is set to release a warning on the clinical use of general anesthetics under the age of 3 years.

What changes in current practice are likely to improve outcomes?

- Owing to differences in physiology and developmental progress between animals and humans, translation of results is difficult.

- So far, clinical studies have showed of a single exposure to anesthesia in childhood has no effect and long term neurocognitive outcome.

- Factors other than anesthesia can also interfere with the normal development: oxygenation, CO_2, blood pressure, hemoglobin, blood glucose, and so on.

Major recommendations

- Maintaining homeostasis is imperative during anesthesia to avoid brain damage that can interfere with short- and long-term development.

- In an attempt to increase perianesthetic safety of infants and toddlers, the Safetots Initiative promotes and encourages maintenance of normalized metabolism and an environment free of anxiety and discomfort (www. Safetots.org).

Summary statement

- Well-conducted studies in animals are needed to better understand the putative mechanism of neurotoxicity, identify neurocognitive outcomes, and identify periods of vulnerability.

Data from Refs.[47,53,57]

REFERENCES

1. Patel P, Sun L. Update on neonatal anesthetic neurotoxicity: insight into molecular mechanisms and relevance to humans. Anesthesiology 2009;110(4):703–8.
2. Creeley C, Dikranian K, Dissen G, et al. Propofol-induced apoptosis of neurones and oligodendrocytes in fetal and neonatal rhesus macaque brain. Br J Anaesth 2013;110(Suppl 1):i29–38.
3. Glatz P, Sandin RH, Pedersen NL, et al. Association of anesthesia and surgery during childhood with long-term academic performance. JAMA Pediatr 2017; 171(1):e163470.
4. O'Leary JD, Janus M, Duku E, et al. A population-based study evaluating the association between surgery in early life and child development at primary school entry. Anesthesiology 2016;125(2):272–9.
5. Graham MR, Brownell M, Chateau DG, et al. Neurodevelopmental assessment in Kindergarten in children exposed to general anesthesia before the age of 4 years: a retrospective matched cohort study. Anesthesiology 2016;125(4): 667–77.
6. Wilder RT, Flick RP, Sprung J, et al. Early exposure to anesthesia and learning disabilities in a population-based birth cohort. Anesthesiology 2009;110(4): 796–804.
7. Backeljauw B, Holland SK, Altaye M, et al. Cognition and brain structure following early childhood surgery with anesthesia. Pediatrics 2015;136(1):e1–12.

8. Ing CH, DiMaggio CJ, Malacova E, et al. Comparative analysis of outcome measures used in examining neurodevelopmental effects of early childhood anesthesia exposure. Anesthesiology 2014;120(6):1319–32.

9. DiMaggio C, Sun LS, Kakavouli A, et al. A retrospective cohort study of the association of anesthesia and hernia repair surgery with behavioral and developmental disorders in young children. J Neurosurg Anesthesiol 2009;21(4):286–91.

10. Bartels M, Althoff RR, Boomsma DI. Anesthesia and cognitive performance in children: no evidence for a causal relationship. Twin Res Hum Genet 2009; 12(3):246–53.

11. Tashiro A, Sandler VM, Toni N, et al. NMDA-receptor-mediated, cell-specific integration of new neurons in adult dentate gyrus. Nature 2006;442(7105):929–33.

12. Ge S, Goh EL, Sailor KA, et al. GABA regulates synaptic integration of newly generated neurons in the adult brain. Nature 2006;439(7076):589–93.

13. Ikonomidou C, Scheer I, Wilhelm T, et al. Brain morphology alterations in the basal ganglia and the hypothalamus following prenatal exposure to antiepileptic drugs. Eur J Paediatr Neurol 2007;11(5):297–301.

14. Istaphanous GK, Ward CG, Nan X, et al. Characterization and quantification of isoflurane-induced developmental apoptotic cell death in mouse cerebral cortex. Anesth Analg 2013;116(4):845–54.

15. Gentry KR, Steele LM, Sedensky MM, et al. Early developmental exposure to volatile anesthetics causes behavioral defects in Caenorhabditis elegans. Anesth Analg 2013;116(1):185–9.

16. Kanungo J, Cuevas E, Ali SF, et al. Ketamine induces motor neuron toxicity and alters neurogenic and proneural gene expression in zebrafish. J Appl Toxicol 2013;33(6):410–7.

17. Jevtovic-Todorovic V, Hartman RE, Izumi Y, et al. Early exposure to common anesthetic agents causes widespread neurodegeneration in the developing rat brain and persistent learning deficits. J Neurosci 2003;23(3):876–82.

18. Rizzi S, Ori C, Jevtovic-Todorovic V. Timing versus duration: determinants of anesthesia-induced developmental apoptosis in the young mammalian brain. Ann N Y Acad Sci 2010;1199:43–51.

19. Olutoye OA, Sheikh F, Zamora IJ, et al. Repeated isoflurane exposure and neuro-apoptosis in the midgestation fetal sheep brain. Am J Obstet Gynecol 2016; 214(4):542.e1-8.

20. Noguchi KK, Johnson SA, Dissen GA, et al. Isoflurane exposure for three hours triggers apoptotoc cell death in neonatal macaque brain. Br J Anaesth 2017; 119(3):524–31.

21. Head BP, Patel HH, Niesman IR, et al. Inhibition of p75 neurotrophin receptor attenuates isoflurane-mediated neuronal apoptosis in the neonatal central nervous system. Anesthesiology 2009;110(4):813–25.

22. Amrock LG, Starner ML, Murphy KL, et al. Long-term effects of single or multiple neonatal sevoflurane exposures on rat hippocampal ultrastructure. Anesthesiology 2015;122(1):87–95.

23. Briner A, De Roo M, Dayer A, et al. Volatile anesthetics rapidly increase dendritic spine density in the rat medial prefrontal cortex during synaptogenesis. Anesthesiology 2010;112(3):546–56.

24. De Roo M, Klauser P, Briner A, et al. Anesthetics rapidly promote synaptogenesis during a critical period of brain development. PLoS One 2009;4(9):e7043.

25. Chen B, Deng X, Wang B, et al. Persistent neuronal apoptosis and synaptic loss induced by multiple but not single exposure of propofol contribute to long-term cognitive dysfunction in neonatal rats. J Toxicol Sci 2016;41(5):627–36.

26. Crompton M. The mitochondrial permeability transition pore and its role in cell death. Biochem J 1999;341:233–49.

27. Green DR, Kroemer G. The pathophysiology of mitochondrial cell death. Science 2004;305(5684):626–9.

28. Yang JC, Cortopassi GA. Induction of the mitochondrial permeability transition causes release of the apoptogenic factor cytochrome c. Free Radic Biol Med 1998;24(4):624–31.

29. Susin SA, Lorenzo HK, Zamzami N, et al. Mitochondrial release of caspase-2 and -9 during the apoptotic process. J Exp Med 1999;189(2):381–94.

30. Li LY, Luo X, Wang X. Endonuclease G is an apoptotic DNase when released from mitochondria. Nature 2001;412(6842):95–9.

31. Suehara T, Morishita J, Ueki M, et al. Effects of sevoflurane exposure during late pregnancy on brain development of offspring mice. Paediatr Anaesth 2016; 26(1):52–9.

32. Popic J, Pesic V, Milanovic D, et al. Propofol-induced changes in neurotrophic signaling in the developing nervous system in vivo. PLoS One 2012;7(4):e34396.

33. Chalon J, Tang CK, Ramanathan S, et al. Exposure to halothane and enflurane affects learning function of murine progeny. Anesth Analg 1981;60(11):794–7.

34. Holliday R. Epigenetics: a historical overview. Epigenetics 2006;1(2):76–80.

35. Neale BM, Kou Y, Liu L, et al. Patterns and rates of exonic de novo mutations in autism spectrum disorders. Nature 2012;(485):242–5.

36. Ibla JC, Hayashi H, Bajic D, et al. Prolonged exposure to ketamine increases brain derived neurotrophic factor levels in developing rat brains. Curr Drug Saf 2009;4(1):11–6.

37. Ju LS, Jia M, Sun J, et al. Hypermethylation of hippocampal synaptic plasticity-related genes is involved in neonatal sevoflurane exposure-induced cognitive impairments in rats. Neurotox Res 2016;29(2):243–55.

38. Wu J, Bie B, Naguib M. Epigenetic manipulation of brain-derived neurotrophic factor improves memory deficiency induced by neonatal anesthesia in rats. Anesthesiology 2016;124(3):624–40.

39. Schenning KJ, Noguchi KK, Martin LD, et al. Isoflurane exposure leads to apoptosis of neurons and oligodendrocytes in 20- and 40-day old rhesus macaques. Neurotoxicol Teratol 2017;60:63–8.

40. Zou X, Liu F, Zhang X, et al. Inhalation anesthetic-induced neuronal damage in the developing rhesus monkey. Neurotoxicol Teratol 2011;33(5):592–7.

41. Zhang X, Liu S, Newport GD, et al. In vivo monitoring of sevoflurane-induced adverse effects in neonatal nonhuman primates using small-animal positron emission tomography. Anesthesiology 2016;125(1):133–46.

42. Zhang X, Liu F, Slikker W Jr, et al. Minimally invasive biomarkers of general anesthetic-induced developmental neurotoxicity. Neurotoxicol Teratol 2017;60: 95–101.

43. Paule MG, Chelonis JJ, Buffalo EA, et al. Operant test battery performance in children: correlation with IQ. Neurotoxicol Teratol 1999;21(3):223–30.

44. Paule MG, Li M, Allen RR, et al. Ketamine anesthesia during the first week of life can cause long-lasting cognitive deficits in rhesus monkeys. Neurotoxicol Teratol 2011;33(2):220–30.

45. Coleman K, Robertson ND, Dissen GA, et al. Isoflurane anesthesia has long-term consequences on motor and behavioral development in infant rhesus macaques. Anesthesiology 2017;126(1):74–84.

46. Warner DO, Chelonis JJ, Paule MG, et al. Performance on the Operant Test Battery in young children exposed to procedures requiring general anaesthesia: the MASK study. Br J Anaesth 2019;122(4):470–9.
47. Hansen HH, Briem T, Dzietko M, et al. Mechanisms leading to disseminated apoptosis following NMDA receptor blockade in the developing rat brain. Neurobiol Dis 2004;16(2):440–53.
48. Clancy B, Darlington R, Finlay B. Translating developmental time across mammalian species. Neuroscience 2001;105(1):7–17.
49. Clancy B, Finlay B, Darlington R, et al. Extrapolating brain development from experimental species to humans. Neurotoxicology 2007;28(5):931–7.
50. Hofacer RD, Deng M, Ward CG, et al. Cell age-specific vulnerability of neurons to anesthetic toxicity. Ann Neurol 2013;73(6):695–704.
51. Hansen TG, Lönnqvist PA. The rise and fall of anaesthesia-related neurotoxicity and the immature developing human brain. Acta Anaesthesiol Scand 2016; 60(3):280–3.
52. Hansen TG, Engelhardt T, Weiss M. The relevance of anesthetic drug-induced neurotoxicity. JAMA Pediatr 2017;171(1):e163481.
53. Weiss M, Vutskits L, Hansen TG, et al. Safe anesthesia for every tot - the SAFETOTS initiative. Curr Opin Anaesthesiol 2015;28(3):302–7.
54. Loepke AW, Istaphanous GK, McAuliffe JJ 3rd, et al. The effects of neonatal isoflurane exposure in mice on brain cell viability, adult behavior, learning, and memory. Anesth Analg 2009;108(1):90–104.
55. Wu B, Yu Z, You S, et al. Physiological disturbance may contribute to neurodegeneration induced by isoflurane or sevoflurane in 14 day old rats. PLoS One 2014;9(1):e84622.
56. Zhou L, Wang Z, Zhou H, et al. Neonatal exposure to sevoflurane may not cause learning and memory deficits and behavioral abnormality in the childhood of Cynomolgus monkeys. Sci Rep 2015;5:11145.
57. Pound P, Bracken MB. Is animal research sufficiently evidence based to be a cornerstone of biomedical research? BMJ 2014;30(348):g3387.
58. Zhang Y, Dong Y, Wu X, et al. The mitochondrial pathway of anesthetic isoflurane-induced apoptosis. J Biol Chem 2010;285(6):4025–37.
59. Boscolo A, Starr JA, Sanchez V, et al. The abolishment of anesthesia-induced cognitive impairment by timely protection of mitochondria in the developing rat brain: the importance of free oxygen radicals and mitochondrial integrity. Neurobiol Dis 2012. https://doi.org/10.1016/j.nbd.2011.12.022.
60. Boscolo A, Milanovic D, Starr JA, et al. Early exposure to general anesthesia disturbs mitochondrial fission and fusion in the developing rat brain. Anesthesiology 2013;118(5):1086–97.

Neurologic Injury in Neonates Undergoing Cardiac Surgery

Dean B. Andropoulos, MD, MHCM[a,b,]*, Ronald Blaine Easley, MD[a,b],
Erin A. Gottlieb, MD[c,d], Ken Brady, MD[e,f]

KEYWORDS

- Neurologic injury • Neonates • Cardiac surgery • Anesthesia

KEY POINTS

- The brain of the neonate with congenital heart disease (CHD) is structurally immature, rendering it more vulnerable to hypoxic ischemic injury including white matter injury.
- 30-40% of neonates with CHD have preoperative MRI brain injury; risk factors include hypoxemia and circulatory instability.
- Intraoperative risk factors for brain injury include extreme hemodilution, prolonged deep hypothermic circulatory arrest, cortical oxyhemoglobin desaturation, and larger exposure to volatile anesthetic agents.
- Early postsurgical indicators of brain injury include EEG seizures; prolonged ICU length of stay is also associated with worse neurodevelopmental outcomes.

INTRODUCTION

As survival after congenital heart surgery in the neonatal period continues to improve and is now greater than 90%,[1] quality of life has become the focus of significant clinical and research efforts. The realization that 25% to 90% of neonates undergoing cardiac surgery have later neurodevelopmental impairment, depending on complexity of

Disclosures: Funding for some of the research described was provided by U.S. National Institutes of Health, Eunice K. Shriver National Institute of Child Health and Development Grant: R21 HD 55501; Charles A. Dana Foundation Brain and Immuno-Imaging Grant 2007; Texas Children's Hospital Anesthesiology Research Fund.
[a] Department of Pediatric Anesthesiology, Perioperative and Pain Medicine, Texas Children's Hospital, Houston, TX, USA; [b] Departments of Anesthesiology and Pediatrics, Baylor College of Medicine, 6551 Main St. E 1940, Houston, TX 77030-3411, USA; [c] Dell Children's Medical Center of Central Texas, Austin, TX, USA; [d] Department of Surgery and Perioperative Care, Dell Medical School at the University of Texas at Austin, 4900 Mueller Blvd., Suite 2H.012C, Austin, TX 78723, USA; [e] Division of Cardiac Anesthesia, Lurie Children's Hospital of Chicago, Chicago, IL, USA; [f] Departments of Anesthesiology and Pediatrics, Northwestern University Feinberg School of Medicine, 225 East Chicago Avenue, Chicago IL 60611, USA
* Corresponding author. 6551 Main Street, E 1940, Houston, TX 77030-3411, USA.
E-mail address: dra@bcm.edu

their heart disease and surgery, as well as genetic factors, has resulted in a large body of new data in the last decade to understand causes as well as treatment strategies (**Fig. 1**).[2] This review focuses on brain injury in neonates undergoing cardiac surgery, emphasizing brain MRI injury findings as structural and microstructural evidence of cellular damage and death in the perioperative period. The authors discuss brain injury according to perioperative time period: prenatal, postnatal preoperative, intraoperative, and postoperative. They then discuss longer-term neurodevelopmental follow-up after neonatal cardiac surgery.

PRENATAL PERIOD

In the past 15 years, brain MRI studies of the prenatal and immediate neonatal periods have demonstrated that the brain in the neonate with congenital heart disease (CHD) is structurally immature, with parameters, such as myelination, cortical infolding, germinal matrix, and bands of migrating glial cells, indicating an average of 4 weeks' delayed maturation in the term infant with complex CHD.[3] Maturation of microstructural indices of cerebral metabolism measured by MRI, including magnetic resonance spectroscopy and diffusion tensor imaging, are also significantly delayed in neonates with transposition of the great arteries (D-TGA) and single-ventricle anatomy.[4] This brain dysmaturity is associated with a greater risk for new brain MRI injury after neonatal cardiac surgery, especially white matter injury (WMI).[5] In utero brain MRI studies suggest alterations in brain oxygen delivery and utilization in children with CHD, especially when oxygenation of the ascending aorta is reduced by the lesion (transposition of the great arteries [TGA], hypoplastic left heart syndrome [HLHS]). Decreased oxygen delivery and utilization in utero are associated with decreased brain volume at term.[6,7] Furthermore, fetal brain MRI studies find a 16% incidence of brain abnormalities in CHD fetuses, including 18% in HLHS and 29% in D-TGA.[8]

CHD is now diagnosed antenatally in as many as 75% or more of cases in many institutions, and trials of fetal therapies have begun in an attempt to improve brain growth and development, and it is hoped, leading to less susceptibility to injury. Pilot data from a maternal hyperoxia trial (9 subjects) showed slower growth and smaller

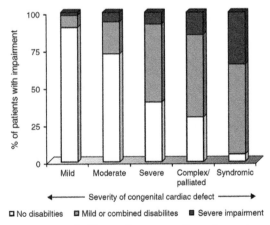

Fig. 1. Gradient between congenital heart disease severity and prevalence of neurodevelopmental impairment. (*From* Wernovsky G. Current insights regarding neurological and developmental abnormalities in children and young adults with complex congenital cardiac disease. Cardiol Young. 2006 Feb;16 Suppl 1:92-104.)

head circumference at birth.[9] A trial of maternal progesterone therapy, designed to assess whether this therapy would hasten maturation of the fetal brain in HLHS and D-TGA, is underway, with no results yet available.[10] Fetal aortic valvuloplasty has been attempted to increase left ventricular size in HLHS; although improving neurodevelopmental outcome was not the primary aim, a neurodevelopmental assessment of 52 patients at an average age of 5 years revealed a very similar pattern of neurodevelopmental delay as patients not undergoing fetal intervention.[11]

Premature delivery is a risk factor for mortality, prolonged hospital course and complications after surgery, and poorer neurodevelopmental outcome.[12,13] The former practice of "elective" delivery at 36 to 38 weeks in CHD fetuses has been demonstrated to be strongly detrimental to outcomes after neonatal cardiac surgery, and current guidelines recommend delivery no sooner than 39 completed weeks gestation unless maternal or fetal indications mandate earlier delivery.

Prenatal diagnosis is associated with a lower risk of postnatal brain injury diagnosed by MRI scanning; in a study of 153 patients with TGA or HLHS, MRI brain injury was present in 48% of those with postnatal diagnosis (44% of the total study population) versus 24% in those with prenatal diagnosis ($P = .003$). In addition, brain development as measured by fractional anisotropy and average diffusion coefficient was better in patients with prenatal diagnosis.[14] The investigators cited lower preoperative oxygen saturation, and higher incidence of acidosis and low cardiac output syndrome in patients with postnatal diagnosis; for example, hemodynamic management is improved in patients with prenatal diagnosis, as the likely explanation for this significant difference.

PRESURGICAL PERIOD

The time from birth to neonatal surgery is a critical period of profound circulatory changes and potential hemodynamic instability that can impair cerebral oxygen delivery and increase the risk for MRI brain injury. Several series of immediate preoperative brain MRI in neonates with CHD document an injury rate of 30% to 40% before surgery (**Figs. 2 and 3**). This injury is predominately WMI, although ischemic stroke is also observed.[5,15–21] Waiting time to neonatal surgery has been associated with WMI in patients with TGA and HLHS.[22,23] Abnormal response of cerebral blood flow (CBF) and metabolism has been documented in these patient groups over the transition period before surgery. Normal (noncardiac disease) subjects have matched increases in both CBF and cerebral metabolic rate for oxygen ($CMRO_2$) over time in the first week of life. Neonates with hypoxia of the ascending aorta show no increase in CBF to match the increase in $CMRO_2$ during this time and a widening $CMRO_2$ deficit (oxygen extraction fraction) each day after birth.[4] A time risk of 3 to 4 days after birth appears to be the time frame beyond which risk of brain injury increases (**Fig. 4**).[24] Anticipatory management consisting of prenatal diagnosis and delivery in a center capable of neonatal cardiac surgery, early institution of prostaglandin E1 where indicated for ductal dependent lesions, and timely diagnostic workup, presurgical planning, and surgery appears to be preferable for reduction of the risk of neurologic injury before surgery.

INTRAOPERATIVE PERIOD

Both interinstitutional and intrainstitutional management of the intraoperative period and cardiopulmonary bypass (CPB) differ profoundly, but several modifiable factors have been studied that can have an effect on neurologic injury and neurodevelopmental outcomes. Several factors have been associated with increased risk of worse neurodevelopmental outcome and are reviewed.

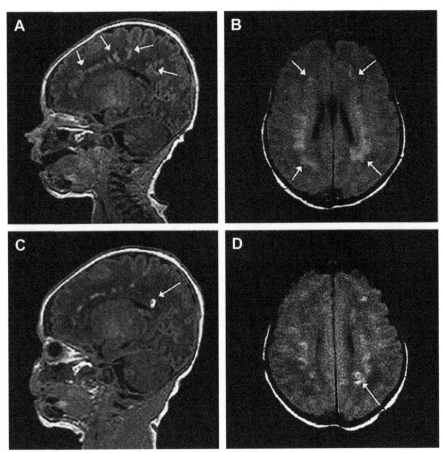

Fig. 2. (A) Preoperative sagittal T1-weighted MRI of a 35-week gestational age infant with hypoplastic left heart syndrome. Significant WMI is present in the periventricular areas (*arrows*). (B) Preoperative axial proton-density T2-weighted image. Note the extensive WMI (*arrows*). (C) Seven-day postoperative T1 sagittal MRI after Norwood stage I palliation. Note the slight improvement to the WMI, but new intraparenchymal/intraventricular hemorrhage and infarction in the atrium near the body of the left lateral ventricle (*arrow*). (D) Proton-density T2-weighted image. Note the WMI and new hemorrhage (*arrow*).

Hematocrit on Bypass

The combined hematocrit trials from Boston Children's Hospital demonstrated that hematocrit less than 24% on bypass for neonates/infants was associated with lower Psychomotor Development Index scores 1 year after surgery.[25] Fifty-six percent of the 271 subjects in these studies underwent deep hypothermic circulatory arrest (DHCA) at 18°C (98% for <45 minutes), and most had periods of low-flow bypass (25% of full flow), also at deep hypothermic temperatures. Full-flow bypass was used at all temperatures except deep hypothermia at 18°C.

Glucose Levels

The Boston Circulatory Arrest Trial assessed perioperative glucose levels and neurodevelopmental outcomes at 1, 4, and 8 years after the neonatal arterial switch operation. Higher glucose levels were not associated with lower

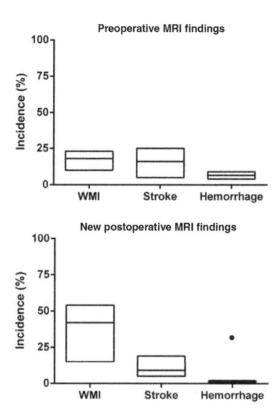

Fig. 3. The incidence of preexisting and new postoperative neurologic injuries diagnosed by brain MRI observed in neonates subjected to CPB. The findings are compiled from 6 reports, 7 centers, and 400 subjects. Median and range are shown with one outlier. (*From* Brady K, Ramamoorthy C, Easley RB, et al. Neurological Monitoring and Outcome. In, Andropoulos DB, Stayer S, Mossad EB, Miller-Hance WC (eds.) Anesthesia for Congenital Heart Disease, 3rd Edition. John wiley & Sons, Inc: Oxford UK, 2015, pp. 230-249.)

neurodevelopmental outcomes; however, they were associated with earlier return of normal electroencephalography (EEG) patterns after surgery. Lower glucose levels tended to predict EEG seizures, but not clinical seizures.[26] Tight glycemic control in the perioperative period was not associated with better neurodevelopmental outcomes at 1 year compared with standard management; however, patients with moderate to severe hypoglycemia from insulin therapy had lower neurodevelopmental outcome scores.[27]

Deep Hypothermic Circulatory Arrest/Regional Cerebral Perfusion

The classic Boston Circulatory Arrest Study demonstrated that DHCA times greater than 41 minutes were associated with lower neurodevelopmental outcomes at age 8 years, with the 95% confidence interval as low as 32 minutes for some tests.[28] Regional cerebral perfusion (RCP) is a perfusion strategy that provides blood flow to the brain while providing a bloodless surgical field for aortic arch reconstruction (**Fig. 5**).[29] With careful titration of RCP flow using near-infrared spectroscopy (NIRS) and transcranial Doppler, 1-year neurodevelopmental outcomes for aortic arch reconstruction surgeries are excellent and likely superior to cohorts using DHCA.[30] However, a recent prospective randomized controlled trial of RCP versus DHCA

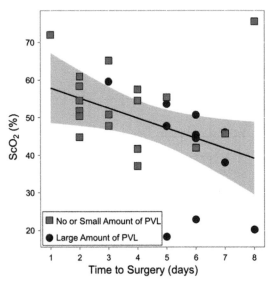

Fig. 4. Preoperative cerebral oxygenation as a function of time-to-surgery in a study of 37 neonates with HLHS.[9] The solid line represents the best-fit line to the data (R2 = 0.17, P = 0.03, slope = −2.7 ± 1.2). The gray ribbon denotes the 95% confidence interval for the mean ScO_2. The symbols represent whether the subject acquired a large amount of new or worsened postoperative periventricular leukomalacia (PVL). (*From* Lynch JM, Gaynor JW, Licht DJ. Brain Injury During Transition in the Newborn With Congenital Heart Disease: Hazards of the Preoperative Period. Semin Pediatr Neurol. 2018 Dec;28:60-65.)

whereby RCP flow was not carefully controlled using neuromonitoring, demonstrated no difference in early postoperative MRI brain injury, or cognitive and motor outcomes at 24 months.[31]

Monitoring

NIRS monitoring remains controversial in some circles; however, recent data suggest that low regional cerebral oxygen saturation (rSO_2) in the period after bypass is associated with lower neurodevelopmental outcome scores at 1 to 2 years.[32,33] There are no published controlled trials of neurodevelopmental outcomes with versus without NIRS monitoring, but physiologic plausibility suggests that monitoring rSO_2 and treating low values (relative 20% below baseline values obtained on room air or absolute rSO_2 of <50%) may be effective to prevent brain injury. **Table 1** displays strategies for monitoring and treating low rSO_2 values.[21]

Anesthetics

There are 2 cohorts that have demonstrated an association of higher volatile anesthetic agent (VAA) exposure during neonatal cardiac surgery with lower neurodevelopmental outcome scores in some domains at age 1 to 4 years. The Philadelphia cohort of 96 HLHS patients demonstrated increasing VAA exposure was associated with lower full-scale IQ, and verbal IQ at age 4 years.[34] The Texas Children's Hospital cohort in 59 neonates undergoing both single-ventricle palliation and 2-ventricle repair demonstrated an association of higher VAA with lower cognitive scores at 1 and 3 years.[35] Whether alternative anesthetic strategies, for example, dexmedetomidine, which is neuroprotective and does not cause neuroapoptosis at usual doses in

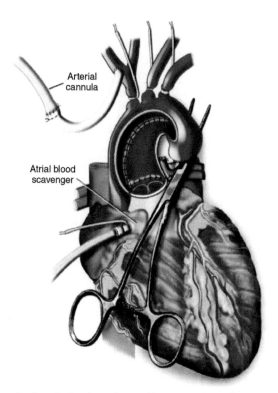

Fig. 5. Selective cerebral perfusion is performed by sewing a graft to the innominate artery and snaring the great vessels. (*From* Pigula FA, Nemoto EM, Griffith BP, Siewers RD. Regional low-flow perfusion provides cerebral circulatory support during neonatal aortic arch reconstruction. J Thorac Cardiovasc Surg. 2000;119:331-9.)

preclinical models, would be associated with improved neurodevelopmental outcome, has yet to be studied.

Other Cardiopulmonary Bypass Approaches

There has only been 1 clinical study of pH versus alpha-stat management on bypass; use of the pH-stat strategy in infants undergoing deep hypothermic CPB was associated with lower postoperative morbidity, shorter recovery time to first electroencephalographic activity, and, in patients with D-transposition, shorter duration of intubation and intensive care unit (ICU) stay.[36] However, at age 1 year, there was no difference in neurodevelopmental testing scores, and at age 2 to 4 years, no differences in development or behavior were noted on parental questionnaires.[37]

Cerebral autoregulation

The neonatal brain requires a minimum arterial blood pressure to regulate blood flow via pressure autoregulation. Autoregulation can be profoundly affected by CPB in neonates, including by hypotension and hypothermia that are often used during cardiac surgery. Mean arterial pressure (MAP) targets during CPB vary widely, from the mid-20s mm Hg during low-flow hypothermic bypass, to the 40- to 60-mm Hg range in some centers. New data from Texas Children's Hospital in neonates document wide individual variability in the lower MAP limit of autoregulation, assessed by cerebral blood volume index derived from NIRS.

Table 1
Potentially modifiable published risk factors for brain injury/lower neurodevelopmental outcome scores after neonatal congenital heart surgery

Time Period	Factor (Example)	Potential Interventions
Prenatal	Brain immaturity: reduced oxygen delivery from ascending aorta Premature delivery	Maternal hyperoxygenation Fetal catheter therapy Maternal progesterone Delay delivery until 39-wk gestation when possible
Presurgical	Hemodynamic instability; hypoxemia; derangement in matching of $CMRO_2$ to CBF	Delivery in cardiac surgical center Early institution of PGE_1 when indicated Anticipatory hemodynamic/ventilatory management Early surgery at 3–4 d when possible
Surgical	Low CPB hematocrit Use and duration of DHCA Use of RCP Abnormal cerebral autoregulation Anesthetic technique Glucose levels Low rSO_2	Maintain >24% Avoid/limit DHCA duration Use RCP with neuromonitoring in lieu of DHCA Higher MAP on bypass: 40–45 mm Hg; real-time autoregulation monitoring (future) Limit volatile anesthetic exposure, ?? dexmedetomidine Maintain adequate serum glucose: 100–200 mg/dL; avoid hypoglycemia Intervene <50%
Postsurgical	EEG seizures ICU length of stay Lack of neurodevelopmental stimulation	EEG monitoring; treat seizures: benzodiazepines, levetiracetam Early extubation Sedation protocols Prevention of infection and hemodynamic deterioration Infant stimulation programs; parental presence
Postnatal and long term	Varying risk of neurodevelopmental impairment	Formal neurodevelopmental assessments/follow-up in early infancy; early intervention where appropriate

Abbreviations: GA, gestational age; PGE_1, prostaglandin E_1.

Prior studies suggesting that neonates do not autoregulate during bypass or during deep hypothermia were confounded by hypotensive management strategies.[38–42] The average lower limit of autoregulation (LLA) for a neonate during CPB ranges from 25 to 45 mm Hg, with a trend upward in the first year of life (**Fig. 6**). Intersubject variability is too great to declare a safe arterial blood pressure for all subjects without real-time monitoring, which is not yet Food and Drug Administration approved. Until the availability of such an NIRS-based monitor in the next few years, it seems prudent to target MAPs on CPB in neonates of 40 to 45 mm Hg during full flow CPB.

Overall incidence of MRI brain injury

Several cohorts of postoperative MRI assessment in neonatal cardiac surgery document an incidence of new MRI injury of 35% to 75%.[5,15–20] This new injury occurs despite application of neuroprotective strategies, such as NIRS monitoring and treatment, higher hematocrits, and RCP in lieu of DHCA. Brain MRI injury in the perioperative period for neonatal CHD surgery has been associated with poorer

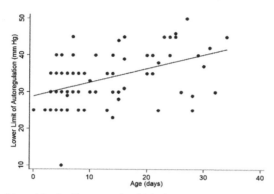

Fig. 6. The upward trend in the first month of life for the average lower limit of autoregulation during cardiopulmonary bypass.

neurodevelopmental outcomes in several cohorts at 1 to 5 years of age.[35,43] Therefore, it would appear that there is significant work ahead to improve brain injury detection and approaches to treatment that could reduce this high incidence of new MRI injury.

Postoperative Period

Postoperative electroencephalography monitoring

Roughly 10% of neonates who have cardiac surgery with CPB have seizures postoperatively, and many of these are clinically silent.[44,45] Neurodevelopmental outcomes are worse in neonates who have seizure after cardiac surgery.[46] One series from Texas Children's Hospital found only 1 brief EEG seizure in 68 neonates; NIRS monitoring was used in this study as well as significant doses of intraoperative and postoperative midazolam so it is not clear whether the significantly lower seizure burden in this study is due to superior brain protection or pharmacologic suppression.[47] The American Clinical Neurophysiology Society recommends continuous EEG monitoring for neonates after cardiac surgery.[48] Despite these recommendations, most centers do not perform continuous EEG monitoring in this setting. Although the identification and treatment of postoperative seizure activity have not yet been demonstrated to mitigate the neurodevelopmental delay associated with seizure activity, additional data about prevention, detection, and treatment of subclinical seizures are warranted, as is appropriate treatment of seizures when they are identified.

Longer duration of ICU length of stay (ICU LOS) has consistently been a significant risk factor for lower neurodevelopmental outcome scores, even after adjusting for other variables, such as cardiac lesion, duration of bypass, MRI brain injury, anesthetic exposure, and low rSO$_2$.[35,49,50] Strategies directed at reducing ICU LOS, such as early weaning and extubation from mechanical ventilation, sedation protocols, early detection of hemodynamic compromise, and prevention of infection and other complications, would appear to be warranted to potentially improve neurodevelopmental outcomes. Environmental enrichment after neonatal surgery, that is, infant stimulation programs, family/parental presence, and so forth, have promise to mitigate some of the effects of neonatal brain injury and to take advantage of neonatal brain plasticity to recover from brain injury.[51]

Postneonatal Period and Long-Term Follow-Up

Because of the widely recognized high risk and incidence of neurodevelopmental outcome problems, it is now the recommendation of all major societies that

Table 2
Causes and treatments of cortical desaturation used at Texas Children's Hospital

Abnormality	Principle	Intervention
Cerebral perfusion pressure	The brain is perfused by pressure, not cardiac output. However, the authors' preference is to treat low pressure with cardiac output support, to avoid excessive vascular resistance and hypoperfusion of the noncerebral vascular beds	During CPB: Increase flow rate and maintain afterload reduction. Vasopressor only if excessive vasoplegia is suspected. Check SVC and aortic cannulae Off CPB: Administer volume judiciously with monitoring of atrial filling pressures. Inotropic support to improve stroke volume. Pacing for bradycardia. Vasopressors when excessive vasoplegia is suspected, and judiciously when volume is not tolerated and/or arrhythmia precludes beta-agonist therapy
Anemia	Low-oxygen-carrying capacity increases vulnerability to watershed WMI. The infant heart has low tolerance for the volume administration of transfusion immediately after bypass	Avoid excessive hemodilution during hypothermia, typically 30%–35%. Blood transfusion and hemofiltration during CPB to a hematocrit >40% at separation. Higher hematocrit at separation allows for a volume-neutral exchange transfusion of platelets if needed
Fever	High brain temperatures increase $CMRO_2$. High global extractions yield low mixed venous oxygen saturations, affecting arterial saturation in infants with mixing lesions	Fevers are treated with antipyretics. Cooling is easily controlled on CPB. After separation and in the ICU, cooling can be accomplished to normothermia when needed with adequate sedation
Hypoxia	Arterial hypoxia in the infant with a mixing lesion must be addressed systematically. Reflex administration of oxygen in this setting can result in systemic hypoperfusion	Lung ventilation and perfusion: tracheal suction, recruitment maneuvers Pulmonary to systemic flow ratio: evaluate for shunt occlusion, pulmonary vascular tone elevation Mixed venous desaturation: see next row
Mixed venous desaturation	Infants with mixing lesions are especially vulnerable to decrements of mixed venous oxygen content. Systemic vascular tone is the most common cause. Excessive work of breathing, agitation, shivering, and fever can contribute to low mixed venous saturation	Alpha-blockade is used for infants during CPB. Afterload reduction with milrinone, nitroprusside, or ACE inhibitors is a preferred first-line therapy after separation from CPB. Intubation, sedation, or paralysis may be necessary in the ICU depending on the acuity. Pressure support trials causing low mixed-venous oxygen saturation and cortical desaturation should be terminated

(continued on next page)

Table 2 (continued)		
Abnormality	Principle	Intervention
Hypocarbia	Arterial CO_2 diffuses freely into the CSF, whereas soluble buffers do not. CBF is increased by acidic CSF (increased CO_2) and decreased by basic CSF (decreased CO_2). CSF buffering over several hours compensates acute changes in CBF caused by arterial CO_2 tension	Whether pH-stat or α-stat methods of measuring arterial CO_2 tension are used, low CBF can be mitigated during CPB by permissive hypercapnia

Abbreviations: ACE, angiotensin-converting enzyme; CSF, cerebral spinal fluid; SVC, superior vena cava.

From Brady K, Ramamoorthy C, Easley RB, et al. Neurological Monitoring and Outcome. In, Andropoulos DB, Stayer S, Mossad EB, Miller-Hance WC (eds.) Anesthesia for Congenital Heart Disease, 3rd Edition. John wiley & Sons, Inc: Oxford UK, 2015, pp. 230-249.

infants undergoing cardiac surgery with bypass have regular, formal neurodevelopmental follow-up testing starting in the first year of life as standard of care.[52] Specific testing over multiple domains, including IQ, speech and language, fine and gross motor control, and executive functioning, should occur at regular intervals, and early developmental intervention should be initiated when deficits are discovered.

SUMMARY

Neurodevelopmental outcomes after neonatal congenital heart surgery are significantly influenced by brain injury detectable by MRI techniques. This brain injury can occur in the prenatal and postnatal periods even before cardiac surgery. Given the significant incidence of new MRI brain injury after cardiac surgery, much work is yet to be done on strategies to detect, prevent, and treat brain injury in the neonatal period in order to optimize longer-term neurodevelopmental outcomes.[53] **Table 2** summarizes the major areas of intervention discussed in this review for prevention and treatment of brain injury in neonatal cardiac surgery.

Best Practices

What is the current practice for neurologic injury in neonates undergoing cardiac surgery?

Best practice/guideline/care path objective(s)

What changes in current practice are likely to improve outcomes?

All of the major recommendations below have potential to improve neurologic outcomes.

Major recommendations

Prenatal period: Achieve accurate prenatal cardiac diagnosis (B), avoid premature delivery (B); deliver in or near tertiary cardiac center (B).[12,13]

Presurgical period: Limit the time presurgery to 3 to 4 days if possible in cyanotic patients (B); consider MRI to assess baseline brain injury status (B).[14,22–24]

Intraoperative period: Maintain hematocrit on bypass 25% or greater (A); do not practice tight glucose control (A); avoid or limit DHCA to 30 minutes (A); use NIRS monitoring and treat low rSO_2 less than 50% (B); maintain MAP on CPB at 40 to 45 mm Hg (B).[25,27,28,32,33,40,41]

Postoperative period: Monitor EEG in high-risk patients and treat seizures (B); limit ICU stay with early extubation and discharge protocols (B); obtain postoperative MRI (B); ensure longer-term follow-up (A).[35,44,45,48,49,52]

Rating for the Strength of the Evidence: A, one or more well-designed randomized controlled trials; B, one or more well-designed prospective observational studies; C, retrospective cohorts or case control studies; D, case reports or expert opinion only.

Bibliographic Source(s): This is an important list of current sources relevant to evidence—see by each recommendation.

REFERENCES

1. The Society of Thoracic Surgeons. Available at: https://www.sts.org/sites/default/files/documents/Fall2018Congenital-STSExecSummary_Neonates.pdf. Accessed April 9, 2019.
2. Wernovsky G. Current insights regarding neurological and developmental abnormalities in children and young adults with complex congenital cardiac disease. Cardiol Young 2006;16(Suppl 1):92–104.
3. Licht DJ, Shera DM, Clancy RR, et al. Brain maturation is delayed in infants with complex congenital heart defects. J Thorac Cardiovasc Surg 2009;137(3):529–36.
4. Miller SP, McQuillen PS, Hamrick S, et al. Abnormal brain development in newborns with congenital heart disease. N Engl J Med 2007;357(19):1928–38.
5. Andropoulos DB, Hunter JV, Nelson DP, et al. Brain immaturity is associated with brain injury before and after neonatal cardiac surgery with high-flow bypass and cerebral oxygenation monitoring. J Thorac Cardiovasc Surg 2010;139(3):543–56.
6. Kaltman JR, Di H, Tian Z, et al. Impact of congenital heart disease on cerebrovascular blood flow dynamics in the fetus. Ultrasound Obstet Gynecol 2005;25:32–6.
7. Sun L, Macgowan CK, Sled JG, et al. Reduced fetal cerebral oxygen consumption is associated with smaller brain size in fetuses with congenital heart disease. Circulation 2015;131:1313–23.
8. Brossard-Racine M, du Plessis A, Vezina G, et al. Brain injury in neonates with complex congenital heart disease: what is the predictive value of MRI in the fetal period? AJNR Am J Neuroradiol 2016;37(7):1338–46.
9. Edwards LA, Lara DA, Sanz Cortes M, et al. Chronic maternal hyperoxygenation and effect on cerebral and placental vasoregulation and neurodevelopment in fetuses with left heart hypoplasia. Fetal Diagn Ther 2018;17:1–13.
10. ClinicalTrials.gov. Available at: https://clinicaltrials.gov/ct2/show/NCT02133573?cond=maternal+progesterone&rank=1;. Accessed April 9, 2019.
11. Laraja K, Sadhwani A, Tworetzky W, et al. Neurodevelopmental outcome in children after fetal cardiac intervention for aortic stenosis with evolving hypoplastic left heart syndrome. J Pediatr 2017;184:130–6.
12. Steurer MA, Baer RJ, Keller RL, et al. Gestational age and outcomes in critical congenital heart disease. Pediatrics 2017;140(4) [pii:e20170999].
13. Sanz JH, Wang J, Berl MM, et al. Executive function and psychosocial quality of life in school age children with congenital heart disease. J Pediatr 2018;202:63–9.
14. Peyvandi S, De Santiago V, Chakkarapani E, et al. Association of prenatal diagnosis of critical congenital heart disease with postnatal brain development and the risk of brain injury. JAMA Pediatr 2016;170(4):e154450.
15. Mahle WT, Tavani F, Zimmerman RA, et al. An MRI study of neurological injury before and after congenital heart surgery. Circulation 2002;106:I109–14.

16. Andropoulos DB, Brady K, Easley RB, et al. Erythropoietin neuroprotection in neonatal cardiac surgery: a phase I/II safety and efficacy trial. J Thorac Cardiovasc Surg 2013;146:124–31.

17. Galli KK, Zimmerman RA, Jarvik GP, et al. Periventricular leukomalacia is common after neonatal cardiac surgery. J Thorac Cardiovasc Surg 2004;127: 692–704.

18. Dent CL, Spaeth JP, Jones BV, et al. Brain magnetic resonance imaging abnormalities after the Norwood procedure using regional cerebral perfusion. J Thorac Cardiovasc Surg 2006;131:190–7.

19. Beca J, Gunn JK, Coleman L, et al. New white matter brain injury after infant heart surgery is associated with diagnostic group and the use of circulatory arrest. Circulation 2013;127:971–9.

20. Block AJ, McQuillen PS, Chau V, et al. Clinically silent preoperative brain injuries do not worsen with surgery in neonates with congenital heart disease. J Thorac Cardiovasc Surg 2010;140:550–7.

21. Brady K, Ramamoorthy C, Easley RB, et al. Chapter 11: neurological monitoring and outcome. In: Andropoulos DB, Stayer S, Mossad EB, et al, editors. Anesthesia for congenital heart disease. 3rd edition. Oxford (United Kingdom): John wiley & Sons, Inc.; 2015. p. 230–49.

22. Lynch JM, Buckley EM, Schwab PJ, et al. Time to surgery and preoperative cerebral hemodynamics predict postoperative white matter injury in neonates with hypoplastic left heart syndrome. J Thorac Cardiovasc Surg 2014;148:2181–8.

23. Petit CJ, Rome JJ, Wernovsky G, et al. Preoperative brain injury in transposition of the great arteries is associated with oxygenation and time to surgery, not balloon atrial septostomy. Circulation 2009;119:709–16.

24. Lynch JM, Gaynor JW, Licht DJ. Brain injury during transition in the newborn with congenital heart disease: hazards of the preoperative period. Semin Pediatr Neurol 2018;28:60–5.

25. Wypij D, Jonas RA, Bellinger DC, et al. The effect of hematocrit during hypothermic cardiopulmonary bypass in infant heart surgery: results from the combined Boston hematocrit trials. J Thorac Cardiovasc Surg 2008;135:355–60.

26. de Ferranti S, Gauvreau K, Hickey PR, et al. Intraoperative hyperglycemia during infant cardiac surgery is not associated with adverse neurodevelopmental outcomes at 1, 4, and 8 years. Anesthesiology 2004;100:1345–52.

27. Sadhwani A, Asaro LA, Goldberg C, et al. Impact of tight glycemic control on neurodevelopmental outcomes at 1 year of age for children with congenital heart disease: a randomized controlled trial. J Pediatr 2016;174:193–8.

28. Wypij D, Newburger JW, Rappaport LA, et al. The effect of duration of deep hypothermic circulatory arrest in infant heart surgery on late neurodevelopment: the Boston Circulatory Arrest Trial. J Thorac Cardiovasc Surg 2003;126:1397–403.

29. Pigula FA, Nemoto EM, Griffith BP, et al. Regional low-flow perfusion provides cerebral circulatory support during neonatal aortic arch reconstruction. J Thorac Cardiovasc Surg 2000;119:331–9.

30. Andropoulos DB, Easley RB, Brady K, et al. Neurodevelopmental outcomes after regional cerebral perfusion with neuromonitoring for neonatal aortic arch reconstruction. Ann Thorac Surg 2013;95:648–54.

31. Algra SO, Jansen NJ, van der Tweel I, et al. Neurological injury after neonatal cardiac surgery: a randomized, controlled trial of 2 perfusion techniques. Circulation 2014;129:224–33.

32. Aly SA, Zurakowski D, Glass P, et al. Cerebral tissue oxygenation index and lactate at 24 hours postoperative predict survival and neurodevelopmental outcome after neonatal cardiac surgery. Congenit Heart Dis 2017;12:188–95.

33. Kussman BD, Wypij D, Laussen PC, et al. Relationship of intraoperative cerebral oxygen saturation to neurodevelopmental outcome and brain magnetic resonance imaging at 1 year of age in infants undergoing biventricular repair. Circulation 2010;122:245–54.

34. Diaz LK, Gaynor JW, Koh SJ, et al. Increasing cumulative exposure to volatile anesthetic agents is associated with poorer neurodevelopmental outcomes in children with hypoplastic left heart syndrome. J Thorac Cardiovasc Surg 2016; 152:482–9.

35. Andropoulos DB, Ahmad HB, Haq T, et al. The association between brain injury, perioperative anesthetic exposure, and 12-month neurodevelopmental outcomes after neonatal cardiac surgery: a retrospective cohort study. Paediatr Anaesth 2014;24:266–74.

36. du Plessis AJ, Jonas RA, Wypij D, et al. Perioperative effects of alpha-stat versus pH-stat strategies for deep hypothermic cardiopulmonary bypass in infants. J Thorac Cardiovasc Surg 1997;114:991–1000.

37. Bellinger DC, Wypij D, du Plessis AJ, et al. Developmental and neurologic effects of alpha-stat versus pH-stat strategies for deep hypothermic cardiopulmonary bypass in infants. J Thorac Cardiovasc Surg 2001;121:374–83.

38. Lynch JM, Ko T, Busch DR, et al. Preoperative cerebral hemodynamics from birth to surgery in neonates with critical congenital heart disease. J Thorac Cardiovasc Surg 2018;156:1657–64.

39. Brady Ken M, Mytar Jennifer O, Lee Jennifer K, et al. Monitoring cerebral blood flow pressure autoregulation in pediatric patients during cardiac surgery. Stroke 2010;41:1957–62.

40. Goswami D, McLeod K, Leonard S, et al. Static cerebrovascular pressure autoregulation remains intact during deep hypothermia. Pediatr Anesth 2017;27: 911–7.

41. Smith B, Vu E, Kibler K, et al. Does hypothermia impair cerebrovascular autoregulation in neonates during cardiopulmonary bypass? Paediatr Anaesth 2017;27: 905–10.

42. Taylor RH, Burrows FA, Bissonnette B. Cerebral pressure-flow velocity relationship during hypothermic cardiopulmonary bypass in neonates and infants. Anesth Analg 1992;74:636–42.

43. Claessens NHP, Algra SO, Ouwehand TL, et al, CHD Lifespan Study Group Utrecht. Perioperative neonatal brain injury is associated with worse school-age neurodevelopment in children with critical congenital heart disease. Dev Med Child Neurol 2018;60(10):1052–8.

44. Naim MY, Gaynor JW, Chen J, et al. Subclinical seizures identified by postoperative electroencephalographic monitoring are common after neonatal cardiac surgery. J Thorac Cardiovasc Surg 2015;150:169–80.

45. Clancy RR, McGaurn SA, Wernovsky G, et al. Risk of seizures in survivors of newborn heart surgery using deep hypothermic circulatory arrest. Pediatrics 2003;111:592–601.

46. Bellinger DC, Wypij D, Rivkin MJ, et al. Adolescents with d-transposition of the great arteries corrected with the arterial switch procedure: neuropsychological assessment and structural brain imaging. Circulation 2011;124:1361–9.

47. Andropoulos DB, Mizrahi EM, Hrachovy RA, et al. Electroencephalographic seizures after neonatal cardiac surgery with high-flow cardiopulmonary bypass. Anesth Analg 2010;110(6):1680–5.

48. Shellhaas RA, Chang T, Tsuchida T, et al. The American Clinical Neurophysiology Society's guideline on continuous electroencephalography monitoring in neonates. J Clin Neurophysiol 2011;28(6):611–7.

49. Newburger JW, Sleeper LA, Bellinger DC, et al. Early developmental outcome in children with hypoplastic left heart syndrome and related anomalies: the single ventricle reconstruction trial. Circulation 2012;125:2081–91.

50. Guerra GG, Robertson CM, Alton GY, et al. Neurotoxicity of sedative and analgesia drugs in young infants with congenital heart disease: 4-year follow-up. Paediatr Anaesth 2014;24:257–65.

51. Fourdain S, St-Denis A, Harvey J, et al, CINC team. Language development in children with congenital heart disease aged 12-24 months. Eur J Paediatr Neurol 2019. https://doi.org/10.1016/j.ejpn.2019.03.002.

52. Marino BS, Lipkin PH, Newburger JW, et al. Neurodevelopmental outcomes in children with congenital heart disease: evaluation and management: a scientific statement from the American Heart Association. Circulation 2012;126:1143–72.

53. Peyvandi S, Latal B, Miller SP, et al. The neonatal brain in critical congenital heart disease: insights and future directions. Neuroimage 2019;185:776–82.

Pharmacology of Common Analgesic and Sedative Drugs Used in the Neonatal Intensive Care Unit

Jamesia Donato, MD[a], Karishma Rao, MD[a],
Tamorah Lewis, MD, PhD[a,b],*

KEYWORDS

• Neonatal • Pharmacology • Sedation • Analgesia • Pain

KEY POINTS

• Neonatal analgesic and sedation drug treatment is challenging because of a rapidly developing target organ.
• Neonatal and infant drug exposure can vary greatly and unpredictably because of development changes in metabolism and metabolic changes related to disease state.
• Multimodal analgesic approaches have the potential to limit exposure to any given drug class and minimize unwanted side effects.
• An increased understanding of pharmacogenetics in the neonatal population provides the opportunity to individualize opiate therapy.

INTRODUCTION

For decades neonatal pain was underrecognized. It was previously believed that the immaturity of the nervous system of neonates protected them from experiencing pain.[1] However, studies have shown that neonates have significant short- and long-term consequences to inadequately treated pain. These consequences include significant hormonal and metabolic stresses[2] and altered responses to pain over time including development of chronic pain syndromes.[1] Anand and colleagues[2]

Disclosure Statement: The authors have nothing to disclose.
[a] Department of Pediatrics, Division of Neonatology, UMKC School of Medicine, Children's Mercy Hospital, 2401 Gillham Road, Kansas City, MO 64108, USA; [b] Division of Clinical Pharmacology, Toxicology and Therapeutic Innovation, Department of Pediatrics, Division of Pediatric Clinical Pharmacology, UMKC School of Medicine, Children's Mercy Hospital, Kansas City, MO, USA
* Corresponding author. Department of Pediatrics, Division of Neonatology, UMKC School of Medicine, Children's Mercy Hospital, 2401 Gillham Road, Kansas City, MO 64108.
E-mail address: trlewis@cmh.edu
twitter: @TamorahLewisMD (T.L.)

Clin Perinatol 46 (2019) 673–692
https://doi.org/10.1016/j.clp.2019.08.004
0095-5108/19/© 2019 Elsevier Inc. All rights reserved.

demonstrated that untreated pain is associated with increased morbidity and mortality. Although it is now understood that treatment of neonatal pain is essential to medical care, there is growing evidence that exposure to certain analgesics and sedatives medications in a critical window of brain development has been associated with poor neurodevelopmental outcomes.[3] Human studies are supported by preclinical models with animal studies providing mechanisms of brain injury including apoptotic neurodegeneration.[4] Hence, one must ensure adequate analgesia and sedation while also minimizing the associated risks.

The treatment of pain in neonates is challenging because the "symptomatic organ" and the drug effect site are in a state of maturation. Neuronal synapses begin to form at 12 weeks of gestation. Electroencephalogram activity is detected around 20 weeks, becoming synchronized by 26 weeks, and demonstrates sleep cycles around 30 weeks.[5] Studies suggest that newborn sensory circuits are more excitable, and their inhibitory pathways mature during the postnatal period. This may suggest that neonates are more susceptible to pain than adults.[6] The delayed maturation of neuroinhibition could be caused by deficiency of neurotransmitters or lack of specific receptors.[7] Newborns have immature neuronal mechanisms limiting their ability to filter sensory stimuli from the periphery and they tend to have exaggerated and generalized responses to these stimuli.[7] Given these differences between the neonatal and more mature brain, it behooves neonatal practitioners to understand the pharmacology of pain and sedation medications, to maximize the benefit to risk ratio in drug therapy.

PHARMACOLOGY OF ANALGESICS IN NEONATES

Neonates are a unique population with regard to drug, metabolism, elimination, and clinical effects. In this section, the pharmacology of different analgesic drugs is described through the lens of these drug properties. Although opiates are the mainstay of pain treatment in the neonatal intensive care unit (NICU), it is important to consider alternatives to opioid analgesics. Use of nonopiates can decrease short- and long-term sequelae including excessive sedation and subsequent withdrawal. In a systematic review performed by Zhu and colleagues,[8] perioperative acetaminophen, nonsteroidal anti-inflammatory drugs (NSAIDs), dexamethasone, ketamine, clonidine, and dexmedetomidine may decrease postoperative pain and opioid consumption in some pediatric surgical populations. More studies that explore these opioid-sparing alternatives should be performed in the preterm and term neonate population to help guide ongoing use, efficacy, and safety with the goal of adequately treating pain in the neonate. Specific drugs discussed in this article along with their mechanism of action, metabolism, and excretion are found for review in **Table 1**.

Nonopioid Analgesics

Acetaminophen

Acetaminophen (*N*-acetyl-p-aminophenol) is a synthetic, nonopioid, centrally acting analgesic used in the treatment of mild to moderate pain in neonates most commonly in the postoperative setting. It is administered by oral, rectal, and intravenous (IV) routes, with the IV route being most commonly used in the postoperative setting. In 2010, IV acetaminophen was first approved by the US Food and Drug Administration for the management of mild to moderate pain, as an adjunctive therapy to opioids in the treatment of moderate to severe pain, and for fever reduction in patients older than 2 years. The precise mechanism of action of acetaminophen is not known; however, it is thought to have a central analgesic effect caused by activation of descending

Table 1
Drug mechanism of action, metabolism, and excretion

Drug	Mechanism of Action	Metabolism	Excretion
Nonopiate analgesics			
Acetaminophen	Activates descending serotonergic inhibitory pathways Inhibits hypothalamic heat-regulating center	Conjugation with glucuronide, conjugation with sulfate (primary in neonates), and oxidation via CYP-450 in the liver	Renal
NSAIDS	Inhibits COX-1 and COX-2	Hepatic biotransformation by CYP-450s CYP2C8, CYP2C9, 2C19 ± glucuronidation	Renal
Opiate analgesics			
Morphine	Opioid receptor agonist	Glucuronidation in the liver (UGT2B7 primary)	Renal
Fentanyl	Opioid receptor agonist	Metabolism by CYP3A4 in the liver	Renal
Remifentanil	Opioid receptor agonist	Tissue and plasma esterases	Renal
Sedatives			
Midazolam	GABA receptor agonist	Hydroxylation by CYP4503A family	Renal
Clonidine	α_2-Agonist	Hydroxylation by CYP2D6	Renal
Dexmedetomidine	α_2-Agonist	Glucuronidation, hydroxylation in the liver	Renal, feces

Abbreviations: COX, cyclooxygenase; CYP, cytochrome; GABA, γ-aminobutyric acid; UGT, uridine diphosphate glucuronosyltransferase.

serotonergic inhibitory pathways in the central nervous system, whereas the antipyretic effect is produced from inhibition of the hypothalamic heat-regulating center. Specifically, in the neonatal population, drug safety is paramount because side effects are intensified in the setting of immature drug metabolism. Acetaminophen has a high therapeutic index making it safe and efficacious in the management of neonatal pain.[9] Acetaminophen has an opioid-sparing effect[10] making it ideal to help balance analgesia.

The pharmacokinetics of IV acetaminophen have been studied in premature neonates. IV administration results in rapid and high plasma concentrations and a clinical analgesic effect within 5 minutes of administration[11] with the maximum concentration occurring near the end of a 15-minute IV infusion. When the IV formulation of acetaminophen is compared with an equivalent oral dose, the maximum concentration is up to 70% higher, whereas overall exposure (area under the concentration time curve [AUC]) is similar.[12] The pharmacokinetic exposure of IV acetaminophen is higher in neonates and infants when compared with older children, adolescents, and adults secondary because of a myriad of factors including but not limited to a higher volume of distribution caused by higher total body water, immature hepatic biotransformation pathways, and diminished protein binding. Pharmacokinetic dosing simulations (interval every 6 hours) in infants and neonates suggest that dose reductions of 33% and 50% in infants 1 month to less than 2 years of age, and in neonates up to 28 days, respectively, produces a pharmacokinetic exposure similar to that observed in older children.

Acetaminophen is widely distributed throughout most body tissues except fat, which may makes it a more ideal analgesic even in small neonates who lack fat stores. Acetaminophen is primarily metabolized in the liver by first-order kinetics and involves three principal pathways: (1) conjugation with glucuronide, (2) conjugation with sulfate (primary in neonates), and (3) oxidation via the cytochrome (CY) P-450 enzyme pathway to form a reactive intermediate metabolite (N-acetyl-p-benzoquinone imine [NAPQI]).[13] Acetaminophen metabolites are mainly cleared renally.[14] Regardless of the route of delivery, the terminal elimination half-life of acetaminophen is approximately 2 to 4 hours in children, adolescents, and adults.[12] It is slightly longer in infants and neonates and is longer still in premature neonates.[9] Maturational effects in acetaminophen metabolism in neonates and infants are well characterized and have demonstrated a limited ability to metabolize acetaminophen via glucuronide.[15] Neonates and infants, therefore, predominantly metabolize acetaminophen via the sulfation pathway, which may help explain reduced clearance.[15]

Acetaminophen has shown opiate-sparing effects in neonates. Following recruitment of 71 neonates and infants undergoing major noncardiac surgery in a randomized, placebo-controlled setting, coadministration of IV paracetamol resulted in a significant reduction (66%) in morphine exposure.[16] More recently, Härmä and colleagues[17] found a similar magnitude effect in preterm neonates (−54% cumulative morphine exposure). In a double-blind, randomized controlled trial, Ceelie and colleagues[16] investigated the utility of IV acetaminophen in infants. The cumulative morphine dose was significantly lower in the acetaminophen group with a median of 121 µg/kg per 48 hours (interquartile range, 99–264) compared with the morphine group with a median of 357 µg/kg per 48 hours (interquartile range, 220–605; P<.001) and is displayed in **Fig. 1**. This finding represents a 66% reduction in

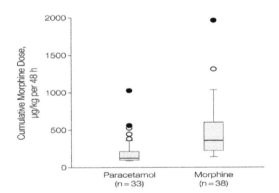

Fig. 1. Cumulative morphine dose for morphine and paracetamol study groups over 48 postoperative hours. Boxes indicate medians (*horizontal lines*) and interquartile ranges; error bars indicate 10th and 90th percentiles. Open black circles indicate outliers with values more than 1.5 times the height of the boxes; solid black circles indicate extreme outliers with values more than three times the height of the boxes. Two extreme outliers were identified in the paracetamol group, the first a boy aged 68 days who underwent surgery for a long-gap esophageal atresia and subsequently needed a chest tube for a pneumothorax and the second a newborn boy with a gastroschisis for which a silo was placed. One extreme outlier was identified in the morphine group, a girl aged 355 days who underwent surgery for a recurrence of a congenital diaphragmatic hernia. (*From* Ceelie I, de Wildt SN, van Dijk M, et al. Effect of intravenous paracetamol on postoperative morphine requirements in neonates and infants undergoing major noncardiac surgery: a randomized controlled trial. JAMA. 2013 Jan 9;309(2):149–54. doi:10.1001/jama.2012.148050; with permission.)

cumulative morphine dosage and thus supports using nonopioid analgesics to improve postoperative pain control and avoid high opioid exposure. In another study by Hong and colleagues,[18] which included 63 children aged 6 to 24 months, acetaminophen had significant fentanyl-sparing effects and also reduced side effects, such as excessive sedation, respiratory depression, constipation, and withdrawal, in pediatric patients in the postoperative setting.

The main side effect of IV acetaminophen in neonates is hepatotoxicity caused by the metabolite NAPQI. NAPQI depletes the liver of glutathione that acts as antioxidant, and directly damages cells in the liver at the mitochondrial level, subsequently resulting in liver failure.[19] Other rarer side effects include bradycardia and hypotension. Based on prospectively collected observations in 72 neonates, only a modest decrease in heart rate (7 bpm) and mean arterial blood pressure (3 mm Hg) following IV paracetamol administration was observed. A minority (9%) of neonates developed hypotension (mean arterial blood pressure < postmenstrual age in weeks, mm Hg).[20]

Nonsteroidal anti-inflammatory drugs

NSAIDS provide another nonopiate for addressing pain in neonates and infants. Although NSAIDS are routinely used in pain management of adults and older children, literature examining the use of NSAIDS for analgesia, antipyresis, and as anti-inflammatory drugs[21] in the neonatal population is lacking because significant safety issues exist. With the advent of selective cyclooxygenase (COX)-2 inhibitors, and increasing demand for opioid-sparing analgesics, the interest in NSAIDS is sharpening.[21]

NSAIDS are one of the pillars and mainstays of therapy for inflammatory pain by reducing prostanoid levels,[22] which contribute to the development of peripheral sensitization through increasing excitability and reducing the pain threshold.[23] The prostanoid system in neonates has the potential to address the inflammatory component of pain but at the risk of other organ injury. Physiologic effects of inhibition of prostaglandin synthesis applicable to neonates include disruption of the sleep cycle, increased risk of pulmonary hypertension, alterations in cerebral blood flow, decreased renal function, disrupted thermoregulation, and alterations in hemostasis balance, among others.[21] NSAIDS inhibit COX-1 and COX-2, which are responsible for converting arachidonic acid into prostaglandins. By inhibiting the COX enzymes, NSAIDs produce analgesic, antipyretic, and/or anti-inflammatory effects. Currently, which COX isoform (COX-1 or COX-2) plays a predominant role in fetal and early neonatal life remains a topic of uncertainty. It is postulated that COX-2 is more upregulated with inflammation and is the main factor playing a role in pain signaling. Oral administration of NSAIDS in neonates results in unpredictable or reduced absorption secondary to irregular gastric emptying, alkaline gastric pH, and decreased intestinal and biliary function.[21] Decrease in muscular blood flow makes intramuscular administration unpredictable and increased skin permeability accelerates drug absorption by the transdermal route.[21] In general, the decreased serum albumin and total protein, the presence of fetal hemoglobin, the increased bilirubin, and reduced adipose tissue in neonates relative to adults results in increased free fraction of drug and a decreased volume of distribution of hydrophobic drugs, such as NSAIDS.[21] Clearance of NSAIDS is reduced in neonates and increased with age. Clearance increases from 2.06 mL/kg/h at 22 to 31 weeks patient-controlled analgesia (PCA)[24] to 9.49 mL/kg/h at 28 weeks PCA[25] to 140 ml/kg/h at 5 years of age.[26]

In a recent meta-analysis by Pacifici,[27] kinetic parameters of ibuprofen were measured in 13 preterm infants with a hemodynamically significant patent ductus arteriosus (gestational age, 28.9 ± 1.9 weeks; birth weight, 1250 ± 460 g) on the 3rd and

5th day of life. Standard doses of ibuprofen were administered on Days 3, 4, and 5. A large degree of interindividual variability was observed in ibuprofen pharmacokinetic parameters. The AUC between 0 and 24 hours after the dose, a marker of drug exposure, decreased significantly from Day 3 to Day 5 of life, indicative of increased clearance.[27] In preterm infants given enteral ibuprofen, the half-life of ibuprofen decreased from 43.1 ± 26.1 hours on the 3rd day of life to 26.8 ± 23.3 hours on the 5th day of life.[28] The half-life is 1.9 ± 0.5 hours in infants 8 to 25 weeks old.[28] This rapid shortening of half-life during neonatal maturation is caused by the rapid increase of CYP2C9 and CYP2C8 hepatic activities.[27]

Ketorolac is another NSAID that has been widely used as an adjunct for improving pain control postoperatively in pediatric and adult patients, but little data exist to support safe use in the neonatal population. Papacci and colleagues[29] assessed postsurgical pain from invasive procedures in spontaneously breathing neonates with chronic lung disease. With administration of IV ketorolac, pain scores (Neonatal Infant Pain Scale) were assessed before and after IV administration of 1 mg/kg of ketorolac and 94.4% of the neonates in the study achieved total pain control. None of these neonates experienced hematologic, renal, or hepatic changes after treatment.[29] In neonates less than 21 days of age, glomerular filtration rate (GFR) is as low as 30 mL/min/1.73 m^2 leading to delayed clearance and resulting in prolonged exposure at a higher volume of distribution.[30] This phenomenon may be more prominent in infants with prematurity.[30]

Important adverse effects to consider when using NSAIDS include gastric irritation that may lead to inflammation and ulceration/erosion; decreased platelet aggregation potentiating the risk for intraventricular hemorrhage (IVH); and lastly decreased GFR leading to acute kidney injury, which has potential to progress to renal failure if unchecked because neonatal clearance is heavily dependent on adequate GFR. These drugs have limited use because of their adverse effects.[31]

Opioid Analgesics

Morphine

Morphine is an opioid and is one of the most frequently used analgesic in NICUs.[30] It acts by binding to mu(μ)-opiate receptors, which are most abundant in the central nervous system where they exert their analgesic effect by stimulating descending inhibitory pathways.[32] Morphine is most commonly used in an oral or IV formulation.

Morphine is primarily metabolized in the liver. It undergoes glucuronidation (uridine diphosphate glucuronosyltransferase [UGT] 2B7 and UGT1A2), sulphation, and oxidation. Sulphation and oxidation are minor pathways in humans.[33] Choonara and colleagues[34] demonstrated that preterm infants even as early as 24 to 25 weeks gestation can metabolize morphine by glucuronidation. The major metabolites of morphine are morphine-3-glucoronide and morphine-6-glucoronide.[34] These metabolites are present in higher concentrations in the plasma than morphine itself.[33] Morphine-6-glucoronide is responsible for additional analgesic effect and morphine-3-glucoronide is considered an inactive metabolite.[34] The plasma concentration of morphine is significantly higher in neonates compared with older populations because of reduced hepatic and renal clearance in this population.[34] In addition, critically ill neonates have large variations in drug levels because of medically impaired hepatic and renal function. Decreased hepatic function leads to decreased metabolism and impairment of morphine clearance. Renal impairment can prolong its half-life and lead to toxicity caused by accumulation.[35]

Adverse effects of morphine include miosis, pruritus, respiratory depression, constipation, increased biliary pressure, urinary retention, and hypotension.[32,36]

Hypotension can occur because of histamine release and associated decrease in systemic vascular resistance.[32] Tolerance and withdrawal are observed with morphine.[37] In a recent randomized controlled trial of morphine for procedural pain in retinopathy of prematurity examinations in preterm infants less than 32 weeks gestation, the study was stopped early (n = 31) because of excessive respiratory depression in the morphine group with no associated analgesic efficacy.[38]

Continuous morphine infusion was studied as part of the NOPAIN trial in comparison with midazolam and placebo. Low-dose morphine reduced the incidence of poor neurologic outcomes in preterm neonates (24% of neonates in the placebo group, 32% in the midazolam group, and 4% in the morphine group; $P = .03$).[39] Interpretation of these results is limited because the sample size was small and limited to only 67 neonates. In a much larger study, the NEOPAIN trial (n = 898), the effect of morphine infusion versus placebo was compared on the composite outcome of death, severe IVH, or periventricular leukomalacia in preterm infants.[40] In intention-to-treat analysis, where many "placebo" infants received open-label morphine, the placebo and morphine groups had similar rates of the composite outcome (26% vs 27%), neonatal death (11% vs 13%), severe IVH (11% vs 13%), and periventricular leukomalacia (9% vs 7%). The more worrisome findings appeared when analyzing only the infants who did not crossover, meaning "placebo" infants received no open-label morphine. In this group, rates of the composite outcome (24% vs 15%; $P = .0338$) and severe IVH (9% vs 3%; $P = .0209$) were significantly higher in the morphine-exposed group. In the cohort of infants who were randomized to placebo infusions, neonates receiving open-label morphine had worse rates of the composite outcome than those not receiving open-label morphine (34% vs 15%; $P<.0001$). Morphine-group neonates receiving open-label morphine were more likely to develop severe IVH (19% vs 9%; $P = .0024$).[40] Taken in sum, the results of these morphine studies in preterm infants warrant extreme caution with use of this drug in the developing brain. Morphine infusions should not be used prophylactically for mechanical ventilation in this age group, and when clinically indicated, using lowest dose possible and weaning off as soon as able decreases infant exposure. A follow-up study of the NEOPAIN cohort[41] concluded that hypotension and preexisting illness were contributors to the morphine-associated morbidity reported in the trial. They urged caution in infants 23 to 26 weeks gestation (most severely immature cerebral autoregulation) and preterm infants with preexisting hypotension.

Fentanyl

Fentanyl is a synthetic opioid also commonly used in NICUs. It is much more potent than morphine (up to 75 times the affinity at the μ-opioid receptor). It is a pure μ-receptor agonist.[42] It has a rapid onset of action and the onset is dependent on the route by which the drug was administered.[43] Given IV, analgesia occurs within 1 to 2 minutes, making it an ideal opiate for acute painful procedures, such as intubation. It can also be administered intranasally in a neonate without IV access (ie, for percutaneously inserted central catheter line insertion) and produces analgesic effect within 5 to 10 minutes. Given its rapid onset of action, short half-life, and lack of significant cardiovascular adverse effects, fentanyl is a popular drug used in infants and neonates during surgical procedures. It also has a shorter duration of action compared with morphine.[44]

Fentanyl undergoes metabolism in the liver[37] by CYP3A4 enzymes[43] and undergoes renal elimination. Koehntop and colleagues[45] studied the pharmacokinetics in 14 neonates undergoing major surgical procedures with ages ranging from less than 1 day old to 14 days old. Fentanyl was given IV, 10 μg/kg (n = 1), 25 μg/kg (n = 4), or 50 µg/kg (n = 9), and plasma concentrations were measured at intervals of up to 18 hours. Plasma concentrations of fentanyl were most appropriately described by a two-compartment model. Fentanyl clearance was 17.94 ± 4.38 mL/kg/min, and terminal elimination half-life was 317 ± 70 minutes.[45]

In a study of 100 neonates,[46] fentanyl pharmacokinetics and efficacy were compared between continuous infusion of 1 µg/kg/h versus IV bolus of 1 µg/kg every 4 hours. Median peak plasma concentration of fentanyl was 3.06 ng/mL versus 0.78 ng/mL in the bolus versus continuous infusion groups. In addition, the bolus group had significantly higher and AUC_{0-24} 19.6 versus 13.2 µg·h/L. Pain scores and adverse effects were comparable between the two regimens. The study concludes that intermittent bolus of fentanyl for analgesia, as compared with continuous infusion, produces wide fluctuations in plasma concentrations and high peak levels

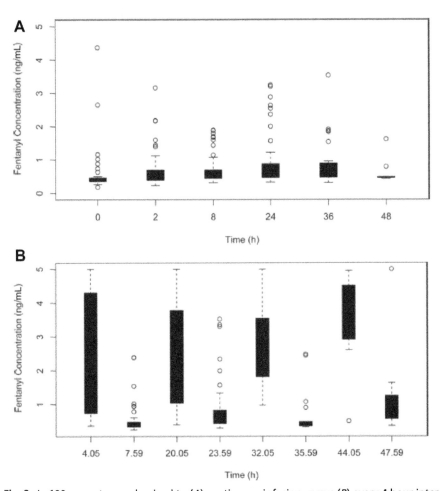

Fig. 2. In 100 neonates randomized to (A) continuous infusion versus (B) every 4 hour intermittent bolus fentanyl, the continuous infusion results in less variable serum concentrations. (*From* Abiramalatha T, Mathew SK, Mathew BS, et al. Continuous infusion versus intermittent bolus doses of fentanyl for analgesia and sedation in neonates: an open-label randomized controlled trial. *Archives of Disease in Childhood - Fetal and Neonatal Edition*. https://doi.org/10.1136/archdischild-2018-315345; with permission.)

(**Fig. 2**). A serum fentanyl concentration of 0.4 ng/mL to 0.6 ng/mL produces adequate analgesia and sedation in neonates.

Fentanyl does not cause as much hemodynamic instability as morphine because it does not cause the release of histamine.[47] Chest wall rigidity is a known and severe adverse effect of bolus IV administration of fentanyl, but this risk is mitigated by slow IV infusion (over 5 minutes), and reversed with naloxone or a temporary paralytic agent (rocuronium). Few cases of laryngospasm have also been reported.[44] The exact mechanism of these adverse effects is not known. Chest wall rigidity and respiratory depression are treated with naloxone[48] or a short-acting paralytic agent, allowing mechanical ventilation by providers. A study by Rey-Santano and colleagues[49] showed that newborn piglets that received fentanyl also demonstrated some degree of chest wall rigidity and depressed brain activity, which were transient. Fentanyl pharmacokinetics in newborn piglets was comparable with human neonates.

Remifentanil

This drug is an ultra-short-acting opioid agent. It is a selective μ-receptor agonist. Its onset of action is about 1 minute with rapid elimination. It is different from other opioids in that it is rapidly metabolized by blood and tissue esterases into an inactive compound that can later undergo renal elimination.[50,51] One study found that remifentanil-based anesthesia did not increase the incidence of apnea in infants undergoing pyloromyotomy when compared with halothane-based anesthesia.[52] Pereira e Silva and colleagues[53] reported that remifentanil was a better option than morphine as a premedication agent before intubation in preterm neonates. In this study, 20 preterm infants 28 to 34 weeks were randomized to preintubation opiate treatment with either morphine, 0.15 mg/kg bolus, versus remifentanil, 1 μg/kg. Both arms also received IV midazolam, 0.2 mg/kg. Intubation conditions, as quantified by a scale, were not "excellent" in any of the morphine-treated infants, compared with 60% of the remifentanil group. A second attempt at intubation was required for none of the remifentanil-treated infants. Remifentanil adverse effects may include hypotension[54] and chest wall rigidity.[55] For remifentanil to be used optimally in the neonatal population, further study is required.

PHARMACOLOGY OF SEDATIVES IN NEONATES

Sedatives alter the level of consciousness and are generally used in conjunction with analgesics.[56] Sedatives are used in various settings in the NICU, for such procedures as endotracheal intubation, in conjunction with analgesics for management of pain and anxiolysis in critically ill infants, during mechanical ventilation, and in postoperative management.[57,58] They also play a role in end-of-life care of the neonate.[59] Although the understanding of the need for pain and sedation management in neonates has evolved over the past few decades[60] with evidence indicating that early pain/agitation is associated with thalamic volume loss and poor neurodevelopmental outcomes,[61] the commonly used sedatives in the NICU are not without risks. Preterm infants are at increased risk of developing adverse events, such as apnea or desaturations in response to sedation/anesthesia.[62] However, the risks of some sedatives extend beyond airway compromise. Midazolam exposure is related to changes in the development of the hippocampus and concern over γ-aminobutyric acid (GABA) agonist exposure in the immature brain. Midazolam was associated with poorer outcomes in a study involving 138 neonates.[3] Therefore, we must be mindful and weigh the risks and benefits of sedative use in every patient and situation because inadequate pain/agitation control and sedative use have been implicated in poor neurodevelopmental outcomes.

Benzodiazepines

Midazolam

Midazolam is a short-acting, water-soluble benzodiazepine. It exerts its sedative effect by binding to GABA receptors.[36] Midazolam can cause anxiolysis, sedation, amnesia, muscle relaxation, but no analgesia.[37] Long-acting benzodiazepines, such as diazepam, are not ideal in preterm and term neonates because of their long elimination half-life and accumulation of N-desmethyldiazepam, which is hypnotic in nature. Midazolam, in contrast, is a short-acting agent with a less active metabolite.[63] High concentrations of midazolam can cause hypotension, bradycardia, and decreased cerebral blood flow velocity.[64]

Midazolam undergoes extensive hydroxylation by members of the CYP-450 family in the liver and then is eliminated by the kidneys.[65] Hepatic and renal function is less mature in preterm infants than full-term neonates. Average parameter values (interpatient percent coefficient of variation) for infants with birth weights 1000 g or less were total systemic clearance of 0.783 mL/min (83%) and volume of distribution of the central compartment of 473 mL (70%). For infants with birth weights more than 1000 g they were as follows: total systemic clearance of 1.24 mL/min (78%) and volume of distribution of the central compartment of 823 mL (43%).[64] The elimination of midazolam in preterm infants 26 to 34 weeks of gestational age and less than 2 weeks of postnatal age is impaired compared with older infants and children because of reduced CYP3A activity and immaturity in renal function at birth.[63,66] There is a large variability in midazolam pharmacokinetics in neonates because of postnatal indomethacin exposure and its effects on volume of distribution and renal function.[66] Burtin and colleagues[67] similarly found that midazolam clearance was higher in neonates older than 39 weeks gestation and noted marked interindividual variability in pharmacokinetics.

α_2-Agonists

Clonidine

Clonidine is an α_2-adrenergic agonist. Activation of the α_2-receptors in the central nervous system decreases sympathetic outflow.[47] Some of the advantages of using clonidine as an adjunct for sedation is that it does not cause the significant respiratory depression observed with opioids. Clonidine can reduce opiate and benzodiazepine requirements.[68] It is also used in the management of neonatal abstinence syndrome[69] (See Kathryn Dee Lizcano MacMillan's article, "Neonatal Abstinence Syndrome: Review of Epidemiology, Care Models and Current Understanding of Outcomes," in this issue). Pontén and colleagues[70] reported that clonidine eliminated ketamine induced apoptosis in a mouse model, so there is increasing evidence that clonidine may have neuroprotective properties against anesthetic exposure. Clonidine is available in oral, IV, intramuscular, transdermal, and rectal preparations.[71] Intranasal administration has been reported in children but not in neonates.[72]

Clonidine undergoes CYP2D6-mediated hydroxylation and renal elimination.[47] About 40% to 60% undergoes biotransformation in the liver and 50% is eliminated unchanged by the kidney. Clearance in infants and neonates is reduced because of immaturity of pathways or renal disease.[71] In a population pharmacokinetic study Xie and colleagues[73] found that clonidine clearance increases after 2 weeks of age and the dose should be increased from 6 μg/kg/d to 9 μg/kg/d for similar drug exposure.

Clonidine adverse effects include hypotension, rebound hypertension, atrioventricular block, bradycardia, and syndrome of inappropriate antidiuretic hormone.[47,69] There are reported cases of postoperative apnea when clonidine was used in caudal or epidural anesthesia in infants.[74–76] Studies have demonstrated similar respiratory depressant effect on a group of adults who received IV clonidine. Although clonidine causes less respiratory depression than opiates, when high levels of sedation are observed, close attention to respiratory status is warranted in infants receiving clonidine.[77]

Dexmedetomidine

Similar to clonidine, dexmedetomidine is a selective α_2-agonist that reduces sympathetic outflow resulting in sedation. Unlike sedative drugs, such as propofol and the benzodiazepines, dexmedetomidine does not act at the GABA receptors. It induces sedation through activation of α_2-receptors in the locus coeruleus and induces a state mimicking natural sleep.[78] Dexmedetomidine can also provide some analgesic effect.[79] In a retrospective study, Dersch-Mills and colleagues[80] performed a review of 38 neonates receiving dexmedetomidine in a medical surgical NICU, including data on duration of use, dose, adverse effects, weaning, and signs of withdrawal. Their study reports potential benefits when dexmedetomidine is used for sedation in neonates, including reduced sedative requirements and earlier enteral feeds.[80] This drug is available in IV and intranasal formulations.[81]

Dexmedetomidine drug is highly protein bound and is almost completely metabolized in the liver by CYP-450 enzyme CYP2A6 and UGT glucuronidation pathways, specifically UGT1A4 and UGT2B10, to inactive metabolites.[82] These metabolites are then excreted in urine (95%) and in feces (4%).[83] Adverse effects include bradycardia and hypotension requiring pressor support in some neonates.[80] It has low risk of related respiratory adverse effects and can be used for procedural sedation in preterm neonates.[81] Use of dexmedetomidine might reduce opioid and benzodiazepine use in a patient and also reduce vasopressor dosing in catecholamine-resistant cardiogenic shock.[84] Withdrawal from dexmedetomidine can pose a challenge and presents as agitation, tremors, and decreased sleep.[85] Chrysostomou and colleagues[86] demonstrated in a phase II/III multicenter trial of dexmedetomidine in preterm and term neonates that it was not associated with any significant adverse events or events requiring medication discontinuation, but that preterm neonates did show decreased plasma clearance and longer elimination half-life.

O'Mara and Weiss[87] reported that because of its sedative properties, dexmedetomidine may have neuroprotective properties in patients with hypoxic ischemic encephalopathy in whom this drug protects the brain from excitotoxicity when used as a sedative agent. Sanders and colleagues[88] demonstrated that dexmedetomidine diminished neuronal injury in vitro in a concentration-dependent fashion and also decreased infarct size in vivo in perinatal hypoxic ischemic encephalopathy rat models. These histopathologic improvements correlated with improved neurologic function. Dexmedetomidine may also have antiapoptotic effects that contribute to its neuroprotective properties. More studies are needed to understand the long-term benefits and effects in the neonatal population. Dexmedetomidine has also shown a role in reducing anesthetic-related injury in animal models.[88]

MULTIMODAL ANALGESIC APPROACHES: THE POWER OF SYNERGY

Multimodal analgesia is a tool used to combine multiple different classes of pain control (environmental, different drug classes) to reduce the exposure to any one class of pain medication, thereby reducing toxicities from high doses of a single drug class. Historically, much of the pharmacologic data to support neonatal analgesia has been extrapolated from adults and older pediatric populations, and there are not many dedicated studies on the multimodal analgesic approach in neonates. Neonatal and infant pain management research faces two major challenges: lack of clear and universally accepted drug end point biomarkers, and the very heterogeneous pharmacokinetics and pharmacodynamics of analgesics in this population.[89] These barriers create challenges when studying one analgesic modality, and are compounded during study of a multimodal analgesic approach. Although these legitimate barriers exist, research must continue to progress to create a body of growing solutions. Loeser[90] proposed a pain model that includes four components: (1) nociception, (2) pain, (3) suffering, and (4) pain behavior. These components are considered when using multimodal pain control. To safely use a synergistic drug model, interactions among different analgesics must be studied more closely. Functional MRI seems a promising method to look for specific brain areas involved in pain processing and the role of analgesics on these pain areas.[89]

The use of paracetamol reduces infant opioid consumption by 66% after major noncardiac surgery.[16] The cumulative median morphine dose in the first 48 hours postoperatively was 121 µg/kg (interquartile range, 99–264) in the paracetamol group and 357 µg/kg (interquartile range, 220–605) in the morphine group.[16] Another study demonstrated a fentanyl-sparing effect of IV paracetamol in infants aged 6 to 24 months following ureteroneocystostomy.[18] In an older pediatric population, Korpela and colleagues[91] showed that a single dose of 40 or 60 mg/kg of rectal acetaminophen has a clear morphine-sparing effect in outpatient surgery for older children, if administered during the induction of anesthesia. A cohort study by Härmä and colleagues[17] found that early administration of paracetamol to very preterm infants decreased morphine administration significantly. Infants in the paracetamol group needed significantly fewer morphine doses per patient than the comparisons, with paracetamol-treated infants requiring 1.78 (standard deviation [SD], 4.56) doses versus control infants requiring 4.35 (SD, 11.53) doses. The paracetamol-exposed had lower cumulative morphine dosage of 0.17 (SD, 0.45) mg/kg versus 0.37 (SD, 0.96) mg/kg.[17]

In a meta-analysis by Maund and colleagues,[92] when paracetamol, NSAIDs, or COX-2 inhibitors were added to PCA morphine, there was a statistically significant reduction in morphine consumption: paracetamol mean difference −6.34 mg, NSAIDs mean difference −10.18, and COX-2 inhibitors mean difference −10.92. Although multicenter double-blind randomized controlled trials are not available to support a synergistic approach to pain control, it is clear that opioid exposure and its subsequent side effects including respiratory depression and withdrawal are lessened with synergistic use of other analgesics. A multimodal approach that allows for synergy among environmental approaches (swaddling, skin to skin), various families of analgesics, and sedatives would be ideal but an enhanced understanding of neonatal pharmacokinetics and pharmacodynamics is needed for medical progress in this area.

PHARMACOGENETICS AND DRUG METABOLISM ONTOGENY

Developmental pharmacology is complex in the neonatal population given large variations in weight, age, and pharmacogenetics that affect pharmacokinetics and pharmacodynamics.[93] With the goal of adequately treating pain in the neonate, one must consider the drug target or receptor, drug transporters, drug metabolizing enzymes, and genetic variability to optimize pain control. Pharmacogenetics can have effects on drug exposure and therefore clinical response. Developmental trajectory (ontogeny) and genetic variability of drug-metabolizing enzymes are interrelated, because one cannot appreciate genetic variability in drug-metabolizing enzyme expression until the protein of interest is sufficiently developmentally expressed. Pharmacogenetic variation may contribute to unpredictable drug exposures given the same weight-based dose of a drug.[94] Although few studies have investigated pharmacogenetics in neonates, we highlight some important data here.

There are examples of potentially clinically actionable pharmacogenetic data in neonates, but more study is required to validate these findings and understand how to incorporate them into clinical care. In neonates, the effect of genetic variation in *CYP2D6* is apparent even in neonates born less than 37 weeks. Tramadol O-demethylation was significantly increased by increasing postmenstrual age and increasing (genetically assigned) *CYP2D6* activity score.[95] In critically ill neonates, genetic variation in the hepatic drug transporter organic cation transporter (OCT)-1 is associated with morphine metabolism (**Fig. 3**).[96] In the study, 85 neonates were genotyped for single-nucleotide polymorphisms in *OCT1* and *UGT2B7*. Morphine clearance was decreased in infants who were homozygous for a loss-of-function mutation in the hepatic transporter required to get circulating morphine into the liver for metabolism. Taking this study into consideration, one may be able to personalize morphine dosing based on genotypically and age-predicted clearance. In neonates randomized to placebo infusion, combined carriage of genetic risk alleles in *OPRM1* and *COMT* were associated with a higher need for rescue morphine during mechanical ventilation.[97]

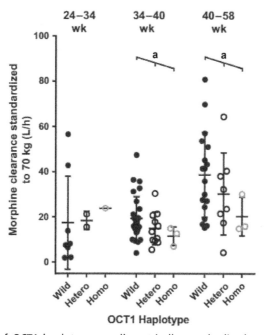

Fig. 3. Influence of OCT1 haplotype on allometrically standardized morphine clearance. Among patients aged 34–40 weeks postmenstrual age (PMA; term) and 40–58 weeks PMA (postterm), loss of function genetic variants of OCT1 are associated with lower morphine clearance values in a decreasing trend (Wild > Hetero > Homo; [a] $P<.05$ both age categories). Hetero, heterozygous; Homo, homozygous; Wild, wild-type. (*From* Hahn D, Emoto C, Euteneuer JC, et al. Influence of OCT1 Ontogeny and Genetic Variation on Morphine Disposition in Critically Ill Neonates: Lessons From PBPK Modeling and Clinical Study. Clin Pharmacol Ther. 2019;105(3):761-768. doi:10.1002/cpt.124; with permission.)

It may be possible to predict which infants are most likely to need opiate for pain while intubated based on genotype.

The current knowledge suggests that individual drug metabolizing isoenzymes can be categorized into one of three classes based on developmental trajectories.[98] A first group of enzymes (eg, CYP3A7, SULT1A3/1A4) are expressed at their highest level in fetal life and their activity decreases and disappears over the first 2 years of life.[98] The second group consists of enzymes (eg, CYP3A5, CYP2C19, SULT1A1) that only display a moderate increase after birth and become more active in later pediatric life. The third group (eg, CYP2D6, CYP3A4, CYP2C9, CYP1A2) displays some increase in the second or third trimester of pregnancy with another relevant increase in phenotypic activity throughout infancy.[98]

Most NSAIDS used in the treatment of pain in the NICU are metabolized by CYP-450 and CYP family of enzymes. Genetic variability in indomethacin metabolism may explain the variability observed in drug exposure and response. Indomethacin is primarily metabolized by the CYP-450 enzyme, CYP2C9, and the serine esterase, carboxylesterase (CES1).[94] Using microsomal and cytosolic fractions from pediatric livers, it has recently been reported that infants aged less than 3 weeks have significantly less CES1 and CES2 than older infants and children.[99] Full expression and thus function of these specific enzymes is indirectly proportional to gestational age and therefore preterm and certainly extremely premature infants have altered metabolism and clearance of NSAIDs.

Acetaminophen undergoes hepatic metabolism through UGT1A1, UGT1A6, SULT1A1, and SULT1A3. The UGT family of transferase enzymes also increases in concentration as gestational age increases, so changing metabolism can affect drug efficacy. The concentration of the SULT family of enzymes is similar between fetal and postnatal livers.[100] Underlying genetic variability among infants in the metabolism of acetaminophen is likely a contributory factor to decreased drug exposure and thus decreased responsiveness in some patients.

GAPS IN KNOWLEDGE

Although well-designed neonatal studies of analgesic and sedation medications are increasingly performed and published, more work needs to be done to fill gaps in knowledge so that there is more precision and accuracy in neonatal analgesic and sedation pharmacology. Researchers and clinicians must be sensitive to the fact that preterm neonates vary dramatically in their drug metabolism from even older infants and certainly from adults. Because of the known and potential effects of development and genetic variability on drug metabolism, basic, translational, and clinical research in neonatal clinical pharmacology is urgently needed, and drug exposure should be considered in trials of pain and sedation medications. As the medical community migrates in a direction of personalized medicine, neonatologists and pediatrician alike have a responsibility to advance evidence-based understanding of the pharmacokinetics and pharmacodynamics of opioid and nonopioid analgesics and sedatives in the neonatal population.

Current literature lacks systematic data on acute perioperative pain management in neonates and mainly focuses on procedural pain management. Data support the efficacy of acetaminophen and NSAIDs, when used as part of a multimodal approach, yet the widespread use of these approaches has not taken hold because of lack of definitive data to support this practice in all neonatal populations. In addition, dose variation and dose individualization studies that account for developmental age and genetically determined rates of drug metabolism are lacking.

Optimal opiate-weaning protocols and opiate-withdrawal algorithms have not been adequately compared. Given the concern for potential long-term deleterious effects

---

Best Practices

What is the current practice for neonatal analgesic and sedation drug therapy?

Best Practice/Guideline/Care Path Objectives
- Use validated pain and sedation scores to guide pharmacologic therapy.
- Opiates are the mainstay of analgesic therapy in most NICUs.

What changes in current practice are likely to improve outcomes?

- Knowledge of the developmental pharmacology of key analgesic and sedation drugs allows increased understanding of the risk-benefit profile.

- Use of a multimodal analgesic approach decreases opiate exposure and minimizes side effects from any single drug class.

- Increased research and implementation of pharmacogenetics and precision therapeutics allows tailoring of analgesic and sedation drug therapy in the NICU.

Major recommendations

- Consider developmental status of drug metabolism when prescribing analgesic and sedative drugs (ie, younger and more preterm infants clear the drugs more slowly and are at increased risk for side effects).

- Consider universal use of nonopiates for analgesic therapy in the postoperative setting. Either acetaminophen or NSAIDs (in the older population) are likely to improve pain control and decrease opiate requirements.

- Consider individual variability in analgesic and sedative dosing requirements. This variability may be developmental, genetic, or environmental (prior drug exposure and tolerance).

Bibliographic Sources: Refs.[8,16,17,96,98]

---

of opiates and benzodiazepines on the developing brain, clinicians as a community can renew research energy and focus on optimal pain control and sedation practices, using modern tools, such as biomarkers, pharmacogenetics, pharmacologic modeling, and implementation science.

ACKNOWLEDGMENTS

This study was funded by NICHD 1K23HD09136201A1 and the Robert Wood Johnson Foundation Harold Amos award Project ID 76230.

REFERENCES

1. Veneziano G, Tobias JD. Chloroprocaine for epidural anesthesia in infants and children. Paediatr Anaesth 2017;27(6):581–90.
2. Anand KJ, Hansen DD, Hickey PR. Hormonal-metabolic stress responses in neonates undergoing cardiac surgery. Anesthesiology 1990;73(4):661–70.
3. Duerden EG, Guo T, Dodbiba L, et al. Midazolam dose correlates with abnormal hippocampal growth and neurodevelopmental outcome in preterm infants. Ann Neurol 2016;79(4):548–59.
4. Young C, Jevtovic-Todorovic V, Qin Y-Q, et al. Potential of ketamine and midazolam, individually or in combination, to induce apoptotic neurodegeneration in the infant mouse brain. Br J Pharmacol 2009;146(2):189–97.

5. Lowery CL, Hardman MP, Manning N, et al. Neurodevelopmental changes of fetal pain. Semin Perinatol 2007;31(5):275–82.

6. Fitzgerald M. The development of nociceptive circuits. Nat Rev Neurosci 2005; 6(7):507–20.

7. Narsinghani U, Anand KJS. Developmental neurobiology of pain in neonatal rats. Lab Anim (NY) 2000;29(9):27–39.

8. Zhu A, Benzon HA, Anderson TA. Evidence for the efficacy of systemic opioid-sparing analgesics in pediatric surgical populations: a systematic review. Anesth Analg 2017;125(5):1569–87.

9. Bertolini A, Ferrari A, Ottani A, et al. Paracetamol: new vistas of an old drug. CNS Drug Rev 2006;12(3–4):250–75.

10. Remy C, Marret E, Bonnet F. Effects of acetaminophen on morphine side-effects and consumption after major surgery: meta-analysis of randomized controlled trials † †Presented in part at the Annual Meeting of the Société Française d'Anesthésie-Réanimation, Paris, April 2004. Br J Anaesth 2005;94(4):505–13.

11. Moller PL, Sindet-Pedersen S, Petersen CT, et al. Onset of acetaminophen analgesia: comparison of oral and intravenous routes after third molar surgery. Br J Anaesth 2005;94(5):642–8.

12. Jahr JS, Lee VK. Intravenous acetaminophen. Anesthesiol Clin 2010;28(4): 619–45.

13. Gelotte CK, Auiler JF, Lynch JM, et al. Disposition of acetaminophen at 4, 6, and 8 g/day for 3 days in healthy young adults. Clin Pharmacol Ther 2007;81(6): 840–8.

14. Morris ME, Levy G. Renal clearance and serum protein binding of acetaminophen and its major conjugates in humans. J Pharm Sci 1984;73(8):1038–41.

15. van Lingen RA, Deinum JT, Quak JM, et al. Pharmacokinetics and metabolism of rectally administered paracetamol in preterm neonates. Arch Dis Child Fetal Neonatal Ed 1999;80(1):F59–63.

16. Ceelie I, de Wildt SN, van Dijk M, et al. Effect of intravenous paracetamol on postoperative morphine requirements in neonates and infants undergoing major noncardiac surgery: a randomized controlled trial. JAMA 2013;309(2):149–54.

17. Härmä A, Aikio O, Hallman M, et al. Intravenous paracetamol decreases requirements of morphine in very preterm infants. J Pediatr 2016;168:36–40.

18. Hong J-Y, Kim WO, Koo BN, et al. Fentanyl-sparing effect of acetaminophen as a mixture of fentanyl in intravenous parent-/nurse-controlled analgesia after pediatric ureteroneocystostomy. Anesthesiology 2010;113(3):672–7.

19. McGill MR, Jaeschke H. Mechanistic biomarkers in acetaminophen-induced hepatotoxicity and acute liver failure: from preclinical models to patients. Expert Opin Drug Metab Toxicol 2014;10(7):1005–17.

20. Allegaert K, Naulaers G. Haemodynamics of intravenous paracetamol in neonates. Eur J Clin Pharmacol 2010;66(9):855–8.

21. Morris JL, Rosen DA, Rosen KR. Nonsteroidal anti-inflammatory agents in neonates. Paediatr Drugs 2003;5(6):385–405.

22. O'Banion MK. Cyclooxygenase-2: molecular biology, pharmacology, and neurobiology. Crit Rev Neurobiol 1999;13(1):45–82.

23. McCleskey EW, Gold MS. Ion channels of nociception. Annu Rev Physiol 1999; 61:835–56.

24. Aranda JV, Varvarigou A, Beharry K, et al. Pharmacokinetics and protein binding of intravenous ibuprofen in the premature newborn infant. Acta Paediatr 1997; 86(3):289–93.

25. Van Overmeire B, Touw D, Schepens PJ, et al. Ibuprofen pharmacokinetics in preterm infants with patent ductus arteriosus. Clin Pharmacol Ther 2001;70(4): 336–43.
26. Scott CS, Retsch-Bogart GZ, Kustra RP, et al. The pharmacokinetics of ibuprofen suspension, chewable tablets, and tablets in children with cystic fibrosis. J Pediatr 1999;134(1):58–63.
27. Pacifici GM. Clinical pharmacology of ibuprofen in preterm infants: a meta-analysis of published data. Med Express 2014;1(2). https://doi.org/10.5935/MedicalExpress.2014.02.02.
28. Sharma PK, Garg SK, Narang A. Pharmacokinetics of oral ibuprofen in premature infants. J Clin Pharmacol 2003;43(9):968–73.
29. Papacci P, De Francisci G, Iacobucci T, et al. Use of intravenous ketorolac in the neonate and premature babies. Paediatr Anaesth 2004;14(6):487–92.
30. Aldrink JH, Ma M, Wang W, et al. Safety of ketorolac in surgical neonates and infants 0 to 3 months old. J Pediatr Surg 2011;46(6):1081–5.
31. Cuzzolin L, Dal Cerè M, Fanos V. NSAID-induced nephrotoxicity from the fetus to the child. Drug Saf 2001;24(1):9–18.
32. Pathan H, Williams J. Basic opioid pharmacology: an update. Br J Pain 2012; 6(1):11–6.
33. Choonara I, Ekbom Y, Lindström B, et al. Morphine sulphation in children. Br J Clin Pharmacol 1990;30(6):897–900.
34. Choonara IA, McKay P, Hain R, et al. Morphine metabolism in children. Br J Clin Pharmacol 1989;28(5):599–604.
35. Altamimi MI, Choonara I, Sammons H. Inter-individual variation in morphine clearance in children. Eur J Clin Pharmacol 2015;71(6):649–55.
36. Brunton L, Chabner B, Knollman B, editors. Goodman & Gilman's the pharmacological basis of therapeutics. 12th edition. New York: McGraw-Hill Education; 2011.
37. Anand KJS. Pharmacological approaches to the management of pain in the neonatal intensive care unit. J Perinatol 2007;27(Suppl 1):S4–11.
38. Hartley C, Moultrie F, Hoskin A, et al. Analgesic efficacy and safety of morphine in the Procedural Pain in Premature Infants (Poppi) study: randomised placebo-controlled trial. Lancet 2018. https://doi.org/10.1016/S0140-6736(18)31813-0.
39. Anand KJ, Barton BA, McIntosh N, et al. Analgesia and sedation in preterm neonates who require ventilatory support: results from the NOPAIN trial. Neonatal outcome and prolonged analgesia in neonates. Arch Pediatr Adolesc Med 1999;153(4):331–8.
40. Anand K, Hall RW, Desai N, et al. Effects of morphine analgesia in ventilated preterm neonates: primary outcomes from the NEOPAIN randomised trial. Lancet 2004;363(9422):1673–82.
41. Hall RW. Morphine, hypotension, and adverse outcomes among preterm neonates: who's to blame? Secondary results from the NEOPAIN trial. Pediatrics 2005. https://doi.org/10.1542/peds.2004-1398.
42. Chen Q, Shang Y, Xu Y, et al. Analgesic effect and pharmacological mechanism of fentanyl and butorphanol in a rat model of incisional pain. J Clin Anesth 2016; 28:67–73.
43. Stanley TH. The fentanyl story. J Pain 2014;15(12):1215–26.
44. Fahnenstich H, Steffan J, Kau N, et al. Fentanyl-induced chest wall rigidity and laryngospasm in preterm and term infants. Crit Care Med 2000;28(3):836–9.
45. Koehntop DE, Rodman JH, Brundage DM, et al. Pharmacokinetics of fentanyl in neonates. Anesth Analg 1986;65(3):227–32.

46. Abiramalatha T, Mathew SK, Mathew BS, et al. Continuous infusion versus intermittent bolus doses of fentanyl for analgesia and sedation in neonates: an open-label randomised controlled trial. Arch Dis Child Fetal Neonatal Ed 2019;104(4): F433–9.

47. Brunton L, Hilal-Dandan R, Bjorn K, editors. Goodman & Gillman's the pharmacological basis of therapeutics. 13th edition. New York: McGraw-Hill Education; 2017.

48. Pacifici GM. Clinical pharmacology of fentanyl in preterm infants. A review. Pediatr Neonatol 2015;56(3):143–8.

49. Rey-Santano C, Mielgo V, Valls-i-Soler A, et al. Evaluation of fentanyl disposition and effects in newborn piglets as an experimental model for human neonates. PLoS One 2014;9(3):e90728.

50. Muellejans B, López A, Cross MH, et al. Remifentanil versus fentanyl for analgesia based sedation to provide patient comfort in the intensive care unit: a randomized, double-blind controlled trial [ISRCTN43755713]. Crit Care 2004;8(1): R1–11.

51. Westmoreland CL, Hoke JF, Sebel PS, et al. Pharmacokinetics of remifentanil (GI87084B) and its major metabolite (GI90291) in patients undergoing elective inpatient surgery. Anesthesiology 1993;79(5):893–903.

52. Galinkin JL, Davis PJ, McGowan FX, et al. A randomized multicenter study of remifentanil compared with halothane in neonates and infants undergoing pyloromyotomy. II. Perioperative breathing patterns in neonates and infants with pyloric stenosis. Anesth Analg 2001;93(6):1387–92.

53. Pereira e Silva Y, Gomez RS, Marcatto J de O, et al. Morphine versus remifentanil for intubating preterm neonates. Arch Dis Child Fetal Neonatal Ed 2007; 92(4):F293–4.

54. Ross AK, Davis PJ, Dear Gd GL, et al. Pharmacokinetics of remifentanil in anesthetized pediatric patients undergoing elective surgery or diagnostic procedures. Anesth Analg 2001;93(6):1393–401, table of contents.

55. de Kort EHM, Hanff LM, Roofthooft D, et al. Insufficient sedation and severe side effects after fast administration of remifentanil during INSURE in preterm newborns. Neonatology 2017;111(2):172–6.

56. Rady MY, Verheijde JL. Uniformly defining continuous deep sedation. Lancet Oncol 2016;17(3):e89.

57. Truog R, Anand KJ. Management of pain in the postoperative neonate. Clin Perinatol 1989;16(1):61–78.

58. Aranda JV, Carlo W, Hummel P, et al. Analgesia and sedation during mechanical ventilation in neonates. Clin Ther 2005;27(6):877–99.

59. Carter BS, Brunkhorst J. Neonatal pain management. Semin Perinatol 2017; 41(2):111–6.

60. Anand KJ, Hickey PR. Pain and its effects in the human neonate and fetus. N Engl J Med 1987;317(21):1321–9.

61. Duerden EG, Grunau RE, Guo T, et al. Early procedural pain is associated with regionally-specific alterations in thalamic development in preterm neonates. J Neurosci 2018;38(4):878–86.

62. Havidich JE, Beach M, Dierdorf SF, et al. Preterm versus term children: analysis of sedation/anesthesia adverse events and longitudinal risk. Pediatrics 2016; 137(3):e20150463.

63. Jacqz-Aigrain E, Daoud P, Burtin P, et al. Pharmacokinetics of midazolam during continuous infusion in critically ill neonates. Eur J Clin Pharmacol 1992;42(3): 329–32.

64. Lee TC, Charles BG, Harte GJ, et al. Population pharmacokinetic modeling in very premature infants receiving midazolam during mechanical ventilation: midazolam neonatal pharmacokinetics. Anesthesiology 1999;90(2):451-7.
65. Jacqz-Aigrain E, Wood C, Robieux I. Pharmacokinetics of midazolam in critically ill neonates. Eur J Clin Pharmacol 1990;39(2):191-2.
66. de Wildt SN, Kearns GL, Hop WC, et al. Pharmacokinetics and metabolism of intravenous midazolam in preterm infants. Clin Pharmacol Ther 2001;70(6): 525-31.
67. Burtin P, Jacqz-Aigrain E, Girard P, et al. Population pharmacokinetics of midazolam in neonates. Clin Pharmacol Ther 1994;56(6):615-25.
68. Carme A, David V, Sergio B, et al. Intravenous clonidine: a useful and safety sedation for critically ill children. Pediatr Res Int J 2018. https://doi.org/10. 23937/2469-5769/1510027.
69. Agthe AG, Kim GR, Mathias KB, et al. Clonidine as an adjunct therapy to opioids for neonatal abstinence syndrome: a randomized, controlled trial. Pediatrics 2009;123(5):e849-56.
70. Pontén E, Viberg H, Gordh T, et al. Clonidine abolishes the adverse effects on apoptosis and behaviour after neonatal ketamine exposure in mice. Acta Anaesthesiol Scand 2012;56(8):1058-65.
71. Potts AL, Larsson P, Eksborg S, et al. Clonidine disposition in children; a population analysis. Paediatr Anaesth 2007;17(10):924-33.
72. Stella MJ, Bailey AG. Intranasal clonidine as a premedicant: three cases with unique indications. Paediatr Anaesth 2008;18(1):71-3.
73. Xie H-G, Cao YJ, Gauda EB, et al. Clonidine clearance matures rapidly during the early postnatal period: a population pharmacokinetic analysis in newborns with neonatal abstinence syndrome. J Clin Pharmacol 2011;51(4):502-11.
74. Lowery R, Zuk J, Polaner DM. Long-term use of clonidine in a critically-ill infant. Paediatr Anaesth 2005;15(8):694-8.
75. Fellmann C, Gerber AC, Weiss M. Apnoea in a former preterm infant after caudal bupivacaine with clonidine for inguinal herniorrhaphy. Paediatr Anaesth 2002; 12(7):637-40.
76. Bouchut JC, Dubois R, Godard J. Clonidine in preterm-infant caudal anesthesia may be responsible for postoperative apnea. Reg Anesth Pain Med 2001; 26(1):83-5.
77. Ooi R, Pattison J, Feldman SA. The effects of intravenous clonidine on ventilation. Anaesthesia 1991;46(8):632-3.
78. Weerink MAS, Struys MMRF, Hannivoort LN, et al. Clinical pharmacokinetics and pharmacodynamics of dexmedetomidine. Clin Pharmacokinet 2017;56(8): 893-913.
79. Su F, Gastonguay MR, Nicolson SC, et al. Dexmedetomidine pharmacology in neonates and infants after open heart surgery. Anesth Analg 2016;122(5): 1556-66.
80. Dersch-Mills DA, Banasch HL, Yusuf K, et al. Dexmedetomidine use in a tertiary care NICU: a descriptive study. Ann Pharmacother 2018. https://doi.org/10. 1177/1060028018812089. 106002801881208.
81. Bua J, Massaro M, Cossovel F, et al. Intranasal dexmedetomidine, as midazolam-sparing drug, for MRI in preterm neonates. Paediatr Anaesth 2018;28(8):747-8.
82. Szumita PM, Baroletti SA, Anger KE, et al. Sedation and analgesia in the intensive care unit: evaluating the role of dexmedetomidine. Am J Health Syst Pharm 2007;64(1):37-44.

83. Gertler R, Brown HC, Mitchell DH, et al. Dexmedetomidine: a novel sedative-analgesic agent. Proc (Bayl Univ Med Cent) 2001;14(1):13–21.
84. Lam F, Bhutta AT, Tobias JD, et al. Hemodynamic effects of dexmedetomidine in critically ill neonates and infants with heart disease. Pediatr Cardiol 2012;33(7): 1069–77.
85. Whalen LD, Di Gennaro JL, Irby GA, et al. Long-term dexmedetomidine use and safety profile among critically ill children and neonates*. Pediatr Crit Care Med 2014;15(8):706–14.
86. Chrysostomou C, Schulman SR, Herrera Castellanos M, et al. A phase II/III, multicenter, safety, efficacy, and pharmacokinetic study of dexmedetomidine in preterm and term neonates. J Pediatr 2014;164(2):276–82.e3.
87. O'Mara K, Weiss MD. Dexmedetomidine for sedation of neonates with HIE undergoing therapeutic hypothermia: a single-center experience. AJP Rep 2018; 8(3):e168–73.
88. Sanders RD, Ma D, Brooks P, et al. Balancing paediatric anaesthesia: preclinical insights into analgesia, hypnosis, neuroprotection, and neurotoxicity. Br J Anaesth 2008;101(5):597–609.
89. Baarslag MA, Allegaert K, Van Den Anker JN, et al. Paracetamol and morphine for infant and neonatal pain; still a long way to go? Expert Rev Clin Pharmacol 2017;10(1):111–26.
90. Loeser JD. Pain and suffering. Clin J Pain 2000;16(2 Suppl):S2–6.
91. Korpela R, Korvenoja P, Meretoja OA. Morphine-sparing effect of acetaminophen in pediatric day-case surgery. Anesthesiology 1999;91(2):442–7.
92. Maund E, McDaid C, Rice S, et al. Paracetamol and selective and non-selective non-steroidal anti-inflammatory drugs for the reduction in morphine-related side-effects after major surgery: a systematic review. Br J Anaesth 2011;106(3): 292–7.
93. Smits A, van den Anker JN, Allegaert K. Clinical pharmacology of analgosedatives in neonates: ways to improve their safe and effective use. J Pharm Pharmacol 2017;69(4):350–60.
94. Lewis TR, Shelton EL, Van Driest SL, et al. Genetics of the patent ductus arteriosus (PDA) and pharmacogenetics of PDA treatment. Semin Fetal Neonatal Med 2018;23(4):232–8.
95. Allegaert K, van Schaik RHN, Vermeersch S, et al. Postmenstrual age and CYP2D6 polymorphisms determine tramadol o-demethylation in critically ill neonates and infants. Pediatr Res 2008;63(6):674–9.
96. Hahn D, Emoto C, Euteneuer JC, et al. Influence of OCT1 ontogeny and genetic variation on morphine disposition in critically ill neonates: lessons from PBPK modeling and clinical study. Clin Pharmacol Ther 2019;105(3):761–8.
97. Matic M, Simons SHP, van Lingen RA, et al. Rescue morphine in mechanically ventilated newborns associated with combined OPRM1 and COMT genotype. Pharmacogenomics 2014;15(10):1287–95.
98. Allegaert K, van de Velde M, van den Anker J. Neonatal clinical pharmacology. Paediatr Anaesth 2014;24(1):30–8.
99. Hines RN, Simpson PM, McCarver DG. Age-dependent human hepatic carboxylesterase 1 (CES1) and carboxylesterase 2 (CES2) postnatal ontogeny. Drug Metab Dispos 2016;44(7):959–66.
100. McGill MR, Jaeschke H. Metabolism and disposition of acetaminophen: recent advances in relation to hepatotoxicity and diagnosis. Pharm Res 2013;30(9): 2174–87.

Assessment of Pain in the Newborn: An Update

Lynne G. Maxwell, MD[a],*, María V. Fraga, MD[b],
Carrie P. Malavolta, MSN, MBE, PNP[c]

KEYWORDS

- Neonate • Pain • Assessment • Pain scales

KEY POINTS

- Many neonatal pain assessment tools are available.
- Although brain-oriented technologies have been explored as more objective indicators of neonatal pain, none are currently ready for clinical implementation.
- Each neonatal intensive care unit should choose a limited number of tools for pain assessment in different populations (full-term, preterm), contexts, and type of pain (procedural, postoperative).
- Nurses should be trained and evaluated for appropriate use of selected tools.
- Pain management protocols using pain score triggers for administration of rescue analgesia should be implemented only with careful oversight to avoid excessive medication administration, which may lead to adverse events such as respiratory depression and/or apnea.

More than 15 million premature infants are born worldwide each year.[1] These infants, along with term neonates who are born ill, compromised either by congenital abnormalities or by peripartum or intrauterine adverse events, spend their first weeks of life hospitalized in the neonatal intensive care unit (NICU) where they are subjected to multiple invasive procedures that are frequently painful. It has been reported that hospitalized infants born at 25 to 42 weeks gestation experienced an average of 14 painful procedures a day during the first 2 weeks of life.[2–4] In addition, many newborns, both premature and term, undergo surgical procedures associated with postoperative pain. Pain is an unpleasant sensory and emotional experience associated with actual or potential tissue damage (International Association for the Study of

This article is an update of an article that originally appeared in Clinics in Perinatology, Volume 40, Issue 3, September 2013.
[a] Anesthesiology and Critical Care, Perelman School of Medicine at the University of Pennsylvania, The Children's Hospital of Philadelphia, 3401 Civic Center Boulevard, Wood 6021, Philadelphia, PA 19104, USA; [b] Perelman School of Medicine, University of Pennsylvania, The Children's Hospital of Philadelphia, 3401 Civic Center Boulevard, Philadelphia, PA 19104, USA; [c] The Children's Hospital of Philadelphia, 3401 Civic Center Boulevard, Philadelphia, PA 19104, USA
* Corresponding author.
E-mail address: maxwell@email.chop.edu

Pain [IASP] Subcommittee on Taxonomy, 1986).[5] As the IASP goes on to state, "The inability to communicate verbally does not negate the possibility that an individual is experiencing pain and is in need of appropriate pain-relieving treatment."[5] Indeed, this circumstance requires caregivers to be knowledgeable about and to implement the most valid and reliable pain assessment tools to optimize pain management in this vulnerable population.

NEURODEVELOPMENTAL CONSIDERATIONS FOR PAIN ASSESSMENT

Although neonates were formerly suspected of having blunted, immature responses to pain, it is now clear that premature and full-term newborns have the neuroanatomic pathways from periphery to cortex required for nociception. In fact, by the 24th week of gestation, painful stimuli are associated with physiologic, hormonal, and metabolic markers of the stress response.[6] Indeed, pain perception and the stress response may be greater in preterm infants because of immaturity of descending inhibitory pathways.

Because the still-developing nervous system of immature preterm neonates differs from term infants, preterm neonates are particularly vulnerable to the effects of pain and stress. The developmental neurobiology of pain confirms that afferent systems are fully functional at 24 weeks gestation; however, the self-regulatory autonomic and neuroendocrine systems that modulate sensory experience may be immature in preterm babies. Development of descending inhibitory pathways is delayed in both neurotransmitter–receptor relationships and in neural connections in the dorsal horn.[7] Tactile threshold is lower, so these infants become sensitized to repeated skin breaking and even tactile stimuli, leading to greater sensitivity to pain during and after this vulnerable period.[8] Careful observation of physiologic and behavioral indicators demonstrates that the sensory, distressing, and disruptive impact of pain is evident in this population; however, recognizing pain and distinguishing it from other conditions remains a challenge. This is especially true because, although infants born at younger gestational ages clearly perceive pain, perhaps to a heightened degree, they do not have the capability to display the full spectrum of pain behavior seen in infants born closer to term, therefore requiring modification of assessment tools to take these differences into account.

IMPLICATIONS OF PAIN EXPERIENCED IN THE NEONATAL PERIOD

Although there are still few empirical data specifically related to long-term effects of early physical pain, studies have shown that newborns, especially preterm infants, are vulnerable to long-term effects, which may lead to permanent changes in brain processing and impaired brain development,[9,10] including altered pain sensitivity and maladaptive behavior later in life.[11,12] A wide spectrum of developmental, learning, and behavioral problems are prevalent among preterm infants, especially in extremely low birth weight (ELBW; <1000 g) neonates. These outcomes are confounded by multiple factors and are in part mediated by neonatal illness, as well as socioeconomic environment. The view that the NICU environment may be a factor in altered development has been expressed for some time, with early repetitive pain interacting with other stressors in the NICU currently viewed as having the most pervasive potential effects.[13,14] After discharge from the NICU, biobehavioral responsivity to invasive skin damage of former ELBW infants was compared with term-born healthy infants at 4 and 8 months corrected age.[15–17] Pain reactivity of ELBW infants at 4 months corrected age did not appear grossly altered. At 8 months, ELBW infants initially showed greater facial response compared with term-born infants but only immediately following finger lance. However, the response of the ELBW infants attenuated rapidly, showing more rapid behavioral and physiologic dampening (less facial and autonomic responses) during recovery. Furthermore, the ELBW infants displayed higher basal resting heart rate, suggesting a possible long-term resetting of autonomic regulation. Conversely, parent rating of their child's pain sensitivity to everyday bumps at 18 months corrected age showed that ELBW toddlers were significantly less reactive to every day pain compared with heavier preterm (1000–2500 g) and term-born infants.[18]

Even infants born at term show persistent effects of pain experienced in the neonatal period. Full-term infants who underwent circumcision without analgesia in the newborn period showed increased pain responses to immunization at 4 to 6 months of age when compared with both female infants and infants who had circumcision with analgesia.[19] These healthy infants do not have the confounders that may affect changes in pain perception and development seen in the premature population. In summary, some studies provide a basis for concern that pain response and behavior may be altered in former preterm infants but potentially confounding factors need to be considered carefully in evaluating human responses beyond infancy because there are multiple sources of stress and influences on neurologic development other than early pain that may contribute to alteration in neurodevelopment.

PAIN ASSESSMENT METHODOLOGY

The gold standard of pain assessment is self-report using validated scales such as a numeric scale or visual analog scale for individuals who are cognitively intact and older than age 8 years, and tools such as the Faces-Revised or Oucher scale for cognitively intact children ages 4 to 8 years.[20] Because neonates are nonverbal, physiologic, behavioral, and biobehavioral indicators are used as a surrogate for self-report. Despite considerable research on the assessment of pain in infants undergoing neonatal intensive care, critical methodological issues remain. Pain assessment in infants becomes even more challenging when typical distress behaviors are confounded by the mechanical ventilation, pharmacologic interventions, and physical restraint inherent to care in the NICU.

PHYSIOLOGIC INDICATORS OF PAIN

Physiologic indicators of pain that are measured by neonatal pain assessment tools are typically relatively noninvasive measures. These include changes in heart rate, respiratory rate, blood pressure, and oxygen saturation.[21] Without the presence of an indwelling arterial catheter, blood pressure measurements via a cuff may be difficult to obtain without inducing discomfort. Use of vital signs alone for pain assessment has been demonstrated to be ineffective due to the inability of neonates to mount a sustained autonomic response to pain and the presence of other factors, such as mechanical ventilation and pharmacologic intervention that may affect vital signs.[22] Physiologic measures may be the only method of assessing pain in infants who are pharmacologically paralyzed or who are severely neurologically impaired. However, it has been suggested that the validity and reliability of these measures are questionable because they are influenced by other physiologic confounders, such as hypovolemia or fever (increased heart rate), or pulmonary parenchymal disease or atelectasis (desaturation, increased work of breathing with grunting).[23]

BEHAVIORAL INDICATORS OF PAIN

Behavioral parameters such as facial activity, crying, body movements, resting positions, fussiness or consolability, and sleeplessness have been the most studied indicators.[21] The ability to assess behavioral indicators may depend on gestational age, mechanical ventilation, and pharmacologic interventions, including sedation and pharmacologic paralysis.[10] The individual parameters in all pain scales used in preterm infants were originally derived from observations of term-born infants. Although preterm infants respond with facial, motor, and physiologic changes, with patterns similar to those seen in term infants, their responses are of smaller magnitude as gestational age decreases,[9,21] and they may have dampened facial responses to repeated invasive procedures. In addition, they may shut down behaviorally to invasive stimuli, leading clinicians to the potentially erroneous conclusion that these infants are not experiencing pain.[24] Furthermore, lack of observation of infants for longer periods of time may fail to capture delayed responses, resulting in underestimation of the need for caregiver intervention.

Currently, no individual physiologic or behavioral indicators reliably and specifically mark the presence of pain in preterm neonates. Moreover, dissociations between physiologic and behavioral responses to painful stimuli are common.[22] For these reasons, reliance on a unidimensional pain index is insufficient.

- Despite awareness of the importance of pain prevention, neonates continue to be exposed to multiple painful procedures daily as part of their routine care in the NICU.
- Currently, no physiologic or behavioral indicators specifically mark the presence of pain in preterm neonates.
- Preterm neonates are vulnerable to long-term effects, which may lead to permanent changes in brain processing, including altered pain sensitivity and maladaptive behavior later in life.

PAIN ASSESSMENT

Accurate assessment of pain is vital to ensure the optimal effectiveness and safety of pain management therapy in neonates who experience pain during the course of their NICU stay. As previously discussed, neonatal pain assessment is complicated because neonates are preverbal and must rely completely on caregivers for pain assessment.[25]

PARENTAL INVOLVEMENT IN PAIN ASSESSMENT

In older preverbal or nonverbal children, parents play an essential role in the pain assessment process because they know their children better than intermittent care providers in the hospital setting. However, the NICU presents some unique challenges in the integration of parent input for pain assessment. Infants in the NICU require frequent painful interventions and are unable to express their discomfort in ways that can be understood by caregivers. This is further complicated by difficulties in finding a balance between effective pain management and avoidance of adverse effects from pain medication.[26] Unfortunately, parents are often an overlooked source of comfort to newborns and usually are excluded from pain management rather than encouraged to contribute to the care of their child. During a prolonged NICU stay, parents may need to return to work. However, even when parents are able to be present, there may be several factors that prevent parents from feeling comfortable providing input on their baby's pain. The high-technology environment and the attributes of the sick infant often interfere with efforts to establish and maintain close proximity. New parents often feel insecure about their babies, and if something unexpected has occurred, such as a premature birth, a term infant with a congenital malformation, or a traumatic birth, parents may feel even further unqualified to assist in providing pain assessment.[27] Furthermore, parents may feel ambivalent: they simply wish to see their baby have minimal pain but not be too sedated. If primary nursing is available for very sick neonates from the onset of care, the primary nurse can assist in providing an accurate description of the baseline for a given infant, as well as in educating parents on what to look for and the continuum between adequate analgesia and oversedation.[28] Parental involvement can also aid the process of learning to parent and assist in the establishment of attachment behaviors, which have been demonstrated to not only enhance parental well-being but also to improve neonatal health outcomes.[29,30]

NEONATAL PAIN ASSESSMENT TOOLS

Because neonates are preverbal and parents may not be able to provide assistance in pain assessment, nurses and other care providers must be well trained in neonatal pain assessment in order to ensure adequate pain management.[28] A large variety of validated neonatal pain-assessment tools has been developed. These tools vary in their combination of physiologic and behavioral measures, as well as whether they take gestational age into account. Additionally, tools have been designed and validated for different types of pain, including procedural, postoperative, acute, and chronic pain.[31] Although more than 40 different neonatal pain assessment tools have been developed,[32] only a few are regularly incorporated into use in most NICUs. Because no comprehensive data exist on those used most commonly, one must infer this from tools used in published studies of neonatal pain. **Table 1** summarizes the features of these commonly used scales according to parameters measured, neonatal population, the painful conditions for which they have been validated, and the scale metric.[28]

Of the commonly used neonatal pain tools listed in **Table 1**:

- Two scales have metric adjustment for prematurity (Premature Infant Pain Profile-Revised [PIPP-R] and Neonatal Pain, Agitation, and Sedation Scale [N-PASS]).
- Other scales have been used in premature infants, although developed in full-term infants.
- Only 1 scale takes sedation into account (N-PASS).

As previously discussed, gestational age can significantly affect the ability of a neonate to mount or display a response to pain, whether through physiologic or behavioral indicators. Historically, neonates have been stratified into groups according to gestational age, birth weight, or postconceptual age (gestational age plus postnatal age). Most neonatal pain scales that make adjustments for prematurity do so using gestational age. Premature infants (younger than 37 weeks) of all gestational ages demonstrate a decreased ability to mount a physiologic response to painful stimuli.[22,25] Multiple factors may influence a premature infant's vital signs, and an increase in heart rate and/or respiratory rate may not be an indicator of pain alone. In addition, very premature infants may be completely unable to demonstrate a change in vital signs due to pain, and the ability to sustain this for any prolonged period of time is markedly diminished.[23] Similarly, the lack of energy reserve present in premature infants of any gestational age may result in an absent or muted behavioral response

Table 1
Summary of neonatal pain assessment tools

Pain Assessment Tool	Gestational Age	Physiologic Components	Behavioral Components	Type of Pain	Adjusts for Prematurity	Scale Metric
Premature Infant Pain Profile-Revised (PIPP-R)[67,68]	26 wk to term	Heart rate, oxygen saturation	Alertness, brow bulge, eye squeeze, nasolabial furrow	Procedural and postoperative	Yes	0–21
Cries, Requires Oxygen, Increased Vital Signs, Expression, Sleeplessness (CRIES)[69]	32–56 wk	Blood pressure, heart rate, oxygen saturation	Cry, expression, sleeplessness	Postoperative	No	0–10
Neonatal Infant Pain Scale (NIPS)[70]	28–38 wk	Breathing pattern	Facial expression, cry, arms, legs, alertness	Procedural	No	0–7
COMFORT (and COMFORTneo)[37,71]	0–3 y (COMFORTneo: 24–42 wk)	Respiratory response, blood pressure, heart rate	Alertness, agitation, physical movements, muscle tone, facial tension	Postoperative (COMFORTneo: prolonged)	No	8–40
Neonatal Facial Coding System (NFCS)[72]	25 wk to term	None	Brow bulge, eye squeeze, nasolabial furrow, open lips, stretch mouth (vertical and horizontal), lip purse, taut tongue, chin quiver	Procedural	No	0–10
Neonatal Pain, Agitation, and Sedation Scale (N-PASS)[35]	0–100 d	Heart rate, respiratory rate, blood pressure, oxygen saturation	Crying or irritability, behavior state, facial expression, extremities or tone	Acute and prolonged pain Also assesses sedation	Yes	Pain: 0–10 Sedation −10–0
Échelle de la Douleur Inconfort Noveau-Né (EDIN; Neonatal Pain and Discomfort) Scale[34]	25–36 wk	None	Facial activity, body movements, quality of sleep, quality of contact with nurses, consolability	Prolonged	No	0–15
Bernese Pain Scale for Neonates (BPSN)[73]	27–41 wk	Respiratory pattern, heart rate, oxygen saturation	Alertness, duration of cry, time to calm, skin color, brow bulge with eye squeeze, posture	Procedural	No	0–27

to painful stimuli.[31] Only 3 commonly used pain scales, the aforementioned PIPP-R and N-PASS, and the Bernese Pain Scale for Neonates (BPSN), have a metric adjustment to account for prematurity; however, other scales have demonstrated validity and reliability in the premature population.[28] The BPSN was recently evaluated with respect to the influence of gestational age on the behavioral components of the score, with the recommendation that the cutoff point increases with increasing gestational age.[32] A recent systematic review of the association of behavioral and physiologic components of pain assessment tools with brain-based indicators of nociception (near-infrared spectroscopy [NIRS] and electroencephalogram [EEG]) found that withdrawal reflex and facial expression were most strongly associated with indicators of nociceptive brain activity, whereas physiologic parameters such as heart rate and oxygen saturation had little correlation.[33]

In addition to gestational age, scales are tested for validity and reliability based on the type of pain that they are designed to assess. These types of pain include procedural, postoperative, acute, and chronic (or prolonged) pain. Additionally, some scales take sedation into account.[28] The presence of agitation or sedation in a neonate can be misinterpreted as pain by those scales that do not take sedation into account.[25] Almost all scales were designed for acute pain, procedural and/or postoperative. The presence of prolonged pain in neonates is much more difficult to assess because neonates may adapt to the presence of prolonged pain from the standpoint of both physiologic and behavioral measures.[34] Only 2 scales have demonstrated validity and reliability for prolonged pain (N-PASS and Échelle de la Douleur Inconfort Noveau-Né [EDIN]),[34,35] but the COMFORTneo scale, based on the COMFORT scale and adapted for use in neonates,[36] has shown promise in measuring prolonged pain in 1 study.[37] Some investigators have suggested the need for a better definition of prolonged pain in newborns.[38]

When choosing specific scales to use for neonatal pain, it is always important to select scales that have been proven validated and reliable, and, if possible, have studies replicating this.[34] There are many challenges to selecting appropriate scales for a given NICU setting. This is because NICU populations are diverse, often made up of premature and term infants; some sedated, paralyzed, and mechanically ventilated infants; and some postsurgical infants. If a given scale relies on an audible cry for assessment, then this scale may not be useable for a sizable portion of the population. As noted previously and in **Table 1**, scales may have demonstrated validity and reliability only for a certain gestational age and a certain type of pain, which makes selecting a single scale for entire NICU population very difficult.[31] Practical considerations also must be factored into scale choice.

As can be seen in **Table 1**, another major difference among tools is the scale metric (the numerical range of possible scores). Although the most commonly used scales in older infants, children, and adults use a 0 to 10 scale, neonatal scales vary widely, with maximum scores ranging from 7 to 40 and minimum scores from 0 to 8. This variability makes the use of tools with disparate scales problematic in a single NICU and may impair education, as well as attempts to compare outcomes for research purposes.

Choosing the best scale, or scales, for a given NICU population will require close examination of the typical patient population for the unit. Scales should be ultimately considered more useful if they are demonstrated to be valid and reliable, if they account for a broad range of gestational ages, and if they have a long track record of use. Even if a scale is determined to be valid and reliable, the feasibility and practical utility must be examined by those who will be using it.[39] If 2 scales are chosen for use on a unit, care providers must be carefully trained and their performance evaluated on an ongoing basis to ensure that they remain consistent among themselves for individual patients. Units may choose to adapt a scale designed for procedural pain to assess pain in all circumstances, but clinicians must constantly assess what they may be missing by not using a scale designed to monitor postoperative pain or in cases of prolonged pain.

NOVEL PHYSIOLOGIC PAIN ASSESSMENT TOOLS AND BIOMARKERS

Despite the plethora of neonatal pain assessment tools, there is no generally agreed on gold standard and there are problems of inconsistency among assessors. Because of the imperfect nature of the various multidimensional neonatal pain assessment tools previously described, more objective, technology-based, autonomic brain and biohormonal measures have been explored as possibly more objective indicators of pain level. These tools include autonomic measures such as heart rate variability[40] and skin conductance, and brain measures such as EEG or NIRS. In addition, hormonal markers of stress, such as cortisol and plasma parameters of oxidative stress, have been evaluated. Holsti and colleagues[41] have referred to this approach as brain-oriented.

Slater and colleagues[42] used NIRS to assess hemodynamic activity over the somatosensory cortex during procedural pain (heel lance) and were the first investigators to find a correlation between cortical hemodynamic and behavioral responses. NIRS works through the differential absorption of infrared light by oxygenated and deoxygenated hemoglobin, with changes in oxygenated hemoglobin absorption reflecting changes in cerebral blood flow that are thought to reflect the regional neural activity that is a measure of pain intensity. There were some painful episodes in which hemodynamic changes were observed in the absence of behavioral changes, suggesting the possibility that pain assessment based on more conventional pain assessment tools may underestimate the pain response in neonates. Subsequent studies by the same investigators and others have confirmed this finding.[43] If the technology is made easier to use in the clinical setting, NIRS may provide a more objective measurement of pain. Implementation of NIRS is problematic because movement and other environmental factors (drug treatment, hemodynamic changes, and respiratory changes) can interfere with accuracy, making its clinical utility questionable.

EEG monitoring measures cortical neuronal activity but isolating cortical evoked responses to pain may require complex time-lock technology, as demonstrated by Slater and colleagues,[44] which may limit its practical implementation. In addition, it may be difficult to distinguish increased cortical somatosensory activity from that related to motor activity, especially in the smallest infants. A recent scoping review of neurophysiologic technologies used for assessment of acute pain in infants suggests that event-related potentials obtained with EEG may have better correlation with noxious painful events than NIRS.[45]

Skin conductance, sometimes referred to as galvanic skin resistance, is related to palm and sole sweating, which reflects increased sympathetic nervous system activity. Changes in frequency and area under the curve have been demonstrated with procedural pain and have been shown to differentiate between pain (heel stick) and stress (alcohol wipe on skin).[46] Gjerstad and colleagues[47] found that an increase in the number of skin conductance fluctuations correlated with an increase in COMFORT score with tracheal suction in intubated children, but sensitivity was impaired by other sources of stress (postoperative pain in the first 24 hours after surgery) and subject to movement artifact. In the setting of postoperative pain in older children, however, skin conductance was found to have low sensitivity and specificity. In the awake patient, measurement was confounded by the nonnoxious factors that affect sympathetic activity, casting doubt on its utility for postoperative pain in neonates.[48]

Cortisol level is a biomarker of pain and stress states that has been used in clinical trial study designs, but it is impractical for real-time pain assessment for treatment decision-making because there is a considerable delay in obtaining the results. Although a past impediment was the need to draw blood for cortisol determination, recent studies have successfully used salivary cortisol samples. Although some studies have found increased serum or salivary cortisol with increased pain and stress, 1 study found a downregulation of serum cortisol response to stress in premature infants with higher exposure to procedural pain in the neonatal period.[49,50] Measures of oxidative stress, such as uric acid and malondialdehyde, have been found to increase after tissue-damaging procedures.[51] These serum markers are not practical real-time measures of pain but may be useful to assess efficacy of pain treatment strategies in a research setting.

Although heart rate and heart rate variability have been proposed as more objective measures of pain, investigators such as Oberlander and Saul[40] have found that medical condition confounders interfere with the utility of heart rate alone as a pain measure and suggest further investigation is needed. Although heart rate alone may not be a reliable indicator of the presence or severity of pain in the neonate, new technologies have been evaluated that use high-frequency analysis for evaluation of the heart rate variability index and the related Newborn Infant Parasympathetic Evaluation Index, which some investigators have suggested might correlate with acute pain.[52] Although preliminary studies suggest some promise, with 1 showing correlation with the presence of prolonged pain,[53] this is another technology whose reliability has not been proven.

A recent study performed in the context of a prospective study evaluating the efficacy of sucrose for procedural pain compared NIRS, skin conductance, salivary cortisol, physiologic parameters, and the Neonatal Facial Coding System (NFCS) as indicators of pain perception in healthy term neonates.[54] The investigators found moderate correlation between salivary cortisol, skin conductance, and NFCS, whereas there was high correlation between NIRS and NFCS. The investigators suggest that there was greater correlation for NIRS because it was more sensitive to a rapid pain response, whereas skin conductance and salivary cortisol changes were reflective of a more prolonged response, which might be more reflective of stress (autonomic response) than pain. These biological and brain-based measures have been used experimentally, are theoretically attractive, and potentially may be more objective measures of pain in neonates and infants than composite pain assessment tools subjectively interpreted by bedside caregivers. However, the lack of standardization and familiarity with these technologies make their use in the clinical setting impractical at this time, therefore clinicians still depend on the pain assessment tools previously described.

PRACTICAL PROBLEMS IN IMPLEMENTATION OF NEONATAL PAIN ASSESSMENT AND ASSESSMENT-BASED TREATMENT

There is no general consensus on a clinical standard for the pain score threshold at which analgesic intervention should be administered. Even in the same infant there is poor correlation between pain score and the presence or absence of analgesic intervention. On the other hand, clinical trials of analgesics frequently establish specific numeric thresholds for different pain interventions, as in the study of intravenous acetaminophen by Ceelie and colleagues.[55] This study design follows on the work of Allegaert and colleagues,[56] who demonstrated that implementation of systematic evaluation of pain (both surgical and nonsurgical), including specific interventions based on pain scores, led to an increase in both amount and duration of prescribed analgesics. A proposed method of improving the link between pain assessment and analgesic intervention involves the incorporation of a pain and discomfort tool (COMFORT) into the computerized order entry system, which was then linked to ordering sufentanil for pain or midazolam for sedation for mechanically ventilated premature infants.[57]

Postoperative studies only rarely link pain scores to specific analgesic treatment, as previously discussed. Franck and colleagues[58] compared 4 pain scales (Children's and Infants' Postoperative Pain Scale [CHIPPS], Cries, Requires Oxygen, Increased Vital Signs, Expression, Sleeplessness [CRIES], COMFORT, and PIPP-R), in addition to urinary and plasma cortisol, in 81 neonates after cardiac surgery. This was done independently from the clinical care of the patient. In this setting, they found that the COMFORT scale performed best with both physiologic and behavioral parameters playing a role, correlating best with both plasma cortisol levels and opioid dose, although the caregivers did not consistently use pain assessment in determining the necessity for analgesic intervention. These investigators point out that "there is no consistent definition or objective measure of the "need for analgesia,"" which may cause bias toward the use of behavioral over physiologic measures or vice versa in intubated, paralyzed patients. This is a fundamental problem in the clinical setting, which is that there is ambiguity in the interface between distress and pain, ambivalence on the part of the caregiver with regard to the beneficial and adverse effects of opioid treatment, and tension between avoiding the adverse effects of untreated pain and the negative consequences of overmedication.[59] Interestingly, a recent study reports that implementation of a neonatal pain and sedation protocol in 2 NICUs resulted in an increase in opiate prescription and pharmacologic interventions.[60] It is difficult even for trained nurses to accurately differentiate pain from other sources of distress, especially in intubated patients. Although nonpharmacologic measures (sucrose-pacifier, swaddling, kangaroo care) have been shown to be efficacious in the procedural pain setting, their utility in the setting of postoperative pain is less clear.

Pain Champions

Many audits of compliance with institutional or unit standards of pain assessment have revealed poor compliance and lack of fidelity in the way the tool was to be applied.[61,62] A recent international prospective observational study investigating neonatal pain assessment practices in 243 European NICUs in 18 countries, where pain guidelines recommend scheduled assessments every 4 to 6 hours, reported that only 10% of neonates received daily assessments of continuous pain.[63] This reveals a significant gap between recommended and actual bedside practices for neonatal pain assessment. For example, de Oliveira showed that there was variability among raters using the PIPP-R score for procedural pain.[64] Raters had difficulty applying the tool, especially with respect to the time required for observation and confusion about the definitions of the behavioral categories. This study identified these factors as a source of confusion and lack of reproducibility of scoring among untrained raters, differentiating the real world clinical setting from the research setting. Franck and Bruce[65] identified multiple issues of interpersonal dynamics and caregiver decision-making that interfere with effective utilization of clinical pain assessment and its relationship to pain treatment. Brahnam and colleagues[66] proposed using facial recognition technology for assessment of neonatal facial pain expressions because it has been observed that health professionals are frequently biased and may over- or under-emphasize elements of the assessment tool. Although utilization of such facial recognition technology may not be practical in the clinical setting, photographs could be used in training caregivers.

Whatever tools are chosen for a given neonatal unit, it is important that the tool be used consistently in a standardized manner. The meticulous training of pain champions or pain assessment superusers may be helpful in ongoing training and assessment of accuracy in implementation of pain assessment tools, as well as in decreasing practice variability between centers.[65]

SUMMARY

Accurate pain assessment in preterm and term neonates in the NICU is of vital importance because of the high prevalence of painful experiences in this population, in the form of both daily procedural pain and postoperative pain. More than 40 tools have been developed to assess pain in neonates that rely on physiologic parameters, behavioral parameters, or both. Each NICU should choose a limited number of tools for pain assessment in different populations (full-term, preterm), contexts, and type of pain (procedural, postoperative). Nurses should be well-trained in the use of selected neonatal pain assessment tools, and ongoing evaluation and reeducation should be implemented to ensure accurate use of these tools. Currently, there is no combination of physiologic and/or behavioral indicators that mark the presence of pain in preterm neonates as reliably and specifically as those validated in full-term infants. This can make pain assessment in preterm neonates particularly challenging. Only 2 pain assessment tools have a metric adjustment to account for prematurity. Preterm neonates are also vulnerable to long-term sequelae of painful experiences, which may lead to permanent changes in brain processing, including altered pain sensitivity and maladaptive behavior later in life. In both term and preterm neonates, parents can be valuable participants in the evaluation of their infant's pain, but they may need reinforcement and education from nurse providers. In the future, brain-oriented technologies may become available to help objectively assess neonatal pain. Future directions include the development of the these technologies and further studies on the optimization of the use of current and future neonatal pain assessment tools and other methods to objectively measure and form the basis of safe and effective treatment of neonatal pain.

Best Practices

What is the current practice for assessment of pain in the neonate?

Best practice, guideline, and care path objectives are implemented.

Pain assessment is essential for the safe and effective management of neonatal pain.

Many neonatal pain assessment tools are available.

Although brain-oriented technologies have been evaluated as more objective indicators of neonatal pain, none are currently ready for clinical implementation.

What changes in current practice are likely to improve outcomes?

Each NICU should choose a limited number of tools for pain assessment in different populations (full-term, preterm) and type of pain (procedural, postoperative).

Nurses should be trained and evaluated for appropriate and consistent use of selected tools.

Pain management protocols using pain score triggers for administration of rescue analgesia should be implemented only with careful oversight to avoid excessive medication administration, which may lead to adverse events such as respiratory depression and/or apnea.

REFERENCES

1. Howson CP, Kinney MV, Lawn JE, editors. March of dimes, PMNCH, Save the children, WHO. Born too soon: the global action report on preterm birth. Geneva (Switzerland): World Health Organization; 2012.
2. Simons SH, Van Dijk M, Anand KS, et al. Do we still hurt newborn babies? A prospective study of procedural pain and analgesia in neonates. Arch Pediatr Adolesc Med 2003;157:1058–64.
3. Carbajal R, Rousset A, Danan C, et al. Epidemiology and treatment of painful procedures in neonates in intensive care units. JAMA 2008;300:60–70.
4. Johnston C, Barrington KJ, Taddio A, et al. Pain in Canadian NICUs. Have we improved over the past 12 years? Clin J Pain 2011;27:225–32.
5. Available at: http://www.iasp-pain.org/terminology?navitemNumber=576#Pain. Accessed March 4, 2019.
6. Lee SJ, Ralston HJ, Drey EA, et al. Fetal pain: a systematic multidisciplinary review of the evidence. JAMA 2005;294:947–54.
7. Beggs S, Fitzgerald M. Development of peripheral and spinal nociceptive systems. In: Anand KJS, Stevens BJ, McGrath PJ, editors. Pain in neonates and infants. 3rd edition. Edinburgh (Scotland): Elsevier; 2007. p. 11–24.
8. Vinall J, Steven PM, Chau V, et al. Neonatal pain in relation to postnatal growth in infants born very preterm. Pain 2012;153:1374–81.
9. Johnston CC, Stevens BJ. Experience in neonatal intensive care unit affects pain response. Pediatrics 1996;98:925–30.
10. Brummelte S, Grunau RVE, Chau V, et al. Procedural pain and brain development in premature infants. Ann Neurol 2012;71:385–96.
11. Anand KJS, Scalzo F. Can adverse neonatal experiences alter brain development and subsequent behavior? Biol Neonate 2000;77:69–82.
12. Taddio A, Katz J. The effects of early pain experience in neonates on pain responses in infancy and childhood. Paediatr Drugs 2005;7:45–57.
13. Anand KJS. Effects of perinatal pain and stress. In: Mayer EA, Saper CB, editors. Progress in brain research, vol. 122. Amsterdam: Elsevier; 2000. p. 117–29.
14. Grunau RE, Holsti L, Peters JWB. Long-term consequences of pain in human neonates. Semin Fetal Neonatal Med 2006;11:268–75.
15. Oberlander TF, Grunau RVE, Pitfield J, et al. The developmental character of cardiac autonomic responses to an acute noxious event in 4- and 8-month old healthy infants. Pediatr Res 1999;45(4 Pt 1):519–25.
16. Grunau RVE, Oberlander TF, Whitfield MF, et al. Pain reactivity in former extremely low birth weight infants at corrected age 8 months compared with term born controls. Infant Behav Dev 2001;24:41–55.
17. Oberlander TF, Grunau RVE, Whitfield MF, et al. Biobehavioral pain responses in former extremely low birth weight infants at four months' corrected age. Pediatrics 2000;105:e6.
18. Grunau RVE, Whitfield MF, Petrie JH. Pain sensitivity and temperament in extremely low- birth-weight premature toddlers and preterm and full-term controls. Pain 1994;58:341–6.
19. Taddio A, Katz J, Ilersich AL, et al. Effect of neonatal circumcision on pain response during subsequent routine vaccination. Lancet 1997;349(9052):599–603.
20. Gaffney A, McGrath PJ, Dick B. Measuring pain in children: developmental and instrument issues. In: Schechter NL, Berde CB, Yaster M, editors. Pain in infants,

children and adolescents. 2nd edition. Philadelphia: Lippincott Williams & Wilkins; 2000. p. 128–41.

21. Craig KD, Whitfield MF, Grunau RVE, et al. Pain in the preterm neonate: behavioral and physiological indices. Pain 1993;52:287–99.

22. Morison SJ, Holsti L, Grunau RVE. Are there developmentally distinct motor indicators of pain in preterm infants? Early Hum Dev 2003;72:131–46.

23. Raeside L. Physiologic measures of assessing infant pain: a literature review. Br J Nurs 2011;20:1370–6.

24. Stevens BJ, Johnston CC, Grunau RVE. Issues of assessment of pain and discomfort in neonates. J Obstet Gynecol Neonatal Nurs 1995;24:849–55.

25. Koeppel R. Assessment and management of acute pain in the newborn. Association of Women's Health, Obstetric and Neonatal Nurses Web Continuing Education Resource; 2007. Available at: https://www.awhonn.org/page/Education. Accessed September 17, 2019.

26. Skene C, Franck L, Curtis P, et al. Parental involvement in neonatal comfort care. J Obstet Gynecol Neonatal Nurs 2012;41(6):786–97.

27. Franck LS, Oulton K, Bruce E. Parental involvement in neonatal pain management: an empirical and conceptual update. J Nurs Scholarsh 2012;44:45–54.

28. Walden M, Gibbins S. Pain assessment and management: guideline for practice. 2nd edition. Glenview (IL): National Association of Neonatal Nurses; 2008. p. 1–29.

29. Siani SA, Dol J, Campbell-Yeo M. Impact of parent-targeted eHealth on parent and infant health outcomes. J Perinat Neonatal Nurs 2017;31(4):332–40.

30. Marfurt-Russenberger K, Axelin A, Kesselring A, et al. The experiences of professionals regarding involvement of parents in neonatal pain management. J Obstet Gynecol Neonatal Nurs 2016;45(5):671–83.

31. Ranger M, Johnston CC, Anand KJ. Current controversies regarding pain assessment in neonates. Semin Perinatol 2007;31:283–8.

32. Schenk K, Stoffel L, Bürgin R, et al. The influence of gestational age in the psychometric testing of the Bernese pain scale for neonates. BMC Pediatr 2019; 19:1380–8.

33. Relland LM, Gehred A, Maitre NL. Behavioral and physiological signs for pain assessment in preterm and term neonates during a nociception specific response: a systematic review. Pediatr Neurol 2019;90:13–23.

34. Debillon T, Zupan V, Ravault N, et al. Development and initial validation of the EDIN scale, a new tool for assessing prolonged pain in preterm infants. Arch Dis Child Fetal Neonatal Ed 2001;85:F36–41.

35. Hummel P, Puchalski M, Creech SD, et al. Clinical reliability and validity of the N-PASS: neonatal pain, agitation and sedation scale with prolonged pain. J Perinatol 2008;28:55–60.

36. Ambuel B, Hamlett KW, Marx CM, et al. Assessing distress in pediatric intensive care environments: the COMFORT scale. J Pediatr Psychol 1992;17:95–109.

37. van Dijk M, Roofthooft DWE, Anand KJ, et al. Taking up the challenge of measuring prolonged pain in (premature) neonates: the COMFORTneo scale seems promising. Clin J Pain 2009;25:607–16.

38. Anand KJS. Defining pain in newborns: need for a uniform taxonomy? Acta Paediatr 2017;106:1438–44.

39. Duhn LJ, Medves JM. A systematic integrative review of infant pain assessment tools. Adv Neonatal Care 2004;4:126–40.

40. Oberlander T, Saul JP. Methodological considerations for the use of heart rate variability as a measure of pain reactivity in vulnerable infants. Clin Perinatol 2002;29:427–43.

41. Holsti L, Grunau RE, Shany E. Assessing pain in preterm infants in the neonatal intensive care unit: moving to a "brain-oriented" approach. Pain Manag 2011;1: 171–9.

42. Slater R, Cantarella A, Franck L, et al. How well do clinical pain assessment tools reflect pain in infants. PLoS Med 2008;5:0928–33.

43. Verriotis M, Fabrizi L, Lee A, et al. Mapping cortical responses to somatosensory stimuli in human infants with simultaneous near-infrared spectroscopy and event-related potential recording. eNeuro 2016;3 [pii:ENEURO.0026-16.2016].

44. Slater R, Worley A, Fabrizi L, et al. Evoked potentials generated by noxious stimulation in the human infant brain. Eur J Pain 2010;14:321–6.

45. Benoit B, Martin-Misener R, Newman A, et al. Neurophysiological assessment of acute pain in infants: a scoping review of research methods. Acta Paediatr 2017; 106:1053–66.

46. de Jesus JA, Tristao RM, Storm H, et al. Heart rate, oxygen saturation, and skin conductance: a comparison study of acute pain in Brazilian newborns. Conf Proc IEEE Eng Med Biol Soc 2011;2011:1875–9.

47. Gjerstad AC, Wagner K, Henrichsen T, et al. Skin conductance versus the modified COMFORT sedation score as a measure of discomfort in artificially ventilated children. Pediatrics 2008;122:e848–53.

48. Choo EK, Magruder W, Montgomery CJ, et al. Skin conductance fluctuations correlate poorly with postoperative self-report pain measures in school-aged children. Anesthesiology 2010;113:175–82.

49. Cong X, Ludington-Hoe SM, Walsh S. Randomized crossover trial of kangaroo care to reduce biobehavioral pain responses in preterm infants. Biol Res Nurs 2011;13:204–16.

50. Grunau RE, Holsti L, Haley DW, et al. Neonatal procedural pain exposure predicts lower cortisol and behavioral reactivity in preterm infants in the NICU. Pain 2005; 113:293–300.

51. Slater L, Asmerom Y, Boskovic DS, et al. Procedural pain and oxidative stress in premature neonates. J Pain 2012;13:590–7.

52. Cremillieux C, Makhlouf A, Pichot V, et al. Objective assessment of induced acute pain in neonatology with the Newborn Infant Parasympathetic Evaluation index. Eur J Pain 2018;22:1071–9.

53. Buyuktiryaki M, Uras N, Okur N, et al. Evaluation of prolonged pain in preterm infants with pneumothorax using heart rate variability analysis and EDIN scores. Korean J Pediatr 2018;61:322–6.

54. Roue J-M, Rioualen S, Gendras J, et al. Multi-modal pain assessment: are near-infrared spectroscopy, skin conductance, salivary cortisol, physiologic parameters and Neonatal Facial Coding System interrelated during venipuncture in healthy, term neonates. J Pain Res 2018;11:2257–67.

55. Ceelie I, de Wildt SN, van Dijk M, et al. Effect of intravenous paracetamol on postoperative morphine requirements in neonates and infants undergoing major noncardiac surgery: a randomized controlled trial. JAMA 2013;309:149–54.

56. Allegaert K, Tibboel D, Naulaers G, et al. Systematic evaluation of pain in neonates: effect on the number of intravenous analgesics prescribed. Eur J Clin Pharmacol 2003;59:87–90.

57. Mazars N, Milesi C, Carbajal R, et al. Implementation of a neonatal pain management module in the computerized physician order entry system. Ann Intensive Care 2012;2:38.
58. Franck LS, Ridout D, Howard R, et al. A comparison of pain measures in newborn infants after cardiac surgery. Pain 2011;152:1758–65.
59. Riddell RP, Racine N. Assessing pain in infancy: the caregiver context. Pain Res Manag 2009;14:27–32.
60. Deindl P, Unterasinger L, Kappler G, et al. Successful implementation of a neonatal pain and sedation protocol at 2 NICUs. Pediatrics 2013;132(1):e211–8.
61. Gradin M, Eriksson M. Neonatal pain assessment in Sweden – a fifteen-year follow up. Acta Paediatr 2010;100:204–8.
62. Akuma AO, Jordan S. Pain management in neonates: a survey of nurses and doctors. J Adv Nurs 2011;68:1288–301.
63. Anand KJS, Eriksson M, Boyle EM, et al. EUROPAIN survey working group of the NeoOpiod Consortium. Acta Paediatr 2017;106(8):1248–59.
64. de Oliveira MVM, de Jesus JAL, Tristao RM. Psychophysical parameters of a multidimensional pain scale in newborns. Physiol Meas 2012;33:39–49.
65. Franck LS, Bruce E. Putting pain assessment into practice: why is it so painful? Pain Res Manag 2009;14:13–20.
66. Brahnam S, Chuang C-F, Sexton RS, et al. Machine assessment of neonatal facial expressions of acute pain. Decis Support Syst 2007;43:1242–54.
67. Stevens BJ, Gibbins S, Yamada J, et al. The premature infant pain profile-revised (PIPP-R): initial validation and feasibility. Clin J Pain 2014;30(3):238–43.
68. Gibbins S, Stevens BJ, Yamada J, et al. Validation of the premature infant pain profile-revised (PIPP-R). Early Hum Dev 2014;90(4):189–93.
69. Krechel SW, Bildner J. CRIES: a new neonatal postoperative pain measurement score. Initial testing of validity and reliability. Paediatr Anaesth 1995;5:53–61.
70. Lawrence J, Alcock D, McGrath P, et al. The development of a tool to assess neonatal pain. Neonatal Netw 1993;12:59–66.
71. van Dijk M, de Boer JB, Koot HM, et al. The reliability and validity of the COMFORT scale as a postoperative pain instrument in 0 to 3-year-old infants. Pain 2000;84:367–77.
72. Grunau RVE, Craig KD. Facial activity as a measure of neonatal pain expression. Adv Pain Res Ther 1990;15:147–55.
73. Cignacco E, Mueller R, Hamers JP, et al. Pain assessment in the neonate using the Bernese pain scale for neonates. Early Hum Dev 2004;78:125–31.

Nonpharmacologic Management of Pain During Common Needle Puncture Procedures in Infants

Current Research Evidence and Practical Considerations: An Update

Carol McNair, RN(EC), MN, PhD(c), NP-Pediatrics, NNP-BC[a],
Marsha Campbell Yeo, RN, PhD NNP-BC[b],
Celeste Johnston, RN, DEd, FCAHS[c,d], Anna Taddio, BScPhm, MSc, PhD[e,*]

KEYWORDS

- Pain • Needle puncture • Neonates • Nonpharmacologic management • Pain relief
- Effectiveness

KEY POINTS

- Medical procedures involving needle puncture are ubiquitous in contemporary health care; they are used to diagnose, treat and monitor medical conditions.
- Cumulatively, infants can be exposed to hundreds of needle procedures over the entire duration of a hospitalization.
- There is sufficient evidence to support the use of nonpharmacologic interventions, particularly breastfeeding, sweet tasting solutions, and skin-to skin care, as primary strategies for pain management during common needle puncture procedures.

INTRODUCTION

Medical procedures involving needle puncture are ubiquitous in contemporary health care; they are used to diagnose, treat, and monitor medical conditions. Healthy infants

This article is an update of an article that originally appeared in Clinics in Perinatology, Volume 40, Issue 3, March 2013.
[a] Nursing and Child Health Evaluative Sciences, The Hospital for Sick Children, 555 University Avenue, Toronto M5G 1X8, Canada; [b] Department of Pediatrics, IWK Health Centre, School of Nursing, Faculty of Health Professions, Dalhousie University, Halifax, Nova Scotia, Canada; [c] Ingram School of Nursing, McGill University, Montreal, Canada; [d] IWK Health Centre, 5850/5980 University Avenue, Halifax B3K 6R8, Canada; [e] Clinical, Social and Administrative Pharmacy, Leslie Dan Faculty of Pharmacy, University of Toronto, Child Health Evaluative Sciences, The Hospital for Sick Children, 144 College Street, Toronto, Ontario M5S 3M2, Canada
* Corresponding author.
E-mail address: anna.taddio@utoronto.ca

undergo about a dozen punctures in their first year of life alone. These procedures routinely include (1) intramuscular injection of vitamin K to prevent hemorrhagic disease, (2) intramuscular and subcutaneous injections of immunizations for vaccine-preventable diseases, and (3) heel lance and/or venipuncture for screening of conditions such as phenylketonuria, hyperbilirubinemia, hypoglycemia, and hypothyroidism. In approximately 10% to 15% of infants hospitalized for medical conditions such as prematurity, congenital anomalies, jaundice, and infection, additional needle puncture procedures are undertaken, such as venous cannulation, to enable administration of nutrition and medication. A list of common needle procedures undertaken in hospitalized infants is displayed in **Box 1**.

Numerous studies have quantified the burden of pain from needle puncture procedures undertaken in hospitalized infants (**Table 1**). Although estimates vary from study to study, research findings continue to demonstrate that sick infants or those delivered preterm routinely experience dozens of procedures per week.[1–3] A recent systematic review demonstrates infants with lower gestational age, lowest birth weights and need for ventilation have the highest number of needle procedures.[3] Cumulatively, infants can be exposed to hundreds of needle procedures over the entire duration of hospitalization.

It is important to treat needle pain in infants, not only to reduce acute distress and suffering, but to also reduce any potential long-term negative impact on brain development and functioning.[11,12] Despite evidence that pain experienced in infancy can have long-standing consequences, pain from needle punctures undertaken in infants remains undertreated.[7,8,13] Nonpharmacologic interventions represent a much more rational approach to minor needle procedures than pharmacologic approaches for managing needle pain in infants.

The past 3 decades witnessed a surge of research investigating the effectiveness of nonpharmacologic methods of pain relief. Recent audits of analgesic practices in hospitalized infants demonstrate that the use of nonpharmacologic interventions surpasses analgesic drugs. In 1 study, the use rate for nonpharmacologic interventions was 18% compared with 2% for pharmacologic interventions.[1] In another study, procedures were more commonly treated with sucrose (14.3%) or other nonpharmacologic interventions (33%) compared with pharmacologic interventions (16%).[2] Studies even more recently conducted in developing countries demonstrated that most infants still underwent painful procedures without any analgesic intervention.[7,8]

Box 1
Needle puncture procedures undertaken in hospitalized infants

Intramuscular injection

Subcutaneous injection

Heel lance

Venipuncture

Venous cannulation

Central line insertion

Arterial puncture

Arterial cannulation

Lumbar puncture

Suprapubic aspiration

No. of Painful Procedures	Period of Time	Total Percentage that Were Needle Punctures	
60.8 per patient	Total stay	70%	Barker & Rutter,[4] 1995
2–10 per day	First 7 d	90%	Johnston et al,[5] 1997
14 per day	First 14 d	15.6%	Simons et al,[6] 2003
12–16 per day	First 14 d	25.6%	Carbajal et al,[2] 2008
0.8 per day	7 d	94%	Johnston et al,[1] 2011
4.3 per day	Total stay	66%	Kyololo et al,[7] 2014
7.5 per patient per day	First 14 d	19.8%	Jeong et al,[8] 2014
11.4 per patient per day	First 14 d	14%	Roofthooft et al,[9] 2014
6.6 per patient per day	Total stay	52.3%	Sposito et al,[10] 2017

Table 1
Epidemiology of procedural pain in infants in intensive care

In a very recent study examining pain management over the entire hospital stay of 242 preterm infants, although improvements in provision of pain treatment from 68% to 84% related to heel lance and intravenous therapy, only 37% of infants undergoing intramuscular injection received any form of pain relief.[14] Audits also demonstrate that organizations with strong pain guidelines for infants can improve the use of nonpharmacologic interventions.[9,15]

This article is an overview of current evidence from systematic reviews for the effectiveness of nonpharmacologic interventions for the management of pain in infants undergoing needle procedures, including swaddling or containment, pacifier or nonnutritive sucking, rocking or holding, breastfeeding and breastmilk, skin-to-skin care, sweet tasting solutions, music therapy, sensorial saturation, and parental presence. In addition, implementation considerations and areas for future research are reviewed.

SWADDLING AND CONTAINMENT

Swaddling and containment are interventions that aim to limit the infant's boundaries, promote self-regulation, and attenuate physiologic and behavioral stress caused by acute pain.[16,17] These interventions are normally differentiated in that swaddling involves wrapping of the infant in a sheet or blanket; limbs flexed; head, shoulders, and hips neutral, without rotation; and hands accessible for exploration[18]; whereas containment refers to restricting the infant's motions by holding or using an arm to place the infant's arms and legs near the trunk to maintain a flexed in utero posture, with limbs placed in body midline.[14] Containment can be achieved using accessories such as rolled blankets or commercially sold neonatal boundaries. Containment provided by a care provider or parent in which they use their hands to a hold the infant in a side lying, flexed fetal-type position is referred to as facilitated tucking.[19] In nonpain conditions, facilitated tucking has been associated with improved duration of sleep, neuromuscular development, and motor organization and reduction in physiologic distress.[20]

Evidence Summary

The effects of swaddling and containment have been examined in both preterm and full-term infants undergoing commonly performed tissue-breaking procedures in the neonatal intensive care unit (NICU). Collectively, 9 studies including infants born at less than 37 weeks and 1 study examining the response of term infants up to 1 month, were reported in a recent systematic review examining the effect of swaddling or tucking on pain-related distress pain reactivity and pain regulation.[17] Additionally, a small meta-analysis of 4 studies conducted in Thailand reports a larger effect of swaddling compared with no intervention on pain scores during heel stick in term infants than in preterm infants.[21] Although swaddling and containment may decrease biobehavioral pain response when compared with no treatment, its effect when compared with other interventions is considerably less and as such should be considered an adjuvant treatment used in combination with one of the more optimal treatments to be discussed elsewhere in this article.[22]

Implementation Considerations

Both containment and swaddling keep the infant in a flexed position and restrain the infant's limbs, decreasing the stress caused by motor disorganization, which is triggered by strong stimuli. It is a simple and feasible intervention that should be provided to infants as an intervention for puncture-related procedural pain. The most limiting factors impacting the clinical usefulness of swaddling relate to (1) the inability to adequately visualize an acutely ill infant, (2) interference with control of body temperature overhead heating units, and (3) possible dislodgment of indwelling catheters or tubing. Conversely, the use of containment either with positional supports or by touch is a feasible option in these circumstances. There have been some issues raised regarding the cost-benefit ratio for the use of facilitated touch provided by neonatal care providers.[23] Swaddling or containment is also generally contraindicated for infants with conditions associated with poor skin integrity, such as extreme prematurity or epidermolysis bullosa.

Research Considerations

The relative effectiveness of the swaddling and containment in infants of different gestational ages requires additional investigation given the lack of studies conducted in full-term infants and older infants. There is some evidence that the effect of swaddling may be very beneficial for infants with a higher gestational age. Swaddled infants with a postconceptional age 31 to 36 weeks seemed to recover physiologic parameters, specifically elevation in arterial oxygen saturation and reduction in heart rate, faster than infants with a postconceptional age of 27 to 31 weeks.[24] To date, no studies have examined the effect of this intervention in older infants up to a year, or the sustained effectiveness of swaddling or containment over ongoing, or across varied procedures. Future research is recommended to fill these knowledge gaps.

PACIFIER AND NON-NUTRITIVE SUCKING
Evidence Summary

In the absence of breastmilk or supplemental infant formula, non-nutritive sucking, generally referred to as the placement of a pacifier or a gloved finger in the infant's mouth to stimulate a sucking response, has been well-studied and reviewed in a recent meta-analysis.[17] The systematic review consisted of the combined effect of 6 studies conducted in preterm infants, 7 in full-term infants, and 1 in infants older than 1 month of age. The authors concluded that there is sufficient evidence that sucking is efficacious when compared with no treatment in reducing pain-related distress reactivity in preterm infants and improving immediate pain-related regulation in preterm and term infants up to 1 month of age.[17]

The mechanism underlying the calming effect of the orotactile stimulation of non-nutritive sucking is unknown. Given the immediate onset of the action and rapid decrease in effect that seems to be associated solely with the action of sucking, it is unlikely to be opioid mediated.[25,26] It may simply be that sensory stimulation derived from sucking blocks the perception of pain or provides distraction. The most likely hypothesis is that sucking enhances the infants' ability to self-regulate their behavioral pain response.[27] Other investigators have found that lower heart rate is associated with non-nutritive sucking[28] and that in nonpain conditions less parasympathetic withdrawal occurs after nipple feeding.[27,29]

Implementation Considerations

For the most part, non-nutritive sucking is a feasible strategy best used as an adjuvant therapy. However, limitations to its use do exist, primarily related to infection risk, most notably in low- to middle-income countries and concerns regarding potential conflict with increasing movement in the Baby Friendly[30] and Neo Baby Friendly Hospital Initiatives.[31] There has however, been recent inclusion of non-nutritive sucking for pain relief as a medical indication that has lessened this concern.[30] Another consideration with non-nutritive sucking is the need for additional care provider support to ensure that the pacifier stays in place in the infant's mouth. This is of primary concern in sick and younger infants. However, given the trend toward family-integrated care, parents are the logical choice to provide this support.[32,33]

Research Considerations

Despite the high quality of studies examining the effectiveness of non-nutritive sucking and pain relief, many questions regarding its use remain unanswered. Although some evidence exists to suggest that longer sucking times (ie, >3 minutes), may be more advantageous, there are insufficient data to confirm or refute this hypothesis.[17] Additionally, as with many nonpharmacologic measures, there is a paucity of literature regarding the effectiveness of non-nutritive sucking in older infants, or the sustained effect across repeated and various tissue breaking and procedures. Sucking-related benefits may be particularly beneficial in older infants during routine immunization injections. Last, very little is known regarding the impact of using non-nutritive sucking for repeated procedural pain on breastfeeding success or the development of oral aversion. Further research is recommended to examine these issues.

ROCKING AND HOLDING
Evidence Summary

Rocking is considered a gentle back and forth motion that stimulates a vestibular response. This movement can be accomplished via simulated means, but in the case of pain relief effectiveness is greater if provided by another person. Holding is defined as the holding of a clothed infant by either a parent or care provider. The research evidence for rocking and holding demonstrates some support for the effectiveness of this intervention as a pain-relieving strategy. In a recent meta-analysis,[17] 2 studies investigated the effect of holding on the pain-related distress pain reactivity of infants after a painful procedure.[34,35] Although rocking or holding without skin contact was not pain relieving, there did seem to be sufficient evidence to recommend its use to enhance pain related regulation when compared with no treatment.[35–37] Separately, in a meta-analysis including infants undergoing immunization, there was some evidence for the effectiveness of holding on decrease injection-related pain and distress, but the mean difference was small and, as such, similar to the treatments described elsewhere in this article, should be considered as adjuvant therapies used in combination with other more effective treatments rather than in isolation.[36]

Research and Implementation Considerations

Given the small number of studies evaluating rocking and holding and the high heterogeneity among them, further investigation is warranted across all age groups. Future studies should attempt to determine the mechanisms underlying the effects of this intervention, specifically with respect to skin contact and familiar presence during holding, which seem to be the salient pain-relieving factors. Also, the extreme importance of understanding better ways to enhance parental involvement as active participants in pain management for their infants cannot be overstated.

BREASTFEEDING AND BREASTMILK
Evidence Summary

There is clear evidence that breastfeeding, when compared with placebo or a no intervention control, effectively decreased pain associated with common needle puncture procedures in infants.[38–41] Results from a recent systematic review conducted by Benoit and colleagues[41] that included 21 studies; 15 evaluated breastfeeding or breastmilk in term infants, and 6 studies in preterm infants showed that direct breastfeeding was more effective than holding, skin-to-skin, and sweet tasting solutions in full-term infants. Breastmilk alone was not as effective.[41] A previous systematic review that included 20 studies (10 pertaining to breastfeeding and 10 investigating supplemental breastmilk) demonstrated that pain scores derived from unidimensional and composite pain assessment tools were generally lower in breastfeeding groups compared with placebo.[38] This review also supported that supplemental breastmilk alone does not seem to be as beneficial as breastfeeding.[38] There seems to be some benefit on heart rate, cry duration, behavioral facial response, and some validated pain assessment tool scores when compared with placebo; however, the cumulative pooled results regarding its pain-relieving effect are inconsistent.[38] A similar systematic review evaluated 10 studies that found breastfeeding was also beneficial in decreasing the pain of vaccinations beyond the neonatal period.[40]

Although the exact mechanism of its pain-relieving effect is unknown, it is most likely related to the combined effects of close proximity of the mother,[25] full ventral skin contact (which may mediate of the release of beta endorphins and oxytocin),[42] sucking, and the effects of other chemicals in milk. The act of breastfeeding may also divert the infant's attention from the painful stimulus.[43]

Implementation Considerations

If a mother is breastfeeding, breastfeeding offers a feasible intervention for pain management that also promotes mother infant bonding and interaction. Limitations to its clinical use include (1) the delayed maturation of the sucking reflex of preterm infants, (2) impaired sucking ability of very sick or critically ill newborns, (3) acceptability of the staff to perform procedures during breastfeeding including, that is, dynamic considerations, availability of the mother, and flexibility of neonatal team to reschedule nonurgent procedures, (4) limitation of use to nursing women, and (5) possible adverse effects.

Little has been reported regarding adverse effects associated with breastmilk administration in younger or sick infants. One study demonstrated sucking in combination with breastmilk in preterm infants was effective in decreasing pain during heel lance.[44] Similarly to sweet tasting agents, the provision of small amounts of breastmilk to a sick or very preterm infant can be associated with episodes of desaturation or choking that are transient and without long-term effect. There are no reports, however, of choking in infants who were breastfed during painful procedures. Practice uptake considerations previously described with respect to implementation of skin-to-skin contact are also applicable to the usefulness of breastfeeding, because there is strong evidence that breastfeeding is effective for needle pain in term infants and infants.

Research Considerations

There is strong evidence that breastfeeding is effective for decreasing needle pain in term infants and infants. There is limited knowledge regarding the sustained effect of breastfeeding across time or in combination with other interventions but there are currently 5 studies comparing these interventions.[41,45] As with pacifier use, there are some concerns that infants may learn to anticipate breastfeeding with an impending painful procedure. Given that breastfeeding is so frequent and painful procedures uncommon or rare, it is unlikely that infants will learn to associate breastfeeding with pain. Nevertheless, this factor has not been evaluated to date and is worthy of future study. In addition, breastmilk is a naturally occurring agent and future research should investigate potential ways to optimize the use of expressed breastmilk for ill or preterm infants unable to breastfeed and undergoing painful procedures.

SKIN-TO-SKIN CARE
Evidence Summary

Ventral skin-to-skin contact between a baby and its mother is commonly referred to as Kangaroo Mother Care owing to its similarity to marsupial mother–infant behavior. Because there may be times in which caregivers other than the mother are holding the infant, it is simply known as kangaroo care or skin-to-skin care. In this paradigm, the infant wearing only a diaper and cap is placed on the mother's bare chest between her breasts and the two are wrapped together with a small blanket, sheet, or a shawl. Typically the mother sits at about a 60° angle.

Although this practice of holding the infant skin-to-skin exists in many cultures, it was specifically used as a facsimile of an incubator in Colombia where there was a shortage of incubators for preterm infants.[46,47] Because it provided warmth from the mother's body and nutrition from her breasts, it was successful as an incubator replacement for some preterm infants. Serendipitously, it was noted that infants in skin-to-skin care were more stable physiologically,[48–50] were in quiet sleep for longer periods of time, and had improved breastfeeding outcomes.[51–53] Since the first study to test this intervention for pain in 2000,[54] altogether 25 studies have been included in a recent systematic review of skin-to-skin care for heel lance, venipuncture, or intramuscular injection in preterm and full-term neonates.[55]

The systematic review demonstrated a reduction on composite pain scores including physiologic and behavioral indicators (eg, Premature Infant Pain Profile, Neonatal Infant Pain Scale). No clear pattern of effects on physiologic (eg, heart rate) and behavioral (eg, facial action) indicators of pain during painful procedures were reported. After painful procedures, skin-to-skin care was associated with more stable regulation.

Given the decrease in pain response, and that skin-to-skin care is a cost-neutral intervention, and that it also facilitates infant regulation and provides warmth and comfort via skin-to-skin contact, it has a clear role in neonatal pain management. At present, skin-to-skin care should be recommended as a nonpharmacologic pain management intervention for common needle procedures in preterm infants and may be considered for full-term infants if breastfeeding is unavailable.

Implementation Considerations

The implementation of skin-to-skin care for procedural pain includes challenges over and above the introduction of change of any kind.[56,57] Some barriers to its implementation are pragmatic; for instance, the dynamics of taking blood from the heel while the infant is in skin-to-skin care and the availability of the mother. The stability of the infant, how it is determined, and the comfort of the staff with putting infants, especially intubated infants with many lines, into skin-to-skin care, as well as the comfort of the staff in doing a procedure in the presence of the parent are issues that involve educational efforts.[56,58] Unit guidelines that are clear and unambiguous are required to determine which infants are eligible for skin-to-skin care during painful procedures and strategies for educating staff and parents regarding how to carry out skin-to-skin care. There are a variety of resources available (eg, educational videos, skin-to-skin care equipment) to facilitate successful skin-to-skin care.[59] For example, a low padded stool, such as an ottoman, can be used for staff to sit on to perform a heel lance. The infant's foot can be gently pulled out from under the wrap around the mother. A more expensive stool with variable height settings will allow for different heights of staff or for different procedures, for example, starting an intravenous line on the scalp. Staff members can participate in choice of a seat and test its settings before actually using it.[56,59]

Regarding issues of feasibility of skin-to-skin care, for nonurgent needle procedures, scheduling can often be done to accommodate the mother's availability. Other caregivers or providers may substitute if mothers are unavailable.[60–62]

Research Considerations

The unanswered questions that remain regarding the use of skin-to-skin care for procedural pain management are numerous. Thus far, all studies have been performed for a single painful event. Studies examining the efficacy of skin-to-skin care over time and over multiple procedures are required to determine if it remains effective or becomes more or less effective over time.[63] The optimal duration of skin-to-skin care before the painful procedure also warrants further examination. How little is needed and if there is a lower and an upper limit to age of effectiveness remain unanswered questions. Although there was a wide range of durations reported in studies included in the review, from 1 to 80 minutes, no direct comparisons were made.[55] The dose may depend on age, and there have been no studies directly comparing infants of different gestational age groups, for example, less than or over 32 weeks.

SWEET TASTING SOLUTION
Evidence Summary

Oral sweet tasting solutions (eg, sucrose in water) are the most widely studied nonpharmacologic intervention for pain management in infants and have been consistently demonstrated to have analgesic effects in infants. Multiple systematic reviews demonstrate a decrease in behavioral pain behaviors in infants given sweet solutions during common needle procedures when compared with placebo water or no intervention,[39,64–66] and sweet tasting solutions are recommended in consensus statements and clinical practice guidelines.[67,68]

Implementation Considerations

Although a variety of sweet tasting chemicals have been evaluated, including natural and artificial, the most widely studied and used in clinical practice is sucrose.[64]

Sucrose is a disaccharide composed of glucose and fructose. Sweet tasting solutions are administered on the infant's tongue with a pacifier, syringe, or cup. Administration with a pacifier stimulates continuous non-nutritive sucking, which may improve effectiveness.[64] Although this systematic review evaluated a variety of doses, a recent randomized controlled trial determined that 0.1 mL of sucrose may be the minimally effective dose across preterm infants.[69]

Previously, as per the systematic review,[64] the usual single dose of sucrose was 0.5 to 2.0 mL of 12% to 24% strength (weight/volume); however, lower doses are typically used in preterm infants (as little as 0.05 mL of 24%) and larger doses in older infants (as much as 10 mL of 25%).[64–66] The onset of action is quick (within seconds), the peak effect occurs at 2 minutes, and the duration of action is up to 10 minutes.[70] Calming effects may last considerably longer than the analgesic effects, as demonstrated by a study of reduced behavioral distress responses during a subsequent handling procedure carried out up to 1 hour afterward.[71]

The mechanism of action by which sweet tasting solution blunts pain responses in infants has not been fully elucidated[70,72]; however, it has been speculated to involve several pathways. One proposed theory is based on the taste-induced release of endogenous opioids; however, other investigators include dopamine and acetylcholine pathways. In addition, sweet tasting solution may induce calming and analgesic effects through non-nutritive sucking and distraction. Of note, a study failed to demonstrate an effect on pain-specific brain activity,[73] questioning whether sucrose is a true analgesic. Behavioral indicators of pain, however, were decreased and, at present, the clinical significance of that study is not known.

Sweet tasting solution is generally well tolerated by infants; adverse effects are rare and transient, and include choking, bradycardia, and oxygen desaturation.[64,74] Data are sparse, however, regarding long-term effects. In 2 multiple dose studies that examined sucrose use over the first 7 and 28 days of life in preterm infants, no differences were reported in neurologic outcomes during the neonatal period.[75,76] However, 1 study suggested that increasing sucrose consumption was associated with worse neurobehavioral development scores.[75,77] A secondary analysis revealed that the cut off of 10 doses over 24 hours differentiated those with decreased neurobehavioral scores.[75] That, however, is the only report of cumulative dose effects and the significance of this result is unknown.

Investigation of the possible adverse effects of repeated exposure to sweet tasting solution in early life is ongoing. Two recent preclinical studies using a mouse model in which they randomly assigned 106 mice to receive sterile water or 24% oral sucrose across 1 of 3 exposures (10 times daily handling, touch, or needle prick) aimed to mimic the NICU context reported that, irrespective of the type of exposure, mice who received repeated doses of 24% oral sucrose had smaller brain volumes[78] and that mice who received repeated 24% oral sucrose during handling in the neonatal period had poorer short-term memory in adulthood compared with mice who received water during handling.[79]

Key issues to be considered when implementing sweet tasting solution analgesia include (1) guidelines for use (including dosing regimen and administration techniques), (2) procedures for ordering, dispensing and documentation, and (3) methods of evaluation. Increased use success may be observed in the presence of the following: a unit guideline, nurse-led ordering, and inclusion of sucrose as part of admission orders.[80] Some centers use commercially available unit-dose products (eg, Tootsweet, SweetEase) and others use pharmacy-compounded bulk preparations. Prepackaged products are more convenient, but individual units need to consider their storage capacities and frequency of use as considerations to which product they choose.

Continual monitoring of clinical response is important to document effectiveness and safety and to allow for individualization of dosing (ie, dose titration to response). Finally, ongoing communication, support, and reinforcement of practices with staff are also critical to ensure continued implementation success. The use of sweet tasting solutions as a soothing technique in nonpain scenarios needs to be discouraged and staff may need reminders to ensure it is not overused.

Research Considerations

Despite the plethora of research with sweet tasting solution, audits of pain management practices demonstrate that sweet tasting solution use varies widely among different practice settings.[64] The variability in use of sweet tasting solution may be due to important knowledge gaps in its pharmacology, including the exact mechanism(s) of action, the relationship between dose and response for infants of different ages and for different procedures, and the long-term effects with repeated use, including potential effects on feeding behaviors. In addition, few trials have evaluated the added benefit of sucrose when coadministered with other nonpharmacologic and pharmacologic analgesics, particularly opioids, as well as contextual factors (eg, unit culture, staffing levels).[81] All of these factors may be contributing to suboptimal use of sweet tasting solution in the clinical setting. Further study of these issues is recommended to optimize its use in infants undergoing needle procedures.

Although there remains little evidence linking sucrose to adverse outcome in human infants, recent reports, despite some limitations in the model, of possible concern in preterm mice,[64,78] warrants further investigation.

MUSIC THERAPY
Evidence Summary

There is some evidence that music therapy may be beneficial in relieving procedural pain in both full-term and preterm infant. Results from a recent review that included 9 randomized trials examining the efficacy of music for pain associated with circumcision and heel lance indicated that newborns exposed to music therapy seem to have greater physiologic stability and diminished pain response.[82]

Research and Implementation Considerations

Owing to the poor quality of some of the studies, a large variation in reported outcomes, and inconsistent findings across procedures, more rigorous trials are needed to confirm or refute the benefits of for pain relief associated with needle puncture. Additionally, although neonatal general recommendations report maintaining a range of 45 to 60 dB,[83] little is known regarding the optimal type or decibel level of the music or potential differences among various gestational age groups.

SENSORIAL SATURATION
Evidence Summary

Sensorial saturation is defined as a multisensorial stimulation consisting of delicate tactile, gustative, auditory, and visual stimuli[84,85] whereby, during the procedure, the infant's attention is attracted by massaging the face, speaking to the infant gently, and instilling a sweet solution on the infant's tongue. Results from systematic review of 8 studies examining the effect of sensorial saturation for pain relief during heel lance, intramuscular injection, and endotracheal suctioning demonstrated that pain scores were lower in the group receiving this intervention.[85]

Implementation Considerations

Sensorial interventions are straightforward and easy to implement. From a cost-effectiveness perspective, one may argue whether the known benefits outweigh added costs of associated with the need for a second care provider. As with many nonpharmacologic interventions, the most logical solution to this concern would be to increase parental involvement.

One hypothesis addressing the beneficial effect of sensorial stimulation, is derived from the Gate Control Theory proposed by Melzack and Wall.[86] Stimuli traveling ascending pathways inhibit the nociceptive signals from painful stimuli through various endogenous mechanisms located along the spino-thalamic tract.[87] The stronger these competing stimuli are, including multiple modalities, the more effective they are in blocking the perception of pain. This finding is in keeping with evidence supporting modalities encompassing multiple stimuli and may help to explain why interventions such as kangaroo care, breastfeeding, or sensorial saturation, which involve tactile, auditory, and olfactory mechanisms are generally more effective than single modalities.

Research Considerations

Many unanswered questions remain related to mechanism of action regarding these interventions and what is the optimal dose—that is, finding the balance between too much and too little stimulation—and potential differences among various gestational age groups. Additionally, future research should focus on ways to educate and enhance parent participation so that parents can lead these interventions.

PARENTAL PRESENCE
Evidence Summary

Researchers began evaluating the impact of parental presence and involvement in their children's care during painful medical procedures and resuscitation using mostly observational studies.[88–91] Researchers developed a body of evidence for the pediatric emergency department and recent systemic reviews demonstrated that almost 90% of parents want the option of participating in their child's procedures and involving parents has no negative effect on emergency staff performing the procedures.[88,90] This work has been extended to the pediatric intensive care unit in a variety of observational studies where both parents and clinicians reported that parental presence during invasive procedures helps the child significantly.[90,91] In this literature, the child's perceptions have not been assessed, although in related studies about immunization pain, children have reported a preference for parents to be present.[90–92]

Overall, parental participation in their infant's general care has shown that, even in the absence of formal parental training about pain, parents can impact the use of pain treatment strategies given to their infants. In 2 separate audits of pain management practices in the NICU, investigators observed greater use of pain treatments if parents were present when procedures were being undertaken.[1,2] Johnston and colleagues[1] found that the presence of parents was associated with an increased use of physical pain treatment strategies or sweet tasting solutions. Similarly, Carbajal and colleagues[2] found parental presence to be one of the factors associated with improved use of specific procedural analgesia. It should be noted, however, that these were observational designs and a causal link cannot be assumed.

In addition to parental presence, parental education may lead to increased use of pain treatment strategies via different mechanisms. Parents may participate in the provision of care, either by providing comfort measures themselves or by advocating for their use with health care providers, who then administer pain treatment interventions. This has been shown across studies whereby parents led use of skin-to-skin contact, facilitated tucking, and breastfeeding.[19,38,55,93]

In 2 subsequent studies,[94,95] including a qualitative study and a randomized controlled trial, parents expressed a desire to be involved in pain management. Eight-five percent of parents (n = 257) in the qualitative study wished to be involved.[94]

These studies clearly demonstrate parents' desire for knowledge about infant pain. When parents have more information, they are more likely to want to participate in comforting their infant.[32–34] In addition, when parents are educated either verbally or with demonstrations about specific interventions, they have shown they will effectively use the intervention during subsequent painful procedures in their infants.[96,97] This has been demonstrated for facilitated tucking and skin-to-skin care.[96–98]

Separately, randomized controlled trials of parent education about pain interventions for infant vaccination have shown that parent-directed education using a video[99,100] and other electronic resources[59,101] increased the use of strategies to reduce pain during infant immunizations and needle-related procedures.[102–104] Giving parents options of various strategies allows parents to choose the strategy they are most comfortable with. Studies that review various parental education strategies support using a wide variety of educational approaches to enhance parental learning.[105–107]

Parents with infants in the NICU have expressed a preference to be present during invasive medical procedures carried out on their infants.[88,94,108–111] In 1 qualitative study, Smith and colleagues[112] showed that parental participation in their infant's care was a critical coping strategy for parents in the NICU. In an randomized controlled trial by Franck and colleagues,[95] parents who received pain specific education were more satisfied than parents in the control group ($P<.01$) and parents who received the booklet expressed interest in being actively involved or present for painful procedures (90% vs 75%; $P<.01$).

There are also data available that have shown that how mothers' respond to their infants' pain experience is linked with how their infant responds to pain in the future.[113–115] Racine and colleagues[115] recently found that a mother's emotional availability can predict an infant's pain-related distress later in infancy. Their longitudinal observational study also showed mothers who had more secure attachment with their infant had infants with lower levels of pain-related distress.[115] These data suggest that engaging parents in the earliest days of their infants' pain management may create this sense of secure attachment and give parents skills to impact their infant's response to pain in later childhood. Moreover, there is some suggestion that a mother's memories of her preterm infant's pain may be associated with later post-traumatic stress symptoms, further emphasizing the importance of optimal pain control to enhance maternal well-being after hospitalization.[116]

Implementation Considerations

All of the pain management interventions discussed in this review are simple and easy to use, yet despite evidence and a variety of practice guidelines,[15,117] studies show that many infants still undergo needle procedures without pain management.[3,7,8] Parents could easily be present and provide all of these interventions to ensure their infant receives appropriate pain management.[14]

Involving parents in providing various nonpharmacologic pain strategies at any age, but especially in infancy, is not a difficult task, yet research shows that many health care providers still do not ask parents to participate or even discuss pain management options with them.[14,92,102,104]

Research Considerations

Further studies evaluating parents' provision of various nonpharmacologic pain management strategies can be a focus of future research. The majority of evidence currently available is with parents using facilitated tucking in NICU, skin-to-skin care, or breastfeeding. Studies with skin-to-skin care are also mostly in the NICU environment, but there are some studies in infants undergoing immunization. Further research with parents' presence or providing pain management in a variety of settings is needed. In addition, ongoing research regarding parental learning is also needed.

COMPARISONS AND COMBINATIONS OF NONPHARMACOLOGIC PAIN MANAGEMENT INTERVENTIONS

There has been increasing research comparing individual nonpharmacologic pain management interventions as well as their combined effects. When compared with a sweet tasting solution (oral sucrose), facilitated tucking alone is not as effective in relieving pain reactivity after a heel lance in very preterm infants.[23,118] However, its use as an adjuvant therapy, in combination with oral sucrose and non-nutritive sucking, seems to be beneficial.[23,119] Similarly, non-nutritive sucking alone when combined with sucrose,[64] 30% glucose,[120] or facilitated tucking[119] seems to be synergistic with respect to lower pain scores, less crying, more stable sleep patterns, and greater physiologic stability. Breastfeeding significantly decreased heart rate elevation and diminished the proportion of crying time, duration of first cry, and total crying time compared with positioning (swaddled and placed in a cot), maternal holding, placebo, pacifier use, no intervention, or oral sucrose group, or both.[38] Pain scores derived from unidimensional and composite pain assessment tools were generally lower in breastfeeding groups compared with positioning, placebo, or oral sucrose group, or both. There is some evidence that, when compared with sweet taste, breastfeeding is at least as effective, may be synergistic, and is potentially superior to sweet taste.[39]

In contrast, although supplemental expressed breastmilk provided in the absence of the mother seems to be of some benefit on heart rate, cry duration, behavioral facial response, and some validated pain assessment tool scores when compared with placebo, this was not the case when compared with sucrose 12.5%, 20%, or 25%. Increases in the heart rate, percentage of time crying, and pain scores were significantly higher in the breastmilk group.[38] Skin-to-skin care has also been studied in combination of other therapies. There were 5 studies that used other treatment controls with skin-to-skin care. One compared enhanced skin-to-skin care that added rocking, singing, and sucking to skin-to-skin care and found no differences in the Premature Infant Pain Profile or time for heart rate to recover.[121] Two studies compared sweet taste and holding (clothed) by female research assistant in full-term infants during heel lance.[35] Duration of crying was decreased by both, with an additive effect in the combination, but facial actions were only decreased with holding.[122]

SUMMARY

There is sufficient evidence to support the use of nonpharmacologic interventions, particularly breastfeeding, sweet tasting solutions, and skin-to skin care as primary strategies for pain management during common needle puncture procedures. They are recommended for managing acute pain and distress in infants during common needle procedures (**Table 2**). Music therapy, sensorial saturation, rocking and holding, swaddling and containment pacifier, and non-nutritive sucking would be considered adjunct

Table 2
Recommended use of non pharmacologic measures for selected needle puncture procedures in infants

Procedure	Sweet Tasting Solution	Breastfeeding	Skin-to-Skin Care	Breastmilk	Swaddling or Containment	Pacifier and non-nutritive sucking	Music Therapy	Sensorial Saturation	Parental Presence	Rocking and Holding
Intramuscular injection	X	X	X	As adjunct	As adjunct	As adjunct	As adjunct	As adjunct	As adjunct	As adjunct
Subcutaneous injection	X	X	X	As adjunct	As adjunct	As adjunct	As adjunct	As adjunct	As adjunct	As adjunct
Heel lance	X	X	X	As adjunct	As adjunct	As adjunct	As adjunct	As adjunct	As adjunct	As adjunct
Venipuncture, venous cannulation	X	X	X	As adjunct	As adjunct	As adjunct	As adjunct	As adjunct	As adjunct	As adjunct

therapies based on current evidence and should be used in combination with breast-feeding, sweet tasting solutions or kangaroo care to ensure adequate management of needle pain. Despite our limited understanding of the underlying mechanisms of actions of nonpharmacologic interventions, there seem to be few documented short-term harms from their use. Similar to pediatric pain management, where distraction techniques are effective in managing painful procedures,[123] the soothing or calming effects of other nonpharmacologic interventions may only be beneficial in this manner.

Some nonpharmacologic interventions are easily implemented (pacifier or non-nutritive sucking, swaddling or containment), whereas others need a collaborative effort (skin-to-skin care, sweet tasting solution). Parents are an untapped resource and should be encouraged to be involved in providing these measures for their infant during painful procedures.[93] It is clear parents want to be involved and, with proper knowledge and support, they can.[82,95,108]

Support from administration and leadership, both formal and informal, are crucial for the implementation of any of these strategies for procedures.[57] Informal leadership is part of the complex concept of unit culture. The culture of the unit must be accepting of any implementation.[81,124]

In summary, needle-related pain is a common experience for infants and as health care professionals; it behooves us to use all possible strategies to mitigate or prevent that pain and its negative consequences. Current research evidence suggests that nonpharmacologic interventions may be used to reduce needle pain.

Best Practices

What is the current practice for managing needle pain for infants?

Best practice, guideline or care path objective
- Provide effective pain management during common needle procedures in infants
- Improve long-term neurologic outcomes by minimizing pain exposures during a key stage of brain development

What changes in current practice are likely to improve outcomes?

- Use effective non pharmacologic strategies to manage pain during needle procedures

Major recommendations

- Sweet tasting solutions, skin-to-skin care, or breastfeeding can be used as primary strategies to manage needle pain in infants

- Swaddling and containment, non-nutritive sucking or pacifier, music therapy, breastmilk, rocking and holding, and sensorial saturation can be used as adjunct treatments with primary strategies to further decrease pain, as appropriate

- Parental presence may also have some adjunct benefit, via direct and indirect promotion of pain mitigation strategy use

Summary

Commonly performed needle procedures in infants (heel lance, immunizations, venous cannulation, venous sampling) should always be undertaken in conjunction with proven nonpharmacologic strategies to minimize pain

Bibliographic Sources: Ref.[17,36,40,51,66]

REFERENCES

1. Johnston C, Barrington K, Taddio A, et al. Pain in Canadian NICUs: have we improved over the past 12 years? Clin J Pain 2011;27:225–32.

2. Carbajal R, Rousset A, Danan C, et al. Epidemiology and treatment of painful procedures in neonates in intensive care units. JAMA 2008;300:60–70. Journal Article. Multicenter Study Research Support, Non-U.S. Gov't.

3. Cruz MD, Fernandes AM, Oliveira CR. Epidemiology of painful procedures performed in neonates: a systematic review of observational studies. Eur J Pain 2016;20:489–98.

4. Barker DP, Rutter N. Exposure to invasive procedures in neonatal intensive care unit admissions. Arch Dis Child Fetal Neonatal Ed 1995;72:F47–8.

5. Johnston CC, Collinge JM, Henderson SJ, et al. A cross-sectional survey of pain and pharmacological analgesia in Canadian neonatal intensive care units. Clin J Pain 1997;13:308–12.

6. Simons SHP, van Dijk M, Anand KS, et al. Do we still hurt newborn babies? Arch Pediatr Adolesc Med 2003;157:1058–964.

7. Kyololo OBM, Stevens B, Gastaldo D, et al. Procedural pain in neonatal units in Kenya. Arch Dis Child Fetal Neonatal Ed 2014;99:F464–7.

8. Jeong IS, Park SM, Lee JM, et al. Perceptions on pain management among Korean nurses in neonatal intensive care units. Asian Nurs Res (Korean Soc Nurs Sci) 2014;8:261–6. Multicenter Study. Research Support, Non-U.S. Gov't.

9. Roofthooft DWE, Simons SHP, Anand KJS, et al. Eight years later, are we still hurting newborn infants? Neonatology 2014;105:218–26.

10. Sposito NPB, Rossato LM, Bueno M, et al. Assessment and management of pain in newborns hospitalized in a neonatal intensive care unit: a cross-sectional study. Rev Lat Am Enfermagem 2017;25:e2931.

11. Brummelte S, Gurnau RE, Chau V, et al. Procedural pain and brain development in premature newborns. Ann Neurol 2012;71:385–96.

12. Walker SM, Franck LS, Fitzgerald M, et al. Long-term impact of neonatal intensive care and surgery on somatosensory perception in children born extremely preterm. Pain 2009;141:79–87.

13. Cong X, Wu J, Vittner D, et al. The impact of cumulative pain/stress on neurobehavioral development of preterm infants in the NICU. Early Hum Dev 2017; 108:9–16.

14. Orovec A, Disher T, Caddell K, et al. Assessment and management of procedural pain during the entire neonatal intensive care unit hospitalization. Pain Manag Nurs 2019. https://doi.org/10.1016/j.pmn.2018.11.061.

15. Lago P, Frigo AC, Baraldi E, et al. Sedation and analgesia practices at Italian neonatal intensive care units: results from the EUROPAIN study. Ital J Pediatr 2017;43:26. Multicenter Study. Observational Study.

16. Huang CM, Tung WS, Kuo LL, et al. Comparison of pain responses of premature infants to the heelstick between containment and swaddling. J Nurs Res 2004; 12:31–40.

17. Pillai Riddell R, Racine N, Turcotte K, et al. Nonpharmacological management of procedural pain in infants and young children: an abridged Cochrane review. Pain Res Manag 2011;16:321–30. Journal Article Research Support, Non-U.S. Gov't Review.

18. Aucott S, Donohue PK, Atkins E, et al. Neurodevelopmental care in the NICU. Ment Retard Dev Disabil Res Rev 2002;8:298–308.

19. Axelin A, Salantera S, Lehtonen L. Facilitated tucking by parents' in pain management of preterm infants-a randomized crossover trial. Early Hum Dev 2006;82:241–7. Randomized Controlled Trial Research Support, Non-U.S. Gov't.

20. van Sleuwen BE, Engelberts AC, Boere-Boonekamp MM, et al. Swaddling: a systematic review. Pediatrics 2007;120:e1097–106.

21. Prasopkittikun T, Tilokskulchai F. Management of pain from heel stick in neonates: an analysis of research conducted in Thailand. J Perinat Neonatal Nurs 2003;17:304–12.
22. Pillai Riddell RR, Racine NM, Turcotte K, et al. Non-pharmacological management of infant and young child procedural pain. Cochrane Database Syst Rev 2011;(10):CD006275. Journal Article. Meta-Analysis. Review.
23. Cignacco E, Axelin A, Stoffel L, et al. Facilitated tucking as a non-pharmacological intervention for neonatal pain relief: is it clinically feasible? ACTA Paediatr 2010;99:1763–5.
24. Fearon I, Kisilevsky BS, Hains SM, et al. Swaddling after heel lance: age-specific effects on behavioral recovery in preterm infants. J Dev Behav Pediatr 1997;18:222–32. Clinical Trial Research Support, Non-U.S. Gov't.
25. Blass EM. Behavioral and physiological consequences of suckling in rat and human newborns. Acta Paediatr Suppl 1994;397:71–6. Review.
26. Blass EM, Watt L. Sucking-and sucrose-induced analgesia in human newborns. Pain 1999;83:611–23.
27. Carbajal R, Chauvet X, Couderc S, et al. Randomized trial of analgesic effects of sucrose, glucose and pacifiers in term neonates. Br Med J 1999;319:1393–7.
28. Blass E, Ciaramitraro V. A new look at some old mechanisms in human newborns: taste and tactile determinants of state, affect, and action. Monogr Soc Res Child Dev 1994;59:1–81.
29. McCain G, Knupp A, Loucas Fontaine J, et al. Heart rate variability responses to nipple feeding for preterm infants with bronchopulmonary dysplasia: three case studies. J Pediatr Nurs 2010;25:215–20.
30. Semenic S, Childerhose JE, Lauriere J, et al. Barriers, facilitators and recommendations related to implementing the Baby-Friendly Initiative (BFI): an integrative review. J Hum Lact 2012;28:317–34.
31. Nyqvist KH, Haggkvist AP, Hansen MN, et al. Expansion of the baby-friendly hospital initiative ten steps to successful breastfeeding into neonatal intensive care: expert group recommendations. J Hum Lact 2013;29:300–9. Practice Guideline.
32. O'Brien K, Robson K, Bracht M, et al. Effectiveness of Family Integrated Care in neonatal intensive care units on infant and parent outcomes: a multicentre, multinational, cluster-randomised controlled trial. Lancet Child Adolesc Health 2018;4:245–54.
33. Gale C. Family integrated care for very preterm infants: evidence for a practice that seems self-evident. Lancet Child Adolesc Health 2018;4:230–1.
34. Carbajal R, Veerapen S, Couderc S, et al. Analgesic effect of breast feeding in term neonates: randomised controlled trial. BMJ 2003;326:13. Clinical Trial Journal Article Randomized Controlled Trial Research Support, Non-U.S. Gov't.
35. Gormally S, Barr RG, Wertheim L, et al. Contact and nutrient caregiving effects on newborn infant pain responses. Dev Med Child Neurol 2001;43:28–38.
36. Taddio A, Ilersich AL, Ipp M, et al. Physical interventions and injection techniques for reducing injection pain during routine childhood immunizations: systematic review of randomized controlled trials and quasi-randomized controlled trials. Clin Ther 2009;31(Suppl 2):S48–76. Journal Article Meta-Analysis Research Support, Non-U.S. Gov't Review.
37. Campos R. Soothing pain-elicited distress in infants with swaddling and pacifiers. Child Development 1989;60:781–92.
38. Shah PS, Herbozo C, Aliwalas LL, et al. Breastfeeding or breast milk for procedural pain in neonates. Cochrane Database Syst Rev 2012;(12):CD004950.

Journal Article Meta-Analysis Research Support, N.I.H., Intramural Research Support, Non-U.S. Gov't. Review.

39. Shah V, Taddio A, Rieder MJ. Effectiveness and tolerability of pharmacologic and combined interventions for reducing injection pain during routine childhood immunizations: systematic review and meta-analyses. Clin Ther 2009;31: S104–51. Review.

40. Harrison D, Reszel J, Bueno M, et al. Breastfeeding for procedural pain in infants beyond the neonatal period. Cochrane Database Syst Rev 2016;(10):CD011248. Meta-Analysis Research Support, Non-U.S. Gov't Review Systematic Review.

41. Benoit B, Martin-Misener R, Latimer M, et al. Breast-feeding analgesia in infants: an update on the current state of evidence. J Perinat Neonatal Nurs 2017;31: 145–59. Meta-Analysis. Review.

42. Hofer M. Hidden regulators in attachment, separation, and loss. Monogr Soc Res Child Dev 1994;59:192–207.

43. Gunnar M. The effects of a pacifying stimulus on behavioural and adrenocortical responses to circumcision in the newborn. J Am Acad Child Psychiatry 1984; 23:34–8.

44. Peng HF, Yin T, Yang L, et al. Non-nutritive sucking, oral breast milk, and facilitated tucking relieve preterm infant pain during heel-stick procedures: a prospective, randomized controlled trial. Int J Nurs Stud 2018;77:162–70. Randomized Controlled Trial.

45. Fallah R, Naserzadeh N, Ferdosian F, et al. Comparison of effect of kangaroo mother care, breastfeeding and swaddling on Bacillus Calmette-Guerin vaccination pain score in healthy term neonates by a clinical trial. J Matern Fetal Neonatal Med 2017;30:1147–50. Randomized Controlled Trial.

46. Charpak N, Ruiz-Pelaez JG, Charpak Y. Rey-Martinez Kangaroo Mother Program: an alternative way of caring for low birth weight infants? One year mortality in a two cohort study. Pediatrics 1994;94:804–10. Comparative Study Research Support, Non-U.S. Gov't.

47. Whitelaw A, Sleath K. Myth of the marsupial mother: home care of very low birth weight babies in Bogota, Colombia. Lancet 1985;1:1206–8. Research Support, Non-U.S. Gov't.

48. Bosque E, Brady J, Afffonso D, et al. Physiological measures of kangaroo versus incubator in a tertiary nursery. J Obstet Gynecol Neonatal Nurs 1995;24:219–26.

49. Ludington-Hoe SM. Evidence-based review of physiologic effects of kangaroo care. Curr Womens Health Rev 2011;7:243–53. Review.

50. Ferber SG, Makhoul IR. Neurobehavioural assessment of skin-to-skin effects on reaction to pain in preterm infants: a randomized, controlled within-subject trial. Acta Paediatr 2008;97:171–6. Journal Article Randomized Controlled Trial.

51. Ferber S, Makhoul I. The effect of skin-to-skin contact (kangaroo care) shortly after birth on the neurobehavioral responses of the term newborn: a randomized, controlled trial. Pediatrics 2004;113:858–65.

52. Furman L, Kennell J. Breastmilk and skin to skin kangaroo care for premature infants. Avoiding bonding failure. Acta Paediatr 2000;89:1280–3.

53. Flacking R, Ewald U, Wallin L. Positive effect of kangaroo mother care on long-term breastfeeding in very preterm infants. J Obstet Gynecol Neonatal Nurs 2011;2011:2.

54. Gray L, Watt L, Blass EM. Skin-to-skin contact is analgesic in healthy newborns. Pediatrics 2000;105:e14. Clinical Trial Journal Article Randomized Controlled Trial Research Support, Non-U.S. Gov't Research Support, U.S. Gov't, P.H.S.

55. Johnston C, Campbell-Yeo M, Disher T, et al. Skin-to-skin care for procedural pain in neonates. Cochrane Database Syst Rev 2017. https://doi.org/10.1002/14651858.CD008435.pub3.

56. Benoit B, Campbell-Yeo M, Johnston C, et al. Staff nurse utilization of kangaroo care as an intervention for procedural pain in preterm infants. Adv Neonatal Care 2016;16:229–38. Clinical Trial Comparative Study.

57. Johnston A. Factors influencing implementation of kangaroo holding in a special care nursery. MCN Am J Matern Child Nurs 2007;32:25–9.

58. Chia P, Sellick K, Gan S. The attitudes and practices of neonatal nurses in the use of kangaroo care. Aust J Adv Nurs 2006;23:20–7.

59. Campbell-Yeo M, Dol J, Disher T, et al. The power of a parent's touch: evaluation of reach and impact of a targeted evidence-based YouTube video. J Perinat Neonatal Nurs 2017;31:341–9.

60. Johnston CC, Campbell-Yeo M, Filion F. Paternal vs maternal kangaroo care for procedural pain in preterm neonates: a randomized crossover trial. Arch Pediatr Adolesc Med 2011;165:792–6. Journal Article Randomized Controlled Trial Research Support, Non-U.S. Gov't.

61. Johnston C, Byron J, Filion F, et al. Alternative female kangaroo care for procedural pain in preterm neonates: a pilot study. Acta Paediatr 2012;101:1147–50. Journal Article. Randomized Controlled Trial. Research Support, Non-U.S. Gov't.

62. Murmu J, Venkatnarayan K, Thapar R, et al. When alternative female Kangaroo care is provided by other immediate postpartum mothers, it reduces postprocedural pain in preterm babies more than swaddling. Acta Paediatr 2017;106: 411–5.

63. Campbell-Yeo M, Johnston C, Benoit B, et al. Trial of repeated analgesia with kangaroo mother care (TRAKC trial). BMC Pediatr 2013;13:182. Journal Article Randomized Controlled Trial. Research Support, Non-U.S. Gov't.

64. Stevens B, Yamada J, Ohlsson A, et al. Sucrose for analgesia in newborn infants undergoing painful procedures. Cochrane Database Syst Rev 2016;(7). CD001069. Available at: http://onlinelibrary.wiley.com/doi/10.1002/14651858.CD001069.pub5/abstract.

65. Harrison D, Yamada J, Adams-Webber T. Sweet tasting solutions for reduction of needle-related procedural pain in children aged one to 16 years. Cochrane Database Syst Rev 2011;(10):CD008408.

66. Harrison D, Beggs S, Stevens B. Sucrose for procedural pain management in infants. Pediatrics 2012;130:918–25.

67. Lago P, Garetti E, Merazzi D, et al. Guidelines for procedural pain in the newborn. Acta Paediatr 2009;98:932–9.

68. Taddio A, Yiu A, Smith R, et al. Variability in clinical practice guidelines for sweetening agents in newborn infants undergoing painful procedures. Clin J Pain 2009;25:153–5.

69. Stevens B, Yamada J, Campbell-Yeo M, et al. The minimally effective dose of sucrose for procedural pain relief in neonates: a randomized controlled trial. BMC Pediatr 2018;18. https://doi.org/10.1186/s12887-018-1026-x.

70. Stevens B, Craig K, Johnston C, et al. Oral Sucrose for procedural pain in infants. Lancet 2011;377:25–6.

71. Taddio A, Shah V, Katz J. Reduced infant response to a routine care procedure after sucrose analgesia. Pediatrics 2009;123:e425–9. Journal Article Randomized Controlled Trial Research Support, Non-U.S. Gov't.

72. Holsti L, Grunau RE. Considerations for using sucrose to reduce procedural pain in preterm infants. Pediatrics 2010;124:1042–7.

73. Slater R, Cornelissen L, Fabrizi L, et al. Oral sucrose as an analgesic drug for procedural pain in newborn infants: a randomized controlled trial. Lancet 2010;376:1225–32.

74. Taddio A, Shah V, Hancock R, et al. Effectiveness of sucrose analgesia in newborns undergoing painful medical procedures. Can Med Assoc J 2008;179: 37–43.

75. Johnston C, Filion F, Snider L, et al. Routine sucrose analgesia during the first week of life in neonates younger than 31 weeks' postconceptual age. Pediatrics 2002;110:523–8.

76. Stevens BRNP, Yamada JRNM, Beyene JP, et al. Consistent management of repeated procedural pain with sucrose in preterm neonates: is it effective and safe for repeated use over time? Clin J Pain 2005;21:543–8 [Article].

77. Johnston C, Filion F, Snider L, et al. How much sucrose is too much sucrose? Pediatrics 2007;119:226.

78. Tremblay S, Ranger M, Chau CMY, et al. Repeated exposure to sucrose for procedural pain in mouse pups leads to long-term widespread brain alterations. Pain 2017;158(8):1586–98.

79. Ranger M, Tremblay S, Chau CMY, et al. Adverse behavioral changes in adult mice following neonatal repeated exposure to pain and sucrose. Front Psychol 2019;9:2394.

80. Lafrak L, Burch K, Caravantes R. Sucrose analgesia: identifying potentially better practices. Pediatrics 2006;119:S197–202.

81. Stevens B, Riahi S, Cardoso R, et al. The influence of context on pain practices in the NICU: perceptions of health care professionals. Qual Health Res 2011;21: 757–70. Research Support, Non-U.S. Gov't.

82. Hartling L, Shaik M, Tjosvold L, et al. Music for medical indications in the neonatal period: a systematic review of randomised controlled trials. Arch Dis Child Fetal Neonatal Ed 2009;94:F349–54.

83. Etzel R, Balk S, Bearer C, et al. Noise: a hazard for the fetus and newborn. Pediatrics 1997;100:724–7.

84. Bellieni CV, Cordelli DM, Marchi S, et al. Sensorial saturation for neonatal analgesia. Clin J Pain 2007;23:219–21. Clinical Trial Comparative Study Journal Article Randomized Controlled Trial.

85. Bellieni CV, Tei M, Coccina F, et al. Sensorial saturation for infants' pain. J Matern Fetal Neonatal Med 2012;25:79–81.

86. Melzack R, Wall P. Pain mechanisms: a new theory. Science 1965;150:971–9.

87. Quirion R. Pain, nociception, and spinal opioid receptors. Prog Neuropsychopharmacol Biol Psychiatry 1984;8:571–9.

88. Power N, Franck L. Parent participation in the care of hospitalized children: a systematic review. J Adv Nurs 2008;62:622–41.

89. Smith RW, Shah V, Goldman RD, et al. Caregiver's response to pain in their children in the emergency department. Arch Pediatr Adolesc Med 2007;161: 578–82.

90. Dingeman S, Mitchell E, Meyer EC, et al. Parent presence during complex invasive procedures and cardiopulmonary resuscitation: a systematic review of the literature. Pediatrics 2007;120:842–54.

91. Curley MAQ, Meyer EC, Scoppettuolo LA, et al. Parent presence during invasive procedures and resuscitation: evaluating a clinical practice change. Am J Respir Crit Care Med 2012;186:1133–9.

92. Taddio A, Shah V, Leung E, et al. Knowledge translation of the HELPinKIDS clinical practice guideline for managing childhood vaccination pain: usability and

knowledge uptake of educational materials directed to new parents. BMC Pediatr 2013;13:23. Clinical Trial Research Support, Non-U.S. Gov't.

93. Campbell-Yeo M, Fernandes A, Johnston C. Procedural pain management for neonates using nonpharmacological strategies: part 2: mother-driven interventions. Adv Neonatal Care 2011;11:312–8 [quiz: 319–20]. Journal Article Review.

94. Franck LS, Allen A, Cox S, et al. Parents' views about infant pain in neonatal intensive care. Clin J Pain 2005;21:133–9.

95. Franck LS, Oulton K, Nderitu S, et al. Parent involvement in pain management for NICU infants: a randomized controlled trial. Pediatrics 2011;128:510–8. Journal Article Multicenter Study Randomized Controlled Trial Research Support, Non-U.S. Gov't.

96. Axelin A, Salantera S, Kirjavainen J, et al. Oral glucose and parental holding preferable to opioid in pain management in preterm infants. Clin J Pain 2009; 25:138–45. Randomized Controlled Trial Research Support, Non-U.S. Gov't.

97. Axelin A, Salanterä S, Lehtonen L. Facilitated tucking by parents in pain management of preterm infants- A randomized crossover trial. Early Hum Dev 2006;82:241–7.

98. Johnston C, Filion F, Campbell-Yeo M, et al. Kangaroo mother care diminishes pain from heel lance in very preterm neonates: a crossover trial. BMC Pediatr 2008;8. https://doi.org/10.1186/1471-2431-8-13.

99. Hillgrove-Stuart J, Pillai Riddell R, Flora DB, et al. Caregiver soothing behaviors after immunization and infant attachment: a longitudinal analysis. J Dev Behav Pediatr 2015;36:681–9. Research Support, Non-U.S. Gov't.

100. Harrison D, Sampson M, Reszel J, et al. Too many crying babies: a systematic review of pain management practices during immunizations on YouTube. BMC Pediatr 2014;14:134. Journal Article Research Support, Non-U.S. Gov't.

101. Stinson J, Gupta A, Dupuis F, et al. Usability testing of an online self-management program for adolescents with cancer. J Pediatr Oncol Nurs 2015;32:70–82.

102. Taddio A, MacDonald NE, Smart S, et al. Impact of a parent-directed pamphlet about pain management during infant vaccinations on maternal knowledge and behavior. Neonatal Netw 2014;33:74–82. Journal Article Research Support, Non-U.S. Gov't.

103. Taddio A, Shah V, Bucci L, et al. Effectiveness of a hospital-based postnatal parent education intervention about pain management during infant vaccination: a randomized control trial. CMAJ 2018;190:E1245–52.

104. Taddio A, Ipp M, Vyas C, et al. Teaching parents to manage pain during infant immunizations: laying the foundation for better pain management practices. Clin J Pain 2014;30:987–94. Journal Article.

105. Ranger M, Grunau RE. Early repetitive pain in preterm infants in relation to the developing brain. Pain Manag 2014;4(1):57–67.

106. Ranger M, Chau CM, Garg A, et al. Neonatal pain-related stress predicts cortical thickness at age 7 years in children born very preterm. PLoS One 2013;8:e76702. Research Support, N.I.H., Extramural Research Support, Non-U.S. Gov't.

107. Richardson B, Falconer A, Shrestha J, et al. Parent-targeted education regarding infant pain management delivered during the perinatal period: a scoping review. Journal of Perinatal and Neonatal Nursing, in press.

108. Franck LS, Oulton KB, Bruce ER. Parental involvement in neonatal pain management: an empirical and conceptual update. J Nurs Scholarsh 2012;44:45–54.

109. Franck L, Cox S, Allen A, et al. Parental concerns and distress about infant pain. Arch Dis Child 2004;89:F71.

110. Franck LS, Scurr K, Couture S. Parent views of infant pain and pain management in the neonatal intensive care unit. Newborn Infant Nurs Rev 2001;1: 106–13.

111. Gale G, Franck LS, Kools S, et al. Parents' perceptions of their infant's pain experience in the NICU. Int J Nurs Stud 2004;41:51–8.

112. Smith VC, Steelfisher GK, Salhi C, et al. Coping with the neonatal intensive care unit experience: parents' strategies and views of staff support. J Perinat Neonatal Nurs 2012;26:343–52.

113. Din Osmun L, Pillai Riddell R, Flora DB. Infant pain-related negative affect at 12 months of age: early infant and caregiver predictors. J Pediatr Psychol 2014;39:23–34. Research Support, Non-U.S. Gov't.

114. Pillai Riddell R, Campbell L, Flora DB, et al. The relationship between caregiver sensitivity and infant pain behaviors across the first year of life. Pain 2011;152: 2819–26. Research Support, Non-U.S. Gov't.

115. Racine NM, Pillai Riddell RR, Flora D, et al. A longitudinal examination of verbal reassurance during infant immunization: occurrence and examination of emotional availability as a potential moderator. Journal of Pediatric Psychology 2012;37(8):935–44.

116. Vinall J, Noel M, Disher T, et al. Memories of infant pain in the neonatal intensive care unit influence posttraumatic stress symptoms in mothers of infants born preterm. Clin J Pain 2018;34:963.

117. Committee on Fetus and Newborn and Section On Anesthesiology and Pain Medicine. Prevention and management of procedural pain in the neonate: an update. Pediatrics 2016;137:e20154271.

118. Campbell-Yeo M. Combining facilitated tucking and non-nutritive sucking appears to promote greater regulation for preterm neonates following heel lance, but does not provide effective pain relief. Invited commentary. Evid Based Nurs 2019;22(1):19.

119. Cignacco EL, Sellam G, Stoffel L, et al. Oral sucrose and facilitated tucking for repeated pain relief in preterms: a randomized controlled trial. Pediatrics 2012; 129:299–308.

120. Mekkaoui N, Issef I, Kabiri M, et al. Analgesic effect of 30% glucose, milk and non-nutritive sucking in neonates. J Pain Res 2012;5:573–7.

121. Johnston CC, Filion F, Campbell-Yeo M, et al. Enhanced kangaroo mother care for heel lance in preterm neonates: a crossover trial. J Perinatology 2009;29: 51–6. Journal Article Randomized Controlled Trial Research Support, Non-U.S. Gov't.

122. Gabriel MAM, de Mendoza BDH, Figueroa LJ, et al. Analgesia with breastfeeding in addition to skin-to-skin contact during heel prick. Arch Dis Child Fetal Neonatal Ed 2013;98:F499–503. Article.

123. Cohen LL. Behavioral approaches to anxiety and pain management for pediatric venous access. Pediatrics 2008;122(Suppl 3):S134–9. Journal Article Review.

124. Kitson A. Recognizing relationships: reflections on evidence-based practice. Nurs Inq 2002;9:179–86.

Epidural and Spinal Anesthesia for Newborn Surgery

Emmett E. Whitaker, MD*, Robert K. Williams, MD

KEYWORDS

- Pediatric anesthesia • Caudal • Spinal • Epidural • Regional anesthesia • Neonate

KEY POINTS

- Neuraxial anesthesia in neonates affords many benefits.
- Serious complications with neuraxial anesthesia in neonates are rare.
- Optimized neuraxial anesthesia in neonates may obviate general anesthesia altogether.
- Safe provision of neuraxial anesthesia in neonates requires that the practitioner be skilled and experienced in neonatal anesthesia.

INTRODUCTION

Neuraxial anesthesia and analgesia are increasingly becoming a routine part of perioperative care in pediatric patients. For many children undergoing surgery, a neuraxial technique can provide excellent postoperative analgesia, dramatically decrease the need for general anesthetics (GA) and opioids, or in some cases eliminate the need for GA altogether. Although the use of neuraxial anesthesia in children is undergoing a resurgence of interest, it is not a new technique. In 1909, Lord Tyrell Gray reported his experience with spinal anesthesia (SA) in 100 patients.[1] Lord Gray became a strong proponent of SA, stating that he found the disadvantages to be "…comparatively trifling when compared with general anesthesia administered under the same conditions." He concluded that "the advantages to be gained by the use of spinal anesthesia have so far impressed me that I am convinced that it will occupy an important place in the surgery of children in the future." As the safety of GA improved during the mid-twentieth century, SA and other neuraxial techniques in children gradually fell into disuse. A landmark report by Abajian and colleagues[2] in 1984 detailed how the use of SA was able to avoid exposure to GA and airway manipulation for

Disclosures: The authors have nothing to disclose.
University of Vermont Larner College of Medicine, Department of Anesthesiology, University of Vermont Medical Center, 111 Colchester Avenue, Burlington, VT 05401, USA
* Corresponding author.
E-mail address: Emmett.Whitaker@UVMHealth.org

surgery in high-risk neonates. Although other reports followed that also suggested several significant benefits to the use of neuraxial anesthesia in children, until recently there had not been a rigorously controlled comparison of the use of GA versus neuraxial anesthesia in children. As a result, Lord Gray's impressions about the advantages of SA in children would not be confirmed until the twenty-first century.

Prompted by concerns over the potential neurotoxicity of GA in young children, a well-controlled, international, multicenter trial examined the use of GA versus awake regional anesthesia in young infants. Although the primary outcome of the study was designed to examine any neurodevelopmental insult from exposure to GA, the investigators also reported several significant benefits to the use of awake regional anesthesia. When compared with their counterparts exposed to GA, awake regional anesthesia infants exhibited less hypotension and early apnea. They also were less likely to have a significant episode of oxygen desaturation postoperatively and slightly shorter times to first feed, while demonstrating lower pain scores in postanesthesia care unit.[3–5]

Neuraxial anesthesia and analgesia have become a common part of perioperative care in pediatric patients, and, as such, an understanding of their implications is paramount for any practitioner caring for neonates. This article focuses on epidural and spinal blockade for surgical procedures in the newborn period. Specific techniques are discussed along with their respective risks and benefits.

RISKS OF GENERAL ANESTHESIA IN NEONATES

Although a complete treatment of the risks of anesthesia in neonates is outside the scope of this review, the benefits of neuraxial anesthesia in neonates cannot be discussed without briefly outlining the risks of GA in this vulnerable population. In recent years, more and more institutions have enacted policies that require all children under the age of 3 years to be cared for by a specialist pediatric anesthesiologist. American College of Surgeons standards recommend that any child under the age of 2 years be cared for by a pediatric anesthesiologist.[6] These policy changes have arisen from several large, well-designed database studies that have shown that perioperative risk in children increases with decreasing age. The rate of intraoperative cardiac arrest in children less than 1 year of age is higher than in children greater than 1 year of age.[7] The rate of intraoperative cardiac arrest in children less than 1 year of age is significantly higher than in elderly (>80 years) patients.[8] Of particular concern is the risk of GA in patients with a history of congenital heart disease.[9] In many cases, the adverse events described in these studies are directly associated with failures in some of the core elements of GA, including airway management, opioid-based pain control, and the effects of GA on neonatal physiology. This inverse relationship between age and perioperative risk when providing anesthesia for neonates continues to make reducing the need for GA or voiding its use altogether more attractive.

Risks associated with opiate therapy in neonates warrants specific mention. Although adequate treatment of surgical pain is an ethical obligation, each practitioner must balance the benefits of parenteral opioids with their inherent risks. In all patients, opioids lead to several adverse effects, including respiratory depression, sedation, pruritus, constipation, bradycardia/hypotension, and apnea. When combined with the residual effects of GA after surgery, significant morbidity and even mortality may result.[10,11] Additionally, opioid tolerance and withdrawal are significant problems in the neonatal intensive care unit (NICU). Administration of opioids in the NICU is common, with 26% of overall neonates receiving opioids. When mechanically ventilated neonates are considered, this number increases to 74%.[12] Perhaps most disturbingly, neonatal exposure to medical opioids is increasing over time.[13] Several unique features of neonatal physiology make accurate dosing of opioids and sedatives difficult in neonates.[14,15] Taken together, these factors may increase the risk of iatrogenically acquired opioid tolerance in NICU patients.[16] Finally, opioid withdrawal is well documented in neonates and may occur after only a few days of opioid therapy.[16] Based on these findings and with ongoing concerns about the risks of GA in young patients, interest in neuraxial techniques continues to grow. This article focuses on epidural and spinal blockade for surgical procedures in the newborn period. Specific techniques are discussed along with their respective risks and benefits.

The ability to perform many surgeries in young patients without the need for GA or sedative medications is of particular importance to contemporary pediatric anesthesia practice, given concerns about the potential neurotoxic effects of anesthetic and sedative medications. This concern was first raised in 1999 when Ikonomidou and colleagues[17] found that antagonism of N-methyl-D-aspartate receptors was associated with widespread neurodegeneration in the juvenile rat brain. As this field developed, the finding of increased neuroapoptosis was replicated in numerous species and with most commonly used anesthetics and sedatives.[18–21] Although the results of recent clinical trials in healthy human children have yielded reassuring results,[3,5,22] uncertainty remains regarding the neurologic effects of anesthesia on the developing brain. As such, avoidance of GA, when possible, is likely to remain desirable to anesthesiologists, surgeons, and parents alike.

DELETERIOUS EFFECTS OF INADEQUATELY TREATED PAIN IN NEONATES

Pain is known to lead to several physiologic perturbations, including hormonal, autonomic, immunologic, and inflammatory effects. Inadequately treated acute pain leads to several deleterious physiologic effects, including altered pain responses in infancy/childhood,[23,24] mechanical hypersensitivity,[25] hyperalgesia,[26] and neurocognitive changes later in life.[27] Additionally, acute pain can lead to neurocellular changes in the brain.[28,29] Repeated inflammatory pain in neonatal rats leads to increased apoptosis in developing neurons[30,31] and poorer neurodevelopmental function in the mature animal.[32] These relationships may be particularly important in the setting of anesthesia and surgery, given that acute pain is almost certainly present, and anesthesiologists must balance the risk of inadequately treated pain with the risks of different analgesic regimens. Recently, Broad and colleagues[29] found that surgery increases neuronal cell death and induces changes in gene expression compared with anesthesia exposure alone, suggesting that pain/nociceptive stimuli may lead to brain injury, even in the setting of GA.

BENEFITS OF NEURAXIAL ANESTHESIA IN NEONATES

Neuraxial anesthesia in neonates is associated with many benefits and advantages compared with GA alone (**Box 1**). As discussed previously, neonates carry the greatest risk of morbidity and mortality with GA. Physiology and organ function in neonates are immature, and as such they are exquisitely sensitive to the effects of opioids and GA.

In the operating room, the immature physiology of neonates actually confers some benefits when neuraxial anesthesia is used. Neuraxial anesthesia provides excellent analgesia and/or surgical anesthesia without causing significant hemodynamic or respiratory compromise, even in patients with significant comorbidities.[4,33–35]

Box 1	
Benefits and risks of neuraxial anesthesia in neonates	
Benefits	**Risks**
• Decreased need for opioids	• Block failure
• Decreased volatile anesthetic requirement	• Infection
• Improved analgesia	• Bleeding
• Decreased cardiovascular and respiratory compromise	• Dural puncture/cerebrospinal fluid leak
	• Intravascular injection
• Decreased need for muscle relaxants	• Seizure
• Decreased need for and duration of mechanical ventilation	• Cardiac arrest
	• Injection site pain
• Earlier return of gastrointestinal function	• Persistent neurologic symptoms
• Potential avoidance of airway instrumentation	• Paralysis
• Earlier return of oral feeding	
• May reduce or eliminate risk of anesthesia-induced neurotoxicity	

Specifically, neuraxial anesthesia allows for reduced volatile anesthetic requirement[36,37] and a reduced need for muscle relaxants.[38] In some cases, neuraxial anesthesia allows for the avoidance of GA altogether, precluding the need for airway instrumentation, systemic sedatives, opioids, airway instrumentation, and even supplemental oxygen.[39] Many infraumbilical procedures can be performed under RA (single-shot caudal anesthesia or SA) with little or no systemic sedation. In cases of SA, Whitaker and colleagues[40] found that in a series of 105 patients, SA alone was sufficient for 85% of cases, with the remaining cases requiring only small doses of dexmedetomidine.

The use of neuraxial anesthesia is also associated with significant postoperative benefits, including decreased early apnea,[41] improved respiratory mechanics,[37,42,43] reduced need for mechanical ventilation,[44,45] earlier return of gastrointestinal function,[42,44,46,47] earlier resumption of oral feeding,[37,41,47–49] attenuated stress response,[50] and perhaps even improved splanchnic perfusion.[49,51] After bladder exstrophy repair in neonates, wound dehiscence was found to be less likely with prolonged neuraxial anesthesia.[52] Beyond the clinical benefits to the patient, SA also is associated with decreased costs related to postoperative monitoring and hospitalization.[53]

RISKS OF NEURAXIAL ANESTHESIA IN NEONATES

Although neuraxial has considerable benefits when used in neonates, it also carries significant risks (see **Box 1**). Nonetheless, available data suggest that even in neonates, neuraxial anesthesia is very safe. One study found only 1 serious complication (meningitis) in a neonate in a series of 2490 cases.[44] The Pediatric Regional Anesthesia Network (PRAN) database has made progress toward a more comprehensive understanding of RA in children. To date, the PRAN investigators have accumulated data, including morbidity and mortality, on more than 100,000 regional blocks in children from 21 pediatric hospitals.[54] In 2012, the PRAN investigators reported the results of regional blocks in 14,917 children. They found no significant morbidity nor mortality in neonates.[55] The PRAN investigators repeated their analysis in 2018, examining more than 100,000 blocks. They found the rate of complications with RA in children to be similar to that seen in adults. Although the investigators analyzed approximately 7 times more blocks, still no complications were observed in neonates.[56] Turning specifically to neuraxial anesthesia, the PRAN investigators quantified complications resulting specifically from caudal blockade in children. Of 18,650 children, 1 neonate suffered a seizure. There were no permanent sequelae nor was there any mortality.[57] The same investigators also studied the safety of indwelling caudal epidural catheters, specifically in neonates. They found the overall incidence of complications to be 13.3 but estimated the risk of serious complications to be 0.3%. Complications in this series were defined as neurologic (paresthesias or a persistent neurologic deficit), local anesthetic (LA) systemic toxicity, infection, vascular (vascular puncture or hematoma), respiratory (pneumothorax or respiratory depression), catheter malfunction, dural puncture, or other. The investigators found that there were no cases of permanent neurologic deficit, 1 case of epidural hematoma, and the rate of severe LA systemic toxicity to be 0.76:10,000. A vast majority of complications were benign catheter malfunctions.[56] Finally, Wong and colleagues[58] found the rate of complications with epidural techniques in neonates to be 4.2%, which was higher than that in infants and small children (1.4% and 0.5%, respectively). Complications in this series included local skin infection, drug error, postdural puncture headache, unrecognized intravascular catheter, unrecognized intrathecal catheter, and several other minor complications that occurred infrequently. Local skin infection or drug error accounted for 59% of complications. One case, however, was a fatal cardiac arrest that was attributed to inadvertent intravascular migration of an epidural catheter and presumed LA systemic toxicity.[58]

Rates of individual complications are difficult to quantify, but some data exist that hint at their incidence. A review of several studies representing approximately 100 institutions found the risk of inadvertent dural puncture to be approximately 1:250 and the risk of seizure to be approximately 1:1250.[44] The risk of other complications (intravascular injection, block failure, infection, and persistent neurologic symptoms), however, remains unclear.

Although neuraxial anesthesia in children, even neonates, has a track record of safety and certainly confers benefits and advantages over GA alone, occasional serious complications can occur.[59] Given the small margin for error when caring for neonates, it is important that a practitioner who possesses the required expertise be performing and managing neuraxial anesthesia in neonatal patients.

ANATOMY OF THE SPINE IN NEONATES

The anatomy of the spine in neonates, compared with older children and adults, has some fundamental differences. First, the bone and connective tissues are immature and soft compared with equivalent structures in adult patients. The rostral/caudal relationships of the spinal cord and the thecal sac also change as a child ages. In neonates and young infants, the conus medullaris ends at approximately the L3 level, whereas in adults it ends at approximately L1. The conus medullaris ascends over the course of the next several months, and, by the age of 1 year, it has reached the L1 level. Similarly, the thecal sac is positioned more caudally (at approximately the S4 level in infants less than 1 year of age). It too ascends over time and typically ends at approximately S2 in children older than 1 year. These features of immature neuraxial anatomy introduce risk of inadvertent spinal cord injury or dural puncture when neuraxial anesthesia is performed in neonates. There is no strict cutoff regarding at how young an age a patient can benefit from neuraxial anesthesia. SA may be of particular benefit to the very young or very premature neonate.[39,60] At the authors'

Box 2
Recommended doses for 0.25% bupivacaine or 0.2% ropivacaine for single-shot caudal anesthesia

Level Desired	Dose
Sacral	0.25 mL/kg
High lumbar	0.5 mL/kg
Low thoracic	1.0 mL/kg

institution, SA is the preferred anesthetic for extremely premature infants (<30 weeks) because it allows avoidance of airway manipulation.

USES OF NEURAXIAL ANESTHESIA IN NEONATES

Neuraxial anesthesia should be considered as a part of the anesthetic (or the sole anesthetic) whenever possible and clinically appropriate.

Epidural Anesthesia

The epidural space is a fat-filled potential space between the ligamentum flavum and the dura mater. Epidural anesthesia and/or analgesia (EA) is produced by injecting medication into the epidural space, usually via a needle or indwelling catheter. The mainstay of this technique is the injection of LA into the epidural space. Although LA is often sufficient to produce adequate anesthesia or analgesia, the addition of many adjuncts has been explored. Epidural clonidine,[61–63] ketamine,[64] fentanyl,[65] morphine,[66] midazolam,[63,67] and dexmedetomidine[68] have been shown to prolong the duration of surgical block and/or analgesia compared with LA alone. In contrast, neostigmine has not been shown to provide any analgesia benefit and may carry significant side effects.[69]

The goal of EA is to render a portion of the body that corresponds to the location of the injection insensate. EA can be performed for any procedure involving the sacral, lumbar, and thoracic regions. Single-shot caudal blockade can be considered for procedures that do not require an indwelling catheter, recognizing that the level of the block is limited by the volume of LA that can be safely administered. Common medications used for single-shot caudal blocks include 0.125% to 0.25% bupivacaine or 0.2% ropivacaine (**Box 2**).

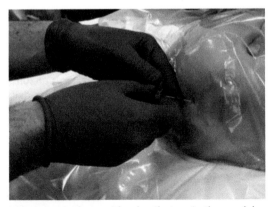

Fig. 1. Approach to placement of an epidural catheter via the caudal approach.

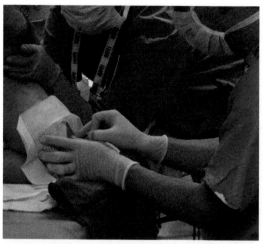

Fig. 2. Awake SA in an infant.

Single-shot caudal blocks typically are administered through a needle designed specifically for caudal blocks or with the assistance of an angiocatheter. When analgesia over a period of days is required, an indwelling catheter can be placed either via the caudal approach, threading the catheter to the desired level (**Fig. 1**) or via the direct lumbar or thoracic approach. Using these techniques, anesthesia and/or analgesia can be provided for most procedures from the midthorax down (eg, gastric tube placement and umbilical herniorraphy).

Spinal Anesthesia

SA has been used for more than 100 years in children and was first described by August Bier[70] in 1899, when he used it for the removal of a tumor from the thigh of an 11-year-old boy. Since then, SA has been used for a multitude of different procedures, either alone or in combination with EA (**Box 3**).

Because the typical neonate has normal spinal anatomy and anatomic landmarks that are easy to palpate, obtaining lumbar puncture is a relatively straightforward procedure in most cases. The authors' practice includes applying an LA cream to the lumbar spine 30 minutes to 45 minutes prior to the procedure. A 22-gauge needle (or 25-gauge needle in the case of extremely small neonates) typically is used to access the intrathecal space. Although the procedure can be performed with the neonate sitting or in the lateral position, it often is easier to reliably identify midline in the sitting position (**Fig. 2**). Due to the remarkable hemodynamic and respiratory

Box 3
Types of surgery potentially amenable to spinal anesthesia

Inguinal hernia repair[71]	Circumcision[40]
Patent ductus arteriosus ligation[72]	Segmental scoliosis surgery[73]
Pyloromyotomy[74]	Peripherally inserted central catheter placement[48]
Gastrostomy/gastroschisis[43]	Achilles tendon lengthening[75]
Colostomy[76]	Ureteral reimplant[77]
Myelomeningocele repair[78]	Anoplasty/rectal biopsy[37]
Hypospadias repair[40]	Bladder augmentation[77]

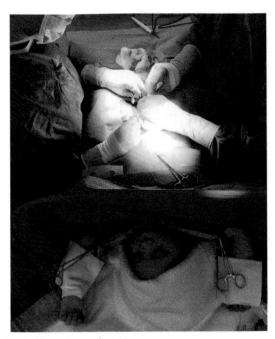

Fig. 3. An unsedated infant asleep after SA.

stability seen with SA in neonates, the procedure often is done prior to placement of a peripheral intravenous catheter. When performed successfully, SA can provide dense surgical anesthesia and motor blockade from the T5-6 dermatome down, allowing the surgeon to operate as high as the upper abdomen.

A feature unique to SA in neonates and infants is that a child usually falls asleep shortly after administration of the SA, even in the absence of systemic sedatives (**Fig. 3**). The etiology of this sedate state is unclear; it has been suggested that deafferentation or lack of somatic input to the reticular activating system may play a role.[79,80]

SUMMARY

Neuraxial anesthesia in neonates is safe and effective. Its use affords several benefits and poses few serious risks. Effective use of neuraxial anesthesia can provide a nearly pain-free perioperative experience for neonates when performed properly. With ongoing concerns about the safety of GA in neonates, the popularity of neuraxial anesthesia in this vulnerable patient population is likely to continue to increase.

REFERENCES

1. Gray HT. A study of spinal anesthesia in children and infants: from a series of 200 cases. Lancet 1909;174(4491):913–7.
2. Abajian JC, Mellish RW, Browne AF, et al. Spinal anesthesia for surgery in the high-risk infant. Anesth Analg 1984;63(3):359–62.
3. McCann ME, de Graaff JC, Dorris L, et al. Neurodevelopmental outcome at 5 years of age after general anaesthesia or awake-regional anaesthesia in infancy

(GAS): an international, multicentre, randomised, controlled equivalence trial. Lancet 2019;393(10172):664–77.

4. McCann ME, Withington DE, Arnup SJ, et al. Differences in blood pressure in infants after general anesthesia compared to awake regional anesthesia (GAS study-a prospective randomized trial). Anesth Analg 2017;125(3):837–45.

5. Davidson AJ, Disma N, de Graaff JC, et al. Neurodevelopmental outcome at 2 years of age after general anaesthesia and awake-regional anaesthesia in infancy (GAS): an international multicentre, randomised controlled trial. Lancet 2016;387(10015):239–50.

6. Surgeons ACo. Optimal resources for children's surgical care v.1 2019. Available at: https://www.facs.org/quality-programs/childrens-surgery/childrens-surgery-verification/standards. Accessed April 1, 2019.

7. Morray JP, Geiduschek JM, Ramamoorthy C, et al. Anesthesia-related cardiac arrest in children: initial findings of the pediatric perioperative cardiac arrest (POCA) registry. Anesthesiology 2000;93(1):6–14.

8. Nunnally ME, O'Connor MF, Kordylewski H, et al. The incidence and risk factors for perioperative cardiac arrest observed in the national anesthesia clinical outcomes registry. Anesth Analg 2015;120(2):364–70.

9. Ramamoorthy C, Haberkern CM, Bhananker SM, et al. Anesthesia-related cardiac arrest in children with heart disease: data from the Pediatric Perioperative Cardiac Arrest (POCA) registry. Anesth Analg 2010;110(5):1376–82.

10. Dahan A, Aarts L, Smith TW. Incidence, reversal, and prevention of opioid-induced respiratory depression. Anesthesiology 2010;112(1):226–38.

11. Morton NS, Errera A. APA national audit of pediatric opioid infusions. Paediatr Anaesth 2010;20(2):119–25.

12. Carbajal R, Eriksson M, Courtois E, et al. Sedation and analgesia practices in neonatal intensive care units (EUROPAIN): results from a prospective cohort study. Lancet Respir Med 2015;3(10):796–812.

13. Lewis T, Erfe BL, Ezell T, et al. Pharmacoepidemiology of opiate use in the neonatal ICU: increasing cumulative doses and iatrogenic opiate withdrawal. J Opioid Manag 2015;11(4):305–12.

14. Bouwmeester NJ, van den Anker JN, Hop WC, et al. Age- and therapy-related effects on morphine requirements and plasma concentrations of morphine and its metabolites in postoperative infants. Br J Anaesth 2003;90(5):642–52.

15. Lynn AM, Nespeca MK, Bratton SL, et al. Intravenous morphine in postoperative infants: intermittent bolus dosing versus targeted continuous infusions. Pain 2000;88(1):89–95.

16. Anand KJ, Hall RW, Desai N, et al. Effects of morphine analgesia in ventilated preterm neonates: primary outcomes from the NEOPAIN randomised trial. Lancet 2004;363(9422):1673–82.

17. Ikonomidou C, Bosch F, Miksa M, et al. Blockade of NMDA receptors and apoptotic neurodegeneration in the developing brain. Science 1999;283(5398):70–4.

18. Zou X, Liu F, Zhang X, et al. Inhalation anesthetic-induced neuronal damage in the developing rhesus monkey. Neurotoxicol Teratol 2011;33(5):592–7.

19. Young C, Jevtovic-Todorovic V, Qin YQ, et al. Potential of ketamine and midazolam, individually or in combination, to induce apoptotic neurodegeneration in the infant mouse brain. Br J Pharmacol 2005;146(2):189–97.

20. Pearn ML, Hu Y, Niesman IR, et al. Propofol neurotoxicity is mediated by p75 neurotrophin receptor activation. Anesthesiology 2012;116(2):352–61.

21. Kodama M, Satoh Y, Otsubo Y, et al. Neonatal desflurane exposure induces more robust neuroapoptosis than do isoflurane and sevoflurane and impairs working memory. Anesthesiology 2011;115(5):979–91.

22. Sun LS, Li G, Miller TL, et al. Association between a single general anesthesia exposure before age 36 months and neurocognitive outcomes in later childhood. JAMA 2016;315(21):2312–20.

23. Taddio A, Katz J, Ilersich AL, et al. Effect of neonatal circumcision on pain response during subsequent routine vaccination. Lancet 1997;349(9052): 599–603.

24. Taddio A, Katz J. The effects of early pain experience in neonates on pain responses in infancy and childhood. Paediatr Drugs 2005;7(4):245–57.

25. Peters CM, Eisenach JC. Contribution of the chemokine (C-C motif) ligand 2 (CCL2) to mechanical hypersensitivity after surgical incision in rats. Anesthesiology 2010;112(5):1250–8.

26. Walker SM, Tochiki KK, Fitzgerald M. Hindpaw incision in early life increases the hyperalgesic response to repeat surgical injury: critical period and dependence on initial afferent activity. Pain 2009;147(1–3):99–106.

27. Bouza H. The impact of pain in the immature brain. J Matern Fetal Neonatal Med 2009;22(9):722–32.

28. Peters JW, Schouw R, Anand KJ, et al. Does neonatal surgery lead to increased pain sensitivity in later childhood? Pain 2005;114(3):444–54.

29. Broad KD, Kawano G, Fierens I, et al. Surgery increases cell death and induces changes in gene expression compared with anesthesia alone in the developing piglet brain. PLoS one 2017;12(3):e0173413.

30. Anand KJ, Garg S, Rovnaghi CR, et al. Ketamine reduces the cell death following inflammatory pain in newborn rat brain. Pediatr Res 2007;62(3):283–90.

31. Duhrsen L, Simons SH, Dzietko M, et al. Effects of repetitive exposure to pain and morphine treatment on the neonatal rat brain. Neonatology 2013;103(1):35–43.

32. Page GG, Blakely WP, Kim M. The impact of early repeated pain experiences on stress responsiveness and emotionality at maturity in rats. Brain Behav Immun 2005;19(1):78–87.

33. Ing C, Sun LS, Friend AF, et al. Adverse events and resource utilization after spinal and general anesthesia in infants undergoing pyloromyotomy. Reg Anesth Pain Med 2016;41(4):532–7.

34. Kachko L, Birk E, Simhi E, et al. Spinal anesthesia for noncardiac surgery in infants with congenital heart diseases. Paediatr Anaesth 2012;22(7):647–53.

35. Ing C, Sun LS, Friend AF, et al. Differences in intraoperative hemodynamics between spinal and general anesthesia in infants undergoing pyloromyotomy. Paediatr Anaesth 2017;27(7):733–41.

36. Willschke H, Machata AM, Rebhandl W, et al. Management of hypertrophic pylorus stenosis with ultrasound guided single shot epidural anaesthesia–a retrospective analysis of 20 cases. Paediatr Anaesth 2011;21(2):110–5.

37. Williams RK, McBride WJ, Abajian JC. Combined spinal and epidural anaesthesia for major abdominal surgery in infants. Can J Anaesth 1997;44(5 Pt 1): 511–4.

38. Brindley N, Taylor R, Brown S. Reduction of incarcerated inguinal hernia in infants using caudal epidural anaesthesia. Pediatr Surg Int 2005;21(9):715–7.

39. Ebert KM, Jayanthi VR, Alpert SA, et al. Benefits of spinal anesthesia for urologic surgery in the youngest of patients. J Pediatr Urol 2019;15(1):49.e1-5.

40. Whitaker EE, Wiemann BZ, DaJusta DG, et al. Spinal anesthesia for pediatric urological surgery: reducing the theoretic neurotoxic effects of general anesthesia. J Pediatr Urol 2017;13(4):396–400.

41. Jones LJ, Craven PD, Lakkundi A, et al. Regional (spinal, epidural, caudal) versus general anaesthesia in preterm infants undergoing inguinal herniorrhaphy in early infancy. Cochrane Database Syst Rev 2015;(6):CD003669.

42. von Ungern-Sternberg BS, Regli A, Frei FJ, et al. The effect of caudal block on functional residual capacity and ventilation homogeneity in healthy children. Anaesthesia 2006;61(8):758–63.

43. Raghavan M, Montgomerie J. Anesthetic management of gastrochisis–a review of our practice over the past 5 years. Paediatr Anaesth 2008;18(11):1055–9.

44. Bosenberg AT, Johr M, Wolf AR. Pro con debate: the use of regional vs systemic analgesia for neonatal surgery. Paediatr Anaesth 2011;21(12):1247–58.

45. Shenkman Z, Hoppenstein D, Erez I, et al. Continuous lumbar/thoracic epidural analgesia in low-weight paediatric surgical patients: practical aspects and pitfalls. Pediatr Surg Int 2009;25(7):623–34.

46. Borgeat A, Aguirre J. Update on local anesthetics. Curr Opin Anaesthesiol 2010; 23(4):466–71.

47. Gerber AC, Weiss M. Awake spinal or caudal anaesthesia in preterms for herniotomies: what is the evidence based benefit compared with general anaesthesia? Curr Opin Anaesthesiol 2003;16(3):315–20.

48. Williams RK, Adams DC, Aladjem EV, et al. The safety and efficacy of spinal anesthesia for surgery in infants: the Vermont Infant Spinal Registry. Anesth Analg 2006;102(1):67–71.

49. Hoehn T, Jetzek-Zader M, Blohm M, et al. Early peristalsis following epidural analgesia during abdominal surgery in an extremely low birth weight infant. Paediatr Anaesth 2007;17(2):176–9.

50. Solak M, Ulusoy H, Sarihan H. Effects of caudal block on cortisol and prolactin responses to postoperative pain in children. Eur J Pediatr Surg 2000;10(4): 219–23.

51. Udassin R, Eimerl D, Schiffman J, et al. Epidural anesthesia accelerates the recovery of postischemic bowel motility in the rat. Anesthesiology 1994;80(4): 832–6.

52. Kost-Byerly S, Jackson EV, Yaster M, et al. Perioperative anesthetic and analgesic management of newborn bladder exstrophy repair. J Pediatr Urol 2008; 4(4):280–5.

53. Sartorelli KH, Abajian JC, Kreutz JM, et al. Improved outcome utilizing spinal anesthesia in high-risk infants. J Pediatr Surg 1992;27(8):1022–5.

54. Pediatric regional anesthesia network. Available at: http://pranetwork.org/. Accessed April 1, 2019.

55. Polaner DM, Taenzer AH, Walker BJ, et al. Pediatric Regional Anesthesia Network (PRAN): a multi-institutional study of the use and incidence of complications of pediatric regional anesthesia. Anesth Analg 2012;115(6):1353–64.

56. Walker BJ, Long JB, Sathyamoorthy M, et al. Complications in pediatric regional anesthesia: an analysis of more than 100,000 blocks from the pediatric regional anesthesia Network. Anesthesiology 2018;129(4):721–32.

57. Suresh S, Long J, Birmingham PK, et al. Are caudal blocks for pain control safe in children? an analysis of 18,650 caudal blocks from the Pediatric Regional Anesthesia Network (PRAN) database. Anesth Analg 2015;120(1):151–6.

58. Wong GK, Arab AA, Chew SC, et al. Major complications related to epidural analgesia in children: a 15-year audit of 3,152 epidurals. Can J Anaesth 2013;60(4): 355–63.

59. Meyer MJ, Krane EJ, Goldschneider KR, et al. Case report: neurological complications associated with epidural analgesia in children: a report of 4 cases of ambiguous etiologies. Anesth Analg 2012;115(6):1365–70.

60. Shenkman Z, Erez I, Freud E, et al. Risk factors for spinal anesthesia in preterm infants undergoing inguinal hernia repair. J Pediatr (Rio J) 2012;88(3):222–6.

61. Akin A, Ocalan S, Esmaoglu A, et al. The effects of caudal or intravenous clonidine on postoperative analgesia produced by caudal levobupivacaine in children. Paediatr Anaesth 2010;20(4):350–5.

62. Lak M, Araghizadeh H, Shayeghi S, et al. Addition of clonidine in caudal anesthesia in children increases duration of post-operative analgesia. Trauma Mon 2012;16(4):170–4.

63. Sanwatsarkar S, Kapur S, Saxena D, et al. Comparative stuNot Found In Databasedy of caudal clonidine and midazolam added to bupivacaine during infraumbilical surgeries in children. J Anaesthesiol Clin Pharmacol 2017;33(2):241–7.

64. Aliena SP, Lini C, Chirayath JJ. Comparison of postoperative analgesic effect of caudal bupivacaine with and without ketamine in Pediatric subumbilical surgeries. J Anaesthesiol Clin Pharmacol 2018;34(3):324–7.

65. Jarineshin H, Fekrat F, Kargar Kermanshah A. Treatment of postoperative pain in pediatric operations: comparing the efficiency of bupivacaine, bupivacaine-dexmedetomidine and bupivacaine-fentanyl for caudal block. Anesth Pain Med 2016;6(5):e39495.

66. Attia J, Ecoffey C, Sandouk P, et al. Epidural morphine in children: pharmacokinetics and CO2 sensitivity. Anesthesiology 1986;65(6):590–4.

67. Krishnadas A, Suvarna K, Hema VR, et al. A comparison of ropivacaine, ropivacaine with tramadol and ropivacaine with midazolam for post-operative caudal epidural analgesia. Indian J Anaesth 2016;60(11):827–32.

68. Trifa M, Tumin D, Tobias JD. Dexmedetomidine as an adjunct for caudal anesthesia and analgesia in children. Minerva Anestesiol 2018;84(7):836–47.

69. Memis D, Turan A, Karamanlioglu B, et al. Caudal neostigmine for postoperative analgesia in paediatric surgery. Paediatr Anaesth 2003;13(4):324–8.

70. Bier A. Experiment regarding the cocainization of the spinal cord. Zentralbl Chir 1899;51:361–9.

71. Webster AC, McKishnie JD, Kenyon CF, et al. Spinal anaesthesia for inguinal hernia repair in high-risk neonates. Can J Anaesth 1991;38(3):281–6.

72. Williams RK, Abajian JC. High spinal anaesthesia for repair of patent ductus arteriosus in neonates. Paediatr Anaesth 1997;7(3):205–9.

73. Dalens BJ, Khandwala RS, Tanguy A. Staged segmental scoliosis surgery during regional anesthesia in high risk patients: a report of six cases. Anesth Analg 1993;76(2):434–9.

74. Islam S, Larson SD, Kays DW, et al. Feasibility of laparoscopic pyloromyotomy under spinal anesthesia. J Pediatr Surg 2014;49(10):1485–7.

75. AlSuhebani M, Martin DP, Relland LM, et al. Spinal anesthesia instead of general anesthesia for infants undergoing tendon Achilles lengthening. Local Reg Anesth 2018;11:25–9.

76. Abreu RA, Vaz FA, Laurino R, et al. Randomized clinical trial comparing spinal anesthesia with local anesthesia with sedation for loop colostomy closure. Arq Gastroenterol 2010;47(3):270–4.

77. Trifa M, Tumin D, Whitaker EE, et al. Spinal anesthesia for surgery longer than 60 min in infants: experience from the first 2 years of a spinal anesthesia program. J Anesth 2018;32(4):637–40.
78. Viscomi CM, Abajian JC, Wald SL, et al. Spinal anesthesia for repair of meningo-myelocele in neonates. Anesth Analg 1995;81(3):492–5.
79. Disma N, Tuo P, Astuto M, et al. Depth of sedation using Cerebral State Index in infants undergoing spinal anesthesia. Paediatr Anaesth 2009;19(2):133–7.
80. Hermanns H, Stevens MF, Werdehausen R, et al. Sedation during spinal anaesthesia in infants. Br J Anaesth 2006;97(3):380–4.

Neonatal Airway Management

Raymond S. Park, MD*, James M. Peyton, MBChB, MRCP, FRCA,
Pete G. Kovatsis, MD, FAAP

KEYWORDS

- Airway management • Neonate • Prematurity • Respiratory physiology • Intubation

KEY POINTS

- Neonates have multiple differences in airway anatomy and physiology that can greatly impact clinical care.
- Premature patients often have associated medical sequelae that should be thoroughly identified before airway interventions.
- Premedication and neuromuscular blockade use have been associated with improved intubation success and decreased complications.
- Videolaryngoscopy has been associated with improved success in tracheal intubation and a decreased risk of complications in neonates.
- Advanced airway management techniques for difficult intubation have lower success rates in smaller patients and assistance from pediatric anesthesia and ENT surgeons should be requested when difficulty is anticipated or experienced.

SPECIFIC ANATOMIC AND PHYSIOLOGIC CONSIDERATIONS FOR NEONATAL AIRWAY MANAGEMENT
Neonatal Airway Anatomy

The anatomy for neonatal airway management presents a diverse set of challenges that contrast sharply to that of the matured airway (**Table 1**). The different challenges begin with the simple yet distinct contrast of the neonatal head relative to the body. In utero and during early childhood, the rapid development of the brain results in a proportionately larger head relative to the body as well as a larger neurocranium (cranial vault and base) to viscerocranium (face) ratio. The relative proportion of the neonatal head compared with the rest of the body is approximately 19%, whereas in the adult the head is only 9%.[1,2] As a result, when the neonate is supine, the head is pushed into flexion (see **Fig. 1**). This flexion often results in upper airway obstruction, difficulty with

Disclosures: Dr P.G. Kovatsis is a medical advisor to Verathon, Inc.
Department of Anesthesiology, Critical Care and Pain Medicine, Boston Children's Hospital, Harvard Medical School, 300 Longwood Avenue, Boston, MA 02115, USA
* Corresponding author.
E-mail address: raymond.park@childrens.harvard.edu

Table 1
Key anatomic aspects of the neonate versus the adult airway

1.	Proportionately larger skull to body and larger cranial vault to face ratios push the head and neck into flexion (**Fig. 1**)
2.	The tongue is proportionately larger relative the oral cavity and occupies more space posteriorly into hypopharynx
3.	The epiglottis is angulated over the laryngeal inlet and onto the laryngeal inlet axis (**Fig. 2**)
4.	The epiglottis is proportionately longer and shaped as a clockwise rotated 'C', inverted 'U' or omega (Ω) (see **Fig. 2**)
5.	The laryngeal inlet axis is angulated anteriorly such that it is directed into the base of tongue
6.	The larynx is more superior with the relative position of vocal cords at C3
7.	The narrowest laryngeal portion is the cricoid cartilage
8.	The aryepiglottic folds are closer to midline and may obscure the vocal cords (see **Fig. 2**)
9.	The arytenoids together with the corniculate and cuneiform cartilages are proportionally larger compared with the size of the laryngeal inlet
10.	The vocal cords are inferiorly inserted at the anterior aspect of the larynx, which results in the anterior commissure angling away from the laryngeal inlet
11.	Pliable laryngeal cartilages are more prone to compression with external manipulation

mask ventilation, and a poor direct laryngoscopic view if the head is not repositioned and stabilized. To optimize the airway, the shoulders should be raised with posterior support and the head shifted to neutral or slightly extended. Overextension of the skull on the neck may result in obstruction as the airway is stretched and then narrowed.

The neonatal larynx has an anterior laryngeal tilt such that its axis is directed into the base of the tongue and the base of the tongue in a neonate occupies more of the

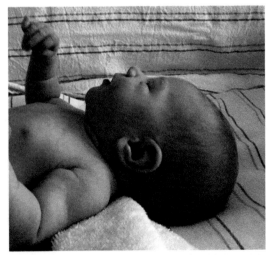

Fig. 1. A healthy neonatal patient. Note the proportionately larger head relative to the body as well as a larger neurocranium (cranial vault and base) to viscerocranium (face) ratio. With appropriate posterior shoulder support, the head does not flex onto the chest. (*Courtesy of* Carolyn Butler, MD, Boston, MA.)

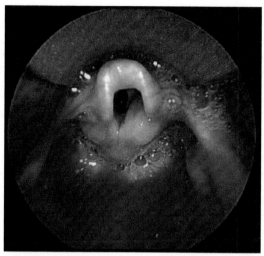

Fig. 2. View on direct laryngoscopy of the neonatal larynx. Note the relative longer, C-shaped epiglottis and the partial obscurement of the posterior laryngeal inlet by the aryepiglottic folds. (*Courtesy of* Gi Soo Lee, MD, EdM, Boston, MA.)

posterior hypopharynx. Therefore, lifting the tongue with jaw thrust and/or placement of an oral or a nasal airway is essential to minimize upper airway obstruction in a sedated or obtunded neonate.

The classical description of the narrowest portion of the neonatal and infant larynx and subglottis is a circumferential cricoid within a funnel shaped larynx.[3] However, this has been questioned in the literature over the last 2 decades.[4–6] Newer investigations have demonstrated the overall shape of the airway to be cylindrical rather than funnel shaped, and that the cricoid cartilage may be elliptical rather than cylindrical.[4,6] A review of the concepts applied in the literature to assess the pediatric larynx concluded that the infant larynx is funnel shaped and the circular or near circular cricoid cartilage remains the narrowest aspect of the larynx,[7] but the debate is far from over.

Neonatal Airway Physiology

Neonates are in constant transition from their former in utero environment, and the physiologic demands of continued growth requires compromise to achieve stability in the face of this ongoing transformation. This compromise between function and growth is manifested in airway and respiratory physiology. Breathing occurs in utero as a part of normal fetal development and transitions at birth to its life-sustaining role. Although the mechanisms causing the onset of breathing at birth are still not fully elucidated, an increase in FiO_2 together with cord clamping are likely key factors initiating rhythmic respirations.[8] Through the birthing process and the onset of physiologic respirations, pulmonary fluid is rapidly expelled via the upper airways and residual pulmonary fluid is transported out through the newly dilated capillaries and lymphatics.[9] As this fluid is moved over the course of hours,[10] lung compliance improves. The neonate needs to generate negative inspiratory pressures in excess of 20 cm H_2O to more than 70 cm H_2O to overcome the initial large surface forces as extrauterine breathing is initiated.[11] With lung expansion, surfactant is discharged into the alveoli to help maintain alveolar stability. To maintain lung volume and essentially, functional residual capacity (FRC), neonates need to expend energy.[9] FRC in adults is the equilibrium between the inward recoil of the lung and the outward recoil of the chest wall, which occurs at end-tidal volume. Owing to the factors detailed in **Box 1**, the calculated FRC or static FRC is incompatible with effective gas exchange.[12] To maintain FRC at levels similar to a supine adult, the neonate truncates exhalation before reaching static FRC, referred to as diaphragmatic braking, which adds, and then maintains extra volume within the respiratory system.[8,13] In addition, intermittent glottic closure using laryngeal adductors during exhalation, referred to as laryngeal braking, provides positive end-expiratory pressure and also helps to maintain neonatal lung volume.[8,13]

Lung volumes in neonates are disproportionately small in relation to body size and their metabolic rate is at least twice that of the adult, resulting in greatly increased ventilatory requirements per unit lung volume. Neonates meets these ventilatory demands through increased respiratory rates.[8,14,15] Dead space volume to tidal volume ratios are similar in adults and neonates. However, given a neonate's very small tidal volume, an increase in dead space results in a greater proportional change, which places further stress on the neonate's respiratory system.

Airway resistance is greater in neonates compared with the older child and adult owing to their small caliber of similar airway generations. Given that resistance is inversely proportional to the radius[4] (or radius[5] during turbulent flow) of the airway, neonates have an increased work of breathing and an increased vulnerability to diseases affecting the airway. Inflammation and secretions have a greater effect on their smaller airways; even a small amount of narrowing results in a significant increase in resistance and work of breathing. Of note, the peripheral airways contribute only a small portion overall to the total airway resistance such that most of the airway resistance is found in the median airways and the extrathoracic airways, particularly the nasal passages.[16,17]

Neonates seem to be more sensitive to irritant and mechanical stimulation of the airway with animal studies, suggesting that they have a period of transient laryngeal hyperexcitability.[8] The protective airway reflexes of coughing and swallowing seen in older children are not consistently seen in neonates. Instead, neonates may instead respond with breath holding, laryngospasm, and central apnea leading to bradycardia.[18–20]

Sedation, anesthesia, or any depressed neurologic status in the neonate may result in marked decrease of FRC as these compensatory mechanisms are diminished or lost. Thus, continuous positive airway pressures and positive end-expiratory pressures are required to improve and then maintain FRC when airway management is instituted.

Box 1
Factors impacting maintenance of FRC in neonates

Pleural pressure is nearly atmospheric in neonates and infants whereas the older child and adults have an average of −5 cm H_2O

Outward recoil of the chest is exceedingly small given a predominately cartilaginous rib cage and less developed muscles of respiration

Inward recoil of the lung is decreased, but only moderately

Even though lung compliance is higher than in an adult, the more significantly decreased outward recoil of the chest wall results an increased risk of volume loss and airway closure, especially when apneic, sedated or with muscle relaxant

Neonates have a transient increase in ventilation when faced with hypoxia, which is soon followed by a sustained ventilatory depression if the hypoxia has not resolved.[8] Of note, even mild hypothermia may abolish the initial transient hyperventilation. This hypoxic depression is often associated with bradycardia and both are exaggerated and persist to an older age in premature infants.[8]

ASSESSMENT AND PREPARATION

Formulating a plan for intubation ideally begins with a thorough review of the patient's medical history and indication for airway intervention. Pertinent medical history includes medications, allergies, last oral intake, gestational age, and relevant medical comorbidities, including any medical issues related to prematurity. With respect to comorbidities, clinicians should be cognizant of specific disease processes that can have implications for neonatal airway management, which may be grouped into anatomic and other nonairway pathophysiology that affect clinical airway management.

Premature neonates commonly have coexisting disease that can significantly impact care and relevant sequelae should be recognized and appropriately integrated into airway management planning. Owing to the immature lung structure and relative lack of surfactant production compared with term neonates, premature patients can develop respiratory distress syndrome, which is characterized by decreased lung compliance, ventilation perfusion mismatch, and increased intrapulmonary shunting. Over time, many of these patients can develop bronchopulmonary dysplasia.[21] Both patients with respiratory distress syndrome and patients with bronchopulmonary dysplasia may have decreased lung compliance and increased airway resistance as well as a need for supplemental oxygen therapy and noninvasive respiratory support such as nasal continuous positive airway pressures. Additionally, patients can have associated pulmonary hypertension,[22,23] which can prevent or limit the neonate's ability to achieve normal cardiovascular circulation and readily revert to a transitional circulation. This factor impacts medication selection and peri-intubation management (**Table 2**). Premature patients also display increased susceptibility toward apneic episodes in the setting of factors such as anesthetic administration and hypoxemia.[24-27] The incidence of patent ductus arteriosus, although uncommon in term neonates, is inversely related to birthweight.[28] Left-to-right shunting associated with patent ductus arteriosus can result in congestive heart failure, decreased cardiac output, and pulmonary congestion. Treatment for circulatory overload generally involves diuretic therapy that can further increase susceptibility to hemodynamic compromise with sedative/hypnotic drug administration.

In addition to prematurity, neonates can be affected by a wide spectrum of congenital or acquired anatomic airway pathologies. Any processes affecting the superficial

Table 2 Common sedation/induction medication and effects on hemodynamics and respiration			
Drug	**HR**	**BP**	**RR**
Fentanyl	Decrease	Same or decrease	Decrease
Ketamine	Same or increase	Same or increase	Same
Midazolam	Decrease	Same or decrease	Decrease
Morphine	Decrease	Same or decrease	Decrease
Propofol	Decrease	Decrease	Decrease

facial anatomy or any portion of the airway, from the nasopharynx and oropharynx to the trachea, should be identified and relevance to airway management considered. Congenital pathology includes conditions such as choanal atresia, laryngeal webs, laryngeal clefts, airway hemangiomas, complete tracheal rings, subglottic cysts, tracheobronchomalacia, laryngomalacia, tracheoesophageal fistulas, or other intraluminal or extraluminal compressive masses such as lymphatic or arteriovenous malformations or vascular rings. A common acquired pathology is subglottic narrowing related to a previous, generally prolonged, intubation that may result in subglottic stenosis in the older neonate or infant.

Providers should also recognize other pathologic conditions that do not directly involve the airway but still significantly impact airway management. For example, abdominal processes such as necrotizing enterocolitis, omphalocele, and gastroschisis may significantly diminish FRC and thus render the patient much more susceptible to hypoxemia in the setting of apnea. In addition to decreasing apneic time to desaturation, abdominal pathology impacts normal gastric emptying and therefore increases the risk of aspiration during airway management. Other conditions such as cervical spine pathology can limit flexion and extension owing to inherent limitations in movement or concern for injury with manipulation. Certain disorders provide challenges to optimal positioning for airway management including, but not limited to, patients with myelomeningocele, encephalocele, and significant hydrocephalus. Last, coexisting cardiac disease can also significantly alter strategies for airway management. Patients who are hemodynamically unstable owing to underlying congenital heart disease or distributive shock may preclude certain premedication or induction regimens and require concurrent hemodynamic management during airway instrumentation. Available electrocardiograms, echocardiograms, and cardiac catheterizations are all part of formulating a plan for airway management. Patients with cardiac disease sensitive to alterations in pulmonary blood flow resulting from changes in respiration such as PDA, tetralogy of Fallot, or pulmonary hypertension need careful planning to maintain appropriate respiratory parameters during active airway management and thereby preserve optimal circulatory balance.

The physical examination should focus on any aspects that would indicate subsequent difficulty with mask ventilation or intubation such as micrognathia or other dysmorphic features. Audible stridor may indicate the presence of subglottic stenosis and obstructed breathing or snoring alerts providers to the possibility of difficult mask ventilation.

Any prior airway management should be reviewed, noting the ability to mask ventilate, the airway techniques attempted, the successful technique and glottic view during each attempt, the providers involved, and any associated challenges or complications.

After completion of the history and physical examination, additional pertinent information and preparation would also include ensuring adequate intravenous access, the availability of suction, and appropriate monitoring. Multiple doses of any anticipated medications should be available as well as appropriate sized airway equipment including endotracheal tubes (ETTs), intubation blades, supraglottic airways (SGA), oral and nasal airways, and adjuncts to facilitate placement such as tongue blades and lubricant jelly. When difficulty is anticipated in managing the airway, appropriate advanced airway equipment and resources should be available before initiating airway management. These resources might include additional skilled providers such as anesthesiologists, otolaryngologists, or providers capable of placing the patient on extracorporeal membrane oxygenation. Most neonatal intubations will occur in the neonatal intensive care unit (NICU) or delivery room. When difficulty is anticipated and the clinical situation allows, consideration should be given to transporting the patient to an operating room. This step allows for additional options for anesthetic and surgical techniques, airway equipment, and a greater concentration of specialized airway clinicians to be available to provide clinical support.

Gastric tubes should be vented before managing the airway to allow egress of gastric insufflation that may occur during mask ventilation. Gastric insufflation can be problematic because it can lead to difficulty with mask ventilation secondary to increased intra-abdominal pressure, causing thoracic impingement as well as increasing the potential for gastroesophageal reflux and pulmonary aspiration. Before proceeding with intubation, arrangements should be made for immediate postintubation care, including ventilators, appropriate sedation medications, and necessary verification of ETT position with ultrasound examination or radiographic imaging such as a chest radiograph.

TECHNIQUES FOR AIRWAY MANAGEMENT

Although endotracheal intubation is usually the airway management technique of choice for neonates presenting to the operating room or those who require prolonged ventilatory support, it is essential that providers be familiar with alternate techniques such as face mask ventilation and SGA placement. Mask ventilation or SGAs may be required as a rescue or stabilizing technique for difficult or failed intubation. SGA or mask ventilation can also be used as an elective method of airway management in situations that do not require prolonged ventilatory support, where there is no concern for aspiration of gastric contents, the airway is accessible, there is low likelihood of device dislodgement, and pulmonary function is relatively intact.

Mask Ventilation

Mask ventilation is a potentially life-saving skill that is the cornerstone of effective airway management. The mask should be sized appropriately to minimize air leak and in general should rest such that the inflatable cushioned portion superiorly encompasses the nose while not covering the eyes, and the inferior border rests on the chin. Whether providing continuous positive airway pressures or positive pressure ventilation, care should be taken to adjust mask and jaw position to optimize oropharyngeal airflow. Ideally, the mouth should be opened and the mandible should be translocated such that the tongue is lifted from the posterior pharyngeal wall and away from the palate. Ideally, pressure on submental tissue should be minimized as this can readily lead to airway obstruction (**Fig. 3**). With proper mask technique, the need for oral airway placement can be minimized. If 2 hands are required for masking, the thumbs are placed over the mask while the index or middle fingers are used to manipulate the mandible. In situations where an oral airway is needed, sizing is carefully assessed because too large of an airway can move the epiglottis posteriorly and worsen obstruction, whereas too small of an airway can push the tongue posteriorly and obstruct the airway. Nasopharyngeal airways can also be useful in relieving airway obstruction. Most nasal airways have an adjustable flange that allows the length of the airway to be changed so that the tip is slightly superior to the glottis. If the length is too long, the tip of the airway can be in the glottis or esophagus, whereas if it is too short, the airway may not have fully bypassed obstructing tissue in the posterior oropharynx. In general, once mask ventilation has been optimized, high airway pressures are not required to effectively ventilate most neonates and are best avoided to prevent gastric insufflation.

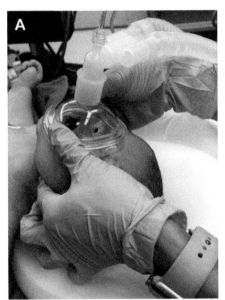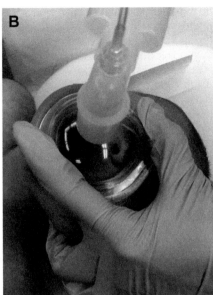

Fig. 3. Technique for 2-handed (*A*) and 1-handed mask (*B*) ventilation. The mouth should be opened and the mandible is translocated such that the tongue is lifted from the posterior pharyngeal wall and away from the palate. Note the avoidance of pressure on submental tissue because this can readily lead to iatrogenic airway obstruction. (*Courtesy of* J. Peyton, MBChB, MRCP, FRCA, Boston, MA.)

Supraglottic Airway

SGA refers to a group of devices that are inserted into the pharynx and can serve as an effective airway management device alone, as a rescue airway device for difficult intubation or mask ventilation, and as a conduit for intubation. Although the terminology laryngeal mask airway (LMA) is often used interchangeably with SGA, LMA refers to a specific brand of SGA (Teleflex LMA), whereas SGA is the more general term for LMA and similar devices. The SGA is positioned in the hypopharynx and surrounds the glottis with a cuff that forms a seal inferiorly at the cricopharyngeus muscle, laterally in the perilaryngeal space and superiorly at the base of the tongue, allowing it to maintain the airway through bypassing oropharyngeal soft tissue (**Fig. 4**). In cases where difficult airway management is anticipated, an SGA can be inserted in an awake neonate with anesthesia administered once an adequate seal and the ability to ventilate is confirmed.[29] SGA in neonates can be used for elective airway management to support ventilation for diagnostic procedures or less often as a part of a general anesthetic in the operating room. It should be noted that SGA are not definitive airways. Compared with endotracheal intubation, SGA are less secure, are generally not suitable for ongoing positive pressure ventilation at higher settings, and do not protect the airway from gastric contents.

To insert an SGA, the mouth is opened and the device is slid against the palate toward the posterior pharyngeal wall until it reaches proper seating position. Lubrication on the SGA surface facilitates placement. Most device manufacturers recommend fully deflating the SGA before insertion, but many times in practice, SGA are inserted without prior deflation. Once the SGA is positioned, it should be inflated if necessary and the inflation pressure adjusted to recommended pressures with a manometer.

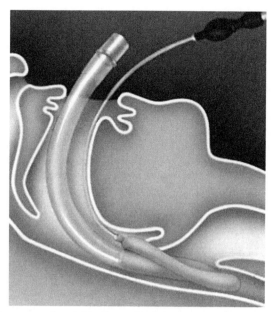

Fig. 4. Correct placement of an SGA. The cuff of the SGA sits in the hypopharynx, the tip occludes the esophagus and the laryngeal opening sitting above the larynx. (*From* Trevisanuto D. The laryngeal mask airway: potential applications in neonates. *Arch Dis Child - Fetal Neonatal Ed*. 2004; with permission.)

Applied positive pressure should result in chest rise and the presence of end-tidal carbon dioxide. In the absence of these findings, it should be assumed that the SGA is positioned incorrectly. In neonates, it is not uncommon for the SGA to be inserted too far, such that the esophagus is fully intubated and distended by the SGA tip, which needs to be withdrawn slightly. The SGA may also further bend the epiglottis over the laryngeal inlet causing significant airway obstruction that may be resolved by repositioning of the SGA and/or the neonate's head and neck position. Alternatively, the tip of the SGA can fold on itself during insertion, preventing effective gas exchange. This can generally be corrected by withdrawing the SGA such that it is no longer folded over and then reinserting it.

Some available SGA have a port specifically meant for gastric venting and suctioning and this can be used after placement to decompress the stomach after prolonged mask ventilation or if there concern for residual gastric contents. These are commonly referred to as second-generation SGA.

Premedication Before Tracheal Intubation

Adverse events associated with tracheal intubation in NICUs occur in approximately 20% of intubations, with severe desaturation in nearly 50% and some sites reporting up to 69%.[30] A large number of clinical trials have demonstrated that the use of premedication before tracheal intubation increases success rates. In particular, the use of sedative medications in combination with neuromuscular blockade has been shown to improve glottic visualization, decrease the number of attempts taken to successfully intubate, and decrease airway trauma.[31–35] Recently, large-scale multicenter intubation registries have been created to gather data on complications associated with airway management in neonates, infants, and children.[30,36,37]

The largest study to date study that examined the use of neuromuscular blockade during neonatal tracheal intubation analyzed 2260 intubations from 11 NICUs, and demonstrated adverse event rates of 23% in patients in whom neuromuscular blockade was not used, compared with only 10% when neuromuscular blockade was used.[38]

Although the weight of evidence supporting the use of sedative premedication and neuromuscular blockade to facilitate tracheal intubation is significant in the general neonatal population, in certain clinical subsets, an unsedated or spontaneously breathing anesthetic technique for intubation may be preferable. This includes patients who may not tolerate the hemodynamic side effects of sedative administration, patients with anticipated difficulty with masking or intubation, and patients who require immediate life-saving intubation that precludes the time necessary to administer sedative medications.

Endotracheal Tube Size

ETT sizing in the neonatal population is largely determined by patient weight and clinical judgment. This can result in a tube being placed initially that may be the wrong size, requiring it to be exchanged. Ideally, the largest tube size should be chosen, such that airway resistance through the ETT is minimized, while limiting undue pressure on the subglottis and trachea. In patients weighing more than 3.0 kg, a 3.0-mm cuffed tube with a low-profile cuff can be considered. For smaller patients, weighing 1.5 to 3.0 kg, a 3.0 -mm uncuffed ETT is generally used, and for patients weighing less than 1.5 kg, a 2.5-mm uncuffed tube is chosen.

Selection of Cuffed Versus Uncuffed Endotracheal Tubes

Traditionally, uncuffed ETT have been used in the neonatal population based on prior understanding of the anatomy of the neonatal airway. As discussed elsewhere in this article, the airway of neonates and young infants had always been described as funnel shaped, with the narrowest portion being the circular, circumferential, nondistensible cricoid cartilage. Therefore, an uncuffed tube with an adequate seal would obviate the need for a cuff. Recent studies have suggested that the cricoid cartilage may be elliptical and wider anteroposteriorly, rather than cylindrical. In this model, a properly sized uncuffed ETT with reasonable leak may still be exerting undue pressure on the transverse tracheal wall at this level.[4,6] In contrast, a smaller diameter cuffed ETT could still provide an adequate seal without exerting excessive pressure on the transverse cricoid. Despite these concerns, there does not seem to be any apparent differences in postextubation stridor among patients intubated with a cuffed versus uncuffed tube both in a study limited to neonates less than 3 kg, and a prospective randomized controlled trial by Weiss and colleagues[39] of more than 2000 young children (average age of <2 years).[40]

Potential advantages to a cuffed ETT include the need for fewer airway manipulations to determine correct tube size, a decreased likelihood of large air leaks, increased protection from aspiration, and less direct airway trauma related to the placement of a smaller ETT compared with similarly sealing, and thus larger, uncuffed ETT. In the study by Weiss and colleagues,[39] the frequency of patients requiring tracheal tube exchanges to find the appropriately sized tube was significantly different between cuffed and uncuffed tubes (2.1% vs 30.8%). Potential disadvantages of a cuffed ETT are associated with the generally smaller ETT diameter than comparable uncuffed ETT. These include greater difficulty with suctioning and increased ventilatory requirements owing to increased resistance with smaller ETT.[41] There is also concern for increased work of breathing during ventilatory weaning, although this may be largely compensated for by appropriate pressure support parameters.[42]

Should a cuffed ETT be used, pressures should be regularly measured and maintained to minimize risk of associated airway trauma owing to excessive cuff inflation (usually <25 cm H_2O).

Nasal Versus Oral Endotracheal Intubation

The choice between nasal and oral ETT placement is largely driven by institutional preference. Nasal tubes are thought to be more secure as well as more comfortable for patients. With prolonged nasal intubation, there is concern for nasal skin breakdown as well as sinusitis owing to obstruction of normal sinus drainage. Nasal intubation can also be associated with epistaxis and trauma during ETT advancement through the nares, and can pose greater technical challenges compared with oral intubation. A Cochrane review evaluating nasal versus oral intubation in newborn infants concluded that there was no clear advantage of nasal versus oral intubation with respect to rates of tube malposition, accidental extubation, tube blockage, reintubation, or and local trauma.[43] In a study analyzing the impact of intubation route on perioperative outcomes in patients presenting for cardiac surgery, in a subgroup analysis of neonatal patients exhibited nasal intubation in 41% of cases.[44] In this neonatal subgroup, nasal intubation was associated with a significant decrease in accidental extubation caused by transesophageal echocardiogram probe manipulation without an associated increased risk of surgical wound infections. This study did not demonstrate any other difference in observed airway complications with respect to route of intubation.

Direct Laryngoscopy

In the neonatal population, direct laryngoscopy (DL) is most commonly performed with a straight blade such as a Miller 0 or Miller 1 blade. Before blade insertion, patients are placed supine with their neck slightly extended. This position serves to align the pharyngeal, oral, and laryngeal axes. Compared with older patients, neonates have a larger occiput and therefore do not generally require a pillow or other device to elevate the head to optimize positioning for laryngoscopy but may require a shoulder elevation to further optimize positioning.

Once positioning is optimized, the patient's mouth is opened and the blade inserted into the mouth. Given the position and angulation of the neonatal larynx along with the posteriorly displaced tongue base, the laryngoscopist should sweep the tongue to the left with the DL blade to create maximal space lateral to the blade and facilitate an unobstructed view of the glottis. If the tongue is not fully swept to the left of the blade, the tongue obstructs the ability to fully see the glottis such that, when the tube is passed toward the glottis, the ETT itself will many times fully obstruct the view of the glottis. In addition, failure to effectively sweep the tongue to the left requires that this thick muscle be displaced anteriorly into the submandibular space. In normal airways, the lack of a tongue sweep may not prevent visualization of the glottis, but it does prevent an optimal view in those neonates with limited submandibular space. The blade is then inserted along the right alveolar groove until the epiglottis is viewed. The epiglottis is subsequently elevated to reveal the glottic opening. In situations where there is difficulty lifting the epiglottis, the blade can alternatively be inserted into the vallecula and with upward and outward force the epiglottis will generally move toward the anterior pharyngeal wall and no longer obstruct the laryngeal view. If there is still epiglottic obstruction of view, external laryngeal manipulation, which in neonates can often be performed using the left fifth finger of the laryngoscopist, can be used to facilitate glottic visualization. The anterior laryngeal angulation as described in the anatomy section often results in the arytenoids appearing to obstruct the pathway of the ETT into the larynx requiring head repositioning and laryngeal manipulation either internally with the blade or externally by an individual's fingers. Together with the inferior insertion of the anterior vocal cord commissure, the laryngeal angulation may make ETT placement challenging even with an adequate view, because the ETT tip may be nearly orthogonal to the anterior laryngeal wall. This causes the ETT tip to abut the anterior wall such that the ETT may not pass easily or at all. This difficulty can be magnified by the fact that, in neonates, the ETT approximates the relative dimension of the larynx resulting in minimal extra space for manipulating the ETT into the subglottis, as can be done in older children and adults.

Videolaryngoscopy

Although DL remains the most commonly chosen technique to perform tracheal intubation in neonates, videolaryngoscopy is becoming increasingly popular. A videolaryngoscope is a device with a video camera positioned at the distal end of the laryngoscope blade, allowing the user to visualize the vocal cords on a video screen. The devices can be classified as having traditional blade design (or nonangulated such as the Storz C-Mac system (Storz, Tuttlingen, Germany), with Miller 0, 1, and 2 blades or Macintosh 0, 1, 2, 3, and 4 blades) or hyperangulated blades, where the laryngoscope blade is curved at an angle ranging between 40° to 80° (such as the Storz C-Mac D-blade or Verathon GlideScope system). The videolaryngoscope systems that use traditional blade designs can also be used to perform DL, meaning an operator can perform both direct, video-assisted DL and pure video laryngoscopy with the same device, using a single intubation attempt. Hyperangulated video laryngoscope blades allow an operator to gain a view of the glottis in situations where it is not possible to align the oral, pharyngeal, and laryngeal axes. The only axis of alignment required to view the glottis is that between the camera and the larynx. This procedure can also be referred to as indirect laryngoscopy.

Videolaryngoscopy use has been associated with improved outcomes during tracheal intubation in the NICU[30] and with decreased rates of adverse outcomes such as severe oxygen desaturation. It improves the laryngeal view compared with DL in children who weigh less than 10 kg.[45] It has also been shown that the use of videolaryngoscopy by inexperienced clinicians can improve first-attempt intubation success rates when the screen is viewed by an instructor during intubation. The instructor can use the view seen on the screen to guide the trainee, and this strategy has been shown to improve intubation success rates by 25%.[46]

Common reasons for failure to intubate the trachea include failure to recognize midline structures and normal anatomy.[47] Nonangulated videolaryngoscopy may also help to teach skills that can be transferred to DL, such as improved anatomic knowledge and recognition of midline structures, that improve the success rate of intubation.[47,48]

In infants who are difficult to intubate, DL has been shown to be a poor technique, with a first-attempt success rates of 4% and an eventual success rate of 22%.[49] Hyperangulated videolaryngoscopy has been shown to have significantly higher success rates when used in neonates with a grade 3 or 4 Cormack and Lehane view at DL.[50]

NICU access to videolaryngoscopy has been limited. A recent UK study demonstrated that only 29% of NICUs have access to videolaryngoscopy, with only 50% having a dedicated difficult airway cart, compared with 55% and 96%, respectively, in pediatric ICUs.[51] However, we believe this number will inevitably increase as the evidence mounts that using videolaryngoscopy is a safe, effective way to improve outcomes associated with tracheal intubation. A recent study examining the factors that NICU fellows identify as important for achieving competency in neonatal intubation revealed that the use of videolaryngoscopy is seen as a major benefit.[52]

AIRWAY MANAGEMENT IN PATIENTS WITH POTENTIAL DIFFICULTY

Neonates represent an extremely high-risk group with respect to difficult airway management. Difficult intubation as defined by the need for more than 3 attempts by a nonresident provider in a multicenter NICU intubation registry occurred in 14% of patients and the odds of severe desaturation in these patients were more than 4-fold higher.[53] In both anticipated and unanticipated difficult intubation in children, patients less than 10 kg have been demonstrated to have higher complication rates than all patients.[36] The reasons for this are multifactorial and include rapid desaturation owing to lower FRC and higher oxygen consumption as well as the generally lower success rates using advanced airway rescue techniques[49,54] compared with adult patients. Difficult airways in children are often anticipated,[36] allowing clinicians opportunity in most cases to develop appropriate plans for initial and rescue airway management strategies. Many patients have airway abnormalities as part of a congenital syndrome that can have other systemic involvement. Assessment should evaluate (1) the ability to mask ventilate and/or use an SGA that can be affected by facial abnormalities or limited mouth opening, (2) issues impacting the ability to place an ETT such as limited mouth opening or choanal atresia, and (3) comorbidities related to any applicable syndrome.

It should again be emphasized that rescue airway techniques have lower success rates in smaller children[49,55] and, therefore, any plans for airway management should anticipate possible failure of a given technique and steps for subsequent management. A combined intubation technique of a flexible fiberscope via an SGA has been shown to have a higher success rate than videolaryngoscopy.[55] This technique is best when used with continuous support of oxygenation and ventilation.[56] All necessary resources, including equipment and personnel, should be prepared and available. Planning for subsequent management in patients who are anticipated to be difficult should involve consultation with pediatric otolaryngologists and pediatric anesthesiologists whenever possible. If clinically feasible, neonates with difficult intubations should be transported to the operating room before the initiation of airway management.

Awake Versus Asleep

If the patient is breathing well without evidence of obstruction or there is obstruction that can be readily bypassed with an airway adjunct (oral/nasal airway, SGA), the patients may receive sedative medications because the expectation is that they can be safely ventilated. For instance, although patients with Robin sequence (**Fig. 5**) readily obstruct from a combination of glossoptosis and micrognathia, they can generally be safely ventilated once the base of the tongue is bypassed with a nasal or oral airway or SGA. If there is concern that the patient cannot be safely ventilated once sedated, the prudent option is to proceed with an awake or minimally sedated, spontaneously breathing technique.

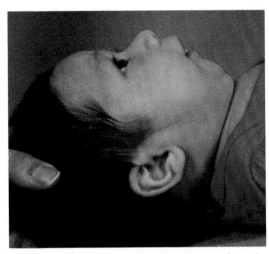

Fig. 5. Patient with Robin sequence characterized by micrognathia, glossoptosis, and associated obstruction to breathing. Robin sequence is one of the most common syndromes associated with difficult intubation in neonatal patients. (*Courtesy of* C. Resnick M.D., D.M.D., Boston, MA)

Neuromuscular Blockade in the Setting of Anticipated Airway Difficulty

If sedative or induction medications are given, clinicians should decide whether to control ventilation and possibly administer muscle relaxants or to preserve spontaneous ventilation. Although spontaneous ventilation does perhaps provide a safety mechanism should airway securement fail, laryngospasm and patient movement can complicate management. Prevention of these complications during spontaneous ventilation requires deep sedation or general anesthesia and medication administration needs careful titration to avoid associated apnea and hemodynamic instability. Selective topicalization of the airway with local anesthetic can minimize reactivity during airway manipulation, although clinicians should be aware of maximum doses of local anesthetics especially in both the full-term and premature neonate. An additional possible advantage of spontaneous ventilation is that patients may not desaturate as readily, possibly leading to less aborted airway attempts owing to desaturation.

If muscle relaxation is administered, movement and laryngospasm are prevented, but controlled ventilation must be maintained at all times. In patients in whom there is concern of complete airway obstruction that cannot be effectively bypassed, muscle relaxation is a relative contraindication because this may precipitate a catastrophic cannot intubate, cannot oxygenate situation. Although apneic oxygenation can prolong time for airway instrumentation,[57,58] airway attempts still may need to be interrupted to provide controlled ventilation to minimize significant increases in alveolar carbon dioxide, particularly in neonates where increases in pulmonary arterial pressures would be detrimental. In addition, prolonged mask ventilation even with modest peak pressures can lead to gastric insufflation that can lead to progressive difficulty in masking.

Techniques for Securing the Difficult Airway

In patients who are anticipated or discovered to have difficult intubation, because complications are associated with increased number of intubation attempts, there should be rapid progression to the most experienced provider to limit overall airway attempts and consideration given to using a technique other than DL for initial airway management or after technique failure. Maintenance of oxygenation can be optimized by providing supplemental oxygen flow in both spontaneously breathing and apneic patients.[57,58] As mentioned, advanced airway rescue techniques have lower success rates in smaller patients, therefore multiple contingencies should be in place in the event of failure with a given technique. In the Pediatric Difficult Airway Registry (PeDI), the most common techniques for airway management were flexible fiberoptic bronchoscopy, videolaryngoscopy and fiberoptic intubation through an SGA.[36]

SUMMARY

Airway management in neonatal patients requires a thorough knowledge of neonatal airway anatomy, respiratory physiology, and clinical implications of commonly occurring comorbidities. Clinicians should have knowledge and competence in basic airway management skills such as mask ventilation, SGA placement, and intubation. In managing the airways of patients who are more medically complex or are anticipated to be difficult to intubate, although providers should be familiar with strategies for management, additional specialized providers should be ideally available to assist with these high-risk cases.

Best Practices

What is the current practice for Neonatal endotracheal intubation

Best practice, guideline, or care path objective(s)
- Decrease morbidity and mortality associated with endotracheal intubation

What changes in current practice are likely to improve outcomes?

- Use of sedative premedication and muscle relaxants before the initial intubation attempt

- Use of videolaryngoscopy for the initial intubation attempt

- Early recognition of difficult intubation and transition to alternate airway techniques and expert assistance

Major recommendations

- Use videolaryngoscopy or video-assisted DL as the initial intubation technique (1B)

- Use sedative premedication and muscle relaxants to optimize intubating conditions in patients with morphologically normal airways (1A)

- In the setting of difficulty intubating, prompt transition to advanced airway techniques and more experienced providers to limit total number of intubation attempts and associated complications (1B)

- If difficulty intubating is anticipated, early involvement of anesthesiology and otolaryngology teams and transfer to the operating room for definitive airway management should be considered (1C)

Bibliographic Source(s): This is important list current sources relevant to evidence. *Data from* Refs.[30–34,36,38,46,49,53]

REFERENCES

1. Orgill DP. Excision and skin grafting of thermal burns. N Engl J Med 2009. https://doi.org/10.1056/nejmct0804451.

2. Burns CH. Nelson textbook of pediatrics. 10th edition. Philadelphia: WB Saunders; 1975.

3. Eckenhoff JE. Some anatomic considerations of the infant larynx influencing endotracheal anesthesia. Anesthesiology 1951. https://doi.org/10.1097/00000542-195107000-00001.

4. Wani TM, Rafiq M, Akhter N, et al. Upper airway in infants—a computed tomography-based analysis. Paediatr Anaesth 2017. https://doi.org/10.1111/pan.13126.

5. Wani TM, Rafiq M, Talpur S, et al. Pediatric upper airway dimensions using three-dimensional computed tomography imaging. Paediatr Anaesth 2017. https://doi.org/10.1111/pan.13116.

6. Litman RS, Weissend EE, Shibata D, et al. Developmental changes of laryngeal dimensions in unparalyzed, sedated children. Anesthesiology 2003. https://doi.org/10.1097/00000542-200301000-00010.

7. Holzki J, Brown KA, Carroll RG, et al. The anatomy of the pediatric airway: has our knowledge changed in 120 years? A review of historic and recent investigations of the anatomy of the pediatric larynx. Paediatr Anaesth 2018. https://doi.org/10.1111/pan.13281.

8. Motoyama E. Respiratory physiology in infants and children. In: Motoyama E, Davis PJ, editors. Smith's anesthesia for infants and children. 7th edition. Philadelphia: Mosby; 2006. p. 12–69.

9. Hooper SB, Te Pas AB, Kitchen MJ. Respiratory transition in the newborn: a three-phase process. Arch Dis Child Fetal Neonatal Ed 2016. https://doi.org/10.1136/archdischild-2013-305704.

10. Blank DA, Omar Farouk Kamlin C, Rogerson SR, et al. Lung ultrasound immediately after birth to describe normal neonatal transition: an observational study. Arch Dis Child Fetal Neonatal Ed 2018. https://doi.org/10.1136/archdischild-2017-312818.

11. Vyas H, Field D, Milner AD, et al. Determinants of the first inspiratory volume and functional residual capacity at birth. Pediatr Pulmonol 1986. https://doi.org/10.1002/ppul.1950020403.

12. Agostoni E. Volume-pressure relationships of the thorax and lung in the newborn. J Appl Physiol 2017. https://doi.org/10.1152/jappl.1959.14.6.909.

13. Mortola JP, Milic E, Noworaj A, et al. Muscle pressure and flow during expiration in infants. Am Rev Respir Dis 1984;129(1):49–53.

14. Schibler A, Hall GL, Businger F, et al. Measurement of lung volume and ventilation distribution with an ultrasonic flow meter in healthy infants. Eur Respir J 2002. https://doi.org/10.1183/09031936.02.00226002.

15. Bancalari E, Clausen J. Pathophysiology of changes in absolute lung volumes. Eur Respir J 1998. https://doi.org/10.1183/09031936.98.12010248.

16. Macklem PT, Mead J. Resistance of central and peripheral airways measured by a retrograde catheter. J Appl Physiol 1967. https://doi.org/10.1152/jappl.1967.22.3.395.

17. Ferris BG, Mead J, Opie LH. Partitioning of respiratory flow resistance in man. J Appl Physiol 1964. https://doi.org/10.1152/jappl.1964.19.4.653.

18. Page M, Jeffery HE. Airway protection in sleeping infants in response to pharyngeal fluid stimulation in the supine position. Pediatr Res 1998. https://doi.org/10.1203/00006450-199811000-00011.

19. Pickens DL, Schefft GL, Thach BT. Pharyngeal fluid clearance and aspiration preventive mechanisms in sleeping infants. J Appl Physiol 1989. https://doi.org/10.1152/jappl.1989.66.3.1164.

20. Thach BT. Some aspects of clinical relevance in the maturation of respiratory control in infants. J Appl Physiol 2008. https://doi.org/10.1152/japplphysiol.01288. 2007.

21. Stoll BJ, Hansen NI, Bell EF, et al. Neonatal outcomes of extremely preterm infants from the NICHD neonatal research network. Pediatrics 2010. https://doi.org/10.1542/peds.2009-2959.

22. Kim DH, Kim HS, Choi CW, et al. Risk factors for pulmonary artery hypertension in preterm infants with moderate or severe bronchopulmonary dysplasia. Neonatology 2011. https://doi.org/10.1159/000327891.

23. Bhat R, Salas AA, Foster C, et al. Prospective analysis of pulmonary hypertension in extremely low birth weight infants. Pediatrics 2012. https://doi.org/10.1542/peds.2011-1827.

24. Rigatto H, Brady JP, de la Torre Verduzco R. Chemoreceptor reflexes in preterm infants: I. The effect of gestational and postnatal age on the ventilatory response to inhalation of 100% and 15% oxygen. Pediatrics 1975;55(5):604–13.

25. Davidson AJ, Morton NS, Arnup SJ, et al. Apnea after awake regional and general anesthesia in infants: the general anesthesia compared to spinal anesthesia study-comparing apnea and neurodevelopmental outcomes, a randomized controlled trial. Anesthesiology 2015. https://doi.org/10.1097/ALN. 0000000000000709.

26. Welborn LG, Rice LJ, Hannallah RS, et al. Postoperative apnea in former preterm infants: prospective comparison of spinal and general anesthesia. Anesthesiology 1990. https://doi.org/10.1097/00000542-199005000-00012.

27. Liu LMP, Cote CJ, Goudsouzian NG. Life-threatening apnea in infants recovering from anesthesia. Anesthesiology 1983. https://doi.org/10.1097/00000542-198312000-00004.

28. Ellison RC, Peckham GJ, Lang P, et al. Evaluation of the preterm infant for patent ductus arteriosus. Pediatrics 1983;71(3):364–72.

29. Templeton TW, Goenaga-Díaz EJ, Runyan CM, et al. A generalized multistage approach to oral and nasal intubation in infants with Pierre Robin sequence: a retrospective review. Paediatr Anaesth 2018. https://doi.org/10.1111/pan.13499.

30. Foglia EE, Ades A, Sawyer T, et al. Neonatal intubation practice and outcomes: an International registry study. Pediatrics 2018. https://doi.org/10.1542/peds. 2018-0902.

31. Lemyre B, Cheng R, Gaboury I. Atropine, fentanyl and succinylcholine for nonurgent intubations in newborns. Arch Dis Child Fetal Neonatal Ed 2009. https://doi.org/10.1136/adc.2008.146068.

32. Dempsey EM, Al Hazzani F, Faucher D, et al. Facilitation of neonatal endotracheal intubation with mivacurium and fentanyl in the neonatal intensive care unit. Arch Dis Child Fetal Neonatal Ed 2006. https://doi.org/10.1136/adc.2005.087213.

33. Roberts KD, Leone TA, Edwards WH, et al. Premedication for nonemergent neonatal intubations: a randomized, controlled trial comparing atropine and fentanyl to atropine, fentanyl, and mivacurium. Pediatrics 2006;118(4):1583–91.

34. Ghanta S, Abdel-Latif ME, Lui K, et al. Propofol compared with the morphine, atropine, and Suxamethonium regimen as induction Agents for neonatal endotracheal intubation: a randomized, controlled trial: in reply. Pediatrics 2007. https://doi.org/10.1542/peds.2007-2352.

35. Carbajal R, Eble B, Anand KJS. Premedication for tracheal intubation in neonates: confusion or controversy? Semin Perinatol 2007. https://doi.org/10.1053/j.semperi.2007.07.006.

36. Fiadjoe JE, Nishisaki A, Jagannathan N, et al. Airway management complications in children with difficult tracheal intubation from the Pediatric Difficult Intubation (PeDI) registry: a prospective cohort analysis. Lancet Respir Med 2016;4(1): 37–48.

37. Nishisaki A, Turner DA, Brown CA, et al. A national emergency airway registry for children: landscape of tracheal intubation in 15 PICUs. Crit Care Med 2013. https://doi.org/10.1097/CCM.0b013e3182746736.

38. Ozawa Y, Ades A, Foglia EE, et al. Premedication with neuromuscular blockade and sedation during neonatal intubation is associated with fewer adverse events. J Perinatol 2019. https://doi.org/10.1038/s41372-019-0367-0.

39. Weiss M, Dullenkopf A, Fischer JE, et al. Prospective randomized controlled multi-centre trial of cuffed or uncuffed endotracheal tubes in small children. Br J Anaesth 2009;103(6):867–73. https://doi.org/10.1093/bja/aep290.

40. Thomas RE, Rao SC, Minutillo C, et al. Cuffed endotracheal tubes in infants less than 3 kg: a retrospective cohort study. Paediatr Anaesth 2018. https://doi.org/10.1111/pan.13311.

41. Thomas R, Rao S, Minutillo C. Cuffed endotracheal tubes in neonates and infants: a survey of practice. Arch Dis Child Fetal Neonatal Ed 2016. https://doi.org/10.1136/archdischild-2015-309241.

42. Thomas J, Weiss M, Cannizzaro V, et al. Work of breathing for cuffed and uncuffed pediatric endotracheal tubes in an in vitro lung model setting. Paediatr Anaesth 2018. https://doi.org/10.1111/pan.13430.

43. Spence K, Barr P. Nasal versus oral intubation for mechanical ventilation of newborn infants. Cochrane Database Syst Rev 2000;(2):CD000948.

44. Greene NH, Jooste EH, Thibault DP, et al. A study of practice behavior for endotracheal intubation site for children with congenital heart disease undergoing surgery: impact of endotracheal intubation site on perioperative outcomes-an analysis of the Society of Thoracic Surgeons Congenital Cardiac Anesthesia Society Database. Anesth Analg 2018. https://doi.org/10.1213/ANE.0000000000003594.

45. Raimann FJ, Cuca CE, Kern D, et al. Evaluation of the C-MAC Miller video laryngoscope sizes 0 and 1 during tracheal intubation of infants less than 10 kg. Pediatr Emerg Care 2017. https://doi.org/10.1097/pec.0000000000001296.

46. O'Shea JE, Thio M, Kamlin CO, et al. Videolaryngoscopy to teach neonatal intubation: a randomized trial. Pediatrics 2015. https://doi.org/10.1542/peds.2015-1028.

47. O'Shea JE, Loganathan P, Thio M, et al. Analysis of unsuccessful intubations in neonates using videolaryngoscopy recordings. Arch Dis Child Fetal Neonatal Ed 2018. https://doi.org/10.1136/archdischild-2017-313628.

48. Parmekar S, Arnold JL, Anselmo C, et al. Mind the gap: can videolaryngoscopy bridge the competency gap in neonatal endotracheal intubation among pediatric trainees? A randomized controlled study. J Perinatol 2017. https://doi.org/10.1038/jp.2017.72.

49. Park R, Peyton JM, Fiadjoe JE, et al. The efficacy of GlideScope ® videolaryngoscopy compared with direct laryngoscopy in children who are difficult to intubate: an analysis from the paediatric difficult intubation registry. Br J Anaesth 2017; 119(5):984–92.

50. Tao B, Liu K, Wang D, et al. Comparison of GlideScope video laryngoscopy and direct laryngoscopy for tracheal intubation in neonates. Anesth Analg 2018. https://doi.org/10.1213/ane.0000000000003637.

51. Foy KE, Mew E, Cook TM, et al. Paediatric intensive care and neonatal intensive care airway management in the United Kingdom: the PIC-NIC survey. Anaesthesia 2018. https://doi.org/10.1111/anae.14359.

52. Brady J, Kovatis K, O'Dea CL, et al. What do NICU fellows identify as important for achieving competency in neonatal intubation? Neonatology 2019;10–6. https://doi.org/10.1159/000494999.

53. Sawyer T, Foglia EE, Ades A, et al. Incidence, impact and indicators of difficult intubations in the neonatal intensive care unit: a report from the National Emergency Airway Registry for Neonates. Arch Dis Child Fetal Neonatal Ed 2019. https://doi.org/10.1136/archdischild-2018-316336.

54. Aziz MF, Brambrink AM, Healy DW, et al. Success of intubation rescue techniques after failed direct laryngoscopy in Adults: a retrospective comparative analysis from the multicenter perioperative outcomes group. Anesthesiology 2016; 125(4):656–66.

55. Burjek NE, Nishisaki A, Fiadjoe JE, et al. Videolaryngoscopy versus fiber-optic intubation through a supraglottic airway in children with a difficult airway: an analysis from the multicenter pediatric difficult intubation registry. Anesthesiology 2017. https://doi.org/10.1097/ALN.0000000000001758.

56. Kovatsis PG. Continuous ventilation during flexible fiberscopic-assisted intubation via supraglottic airways. Paediatr Anaesth 2016. https://doi.org/10.1111/pan.12863.

57. Riva T, Pedersen TH, Seiler S, et al. Transnasal humidified rapid insufflation ventilatory exchange for oxygenation of children during apnoea: a prospective randomised controlled trial. Br J Anaesth 2018;120(3):592–9.

58. Humphreys S, Lee-Archer P, Reyne G, et al. Transnasal humidified rapid-insufflation ventilatory exchange (THRIVE) in children: a randomized controlled trial. Br J Anaesth 2017;118(2):232–8.

Effects of Vasoactive Medications and Maternal Positioning During Cesarean Delivery on Maternal Hemodynamics and Neonatal Acid–Base Status

Allison Lee, MD, MS[a],*,
Warwick Ngan Kee, BHB, MBChB, MD, FANZCA, FHKCA, FHKAM
(Anaesthesiology)[b]

KEYWORDS

- Uteroplacental perfusion • Neonatal acidemia • Peripartum hemodynamics
- Maternal hypotension • Left uterine displacement • Aortocaval compression
- Cesarean delivery

KEY POINTS

- Adequacy of uteroplacental blood flow is the key determinant of exchange of oxygen, nutrients and waste between mother and fetus.
- Placental blood flow is highly dependent on maternal blood pressure because there is limited autoregulation of the placental circulation.
- During the peripartum period, maternal hypotension may occur secondary to the effects of anesthesia, hypovolemia (eg, due to hemorrhage), and aortocaval compression.
- Optimizing maternal hemodynamics during the peripartum period requires optimal selection and use of intravenous fluids and vasopressors, and optimizing maternal positioning to limit vena caval compression.

INTRODUCTION

Acute events during the peripartum period and their management during anesthesia can significantly contribute to the neonate's acid-base status at birth. Maternal hemodynamics, fluid management, choice of vasopressor, maternal positioning and

Disclosure Statement: The authors have nothing to disclose.
[a] Department of Anesthesiology, Columbia University Medical Center, Columbia University, 630 West 168th Street PH-5, New York, NY 10032, USA; [b] Department of Anesthesiology, Sidra Medicine, Al Gharrafa Street, Ar-Rayyan, Doha, Qatar
* Corresponding author.
E-mail address: al3196@cumc.columbia.edu

Clin Perinatol 46 (2019) 765–783
https://doi.org/10.1016/j.clp.2019.08.009
0095-5108/19/© 2019 Elsevier Inc. All rights reserved.

anesthesia technique influence neonatal outcomes, primarily via their impact on the adequacy of uteroplacental blood flow, which is central to the transplacental exchange of oxygen, nutrients and waste between mother and fetus. Acid-base status is commonly used as a measure of neonatal outcome because it is objective and can be easily and routinely performed.

UTEROPLACENTAL CIRCULATION

Over the course of pregnancy, adaptations in blood flow to the uterus take place. Blood flow markedly increases from pre-pregnancy levels of 50 to 100 mL/min to 700 to 900 mL/min at term (approximately 12% of maternal cardiac output).[1] Major contributions are derived from both the uterine and ovarian arteries; in rhesus monkeys it has been estimated that the ovarian arteries supply half the blood flow to the upper one-third of the uterus, with the remainder (83%) supplied by the uterine arteries.[2] Regionally, increased common iliac artery blood flow is associated with concomitantly decreased external iliac artery blood flow, which essentially represents a "steal" phenomenon resulting in preferential distribution of pelvic blood flow to the uterus.[3] In primates at term, 80% - 90% of blood flow to the uterus supplies the placenta, with the remainder perfusing the myometrium and non-placental endometrium.[4] Placental and non-placental circulations differ anatomically and functionally, particularly with respect to the regulation of blood flow and the effects of uterine contractions.[4]

The placental circulation is a low-resistance circulation, thought to resemble an arteriovenous shunt, with oxygenated maternal blood from spiral arteries bathing trophoblastic villi, and blood from the basal plate returning via collecting veins.[3] A rich fetal capillary network supplies trophoblastic villi, representing a surface area of 12 - 14 m^2 at term.[5] Functionally, the placenta behaves as a "venous equilibrator" whereby umbilical venous blood oxygen tension approximates that of the maternal uterine veins.[6] Studies in both animals and humans indicate that under normal conditions, blood flow exceeds the minimum necessary to meet fetal oxygen demand, creating a large safety margin[7]; in circumstances of decreased uterine blood flow, decreased oxygen delivery can be compensated for by increased oxygen extraction within limits in healthy fetuses without the occurrence of significant acidosis.[8]

The placental circulation is considered to be maximally dilated with limited capacity for autoregulation with the result that placental blood flow is highly dependent on maternal blood pressure.[9] Decreases in uterine arterial pressure may result from aortic compression, hypovolemia (eg, hemorrhage), drug-induced hypotension and sympathetic blockade. Increases in uterine venous pressure may occur with vena caval compression, uterine contractions, and skeletal muscle hypertonus (such as during seizures or the Valsalva maneuver). Increased uterine vascular resistance may occur from the effects of endogenous and exogenous vasoconstrictors and local anesthetics in high concentration.[10] During labor, uterine contractions create intermittent cyclical decreases in perfusion with the result that pH decreases and Pco_2 and base deficit increase (about 1 mmol/L per hour during the second stage of labor).[11]

INTERPRETATION OF UMBILICAL CORD BLOOD GASES

Paired umbilical arterial and venous gas analysis gives insight into the course of events leading up to delivery. Values are influenced by parity, gestational age, breech presentation, multiple gestation, and mode of delivery, and are correlated with the duration of labor and the uterine-incision-to-delivery interval during cesarean delivery.[11,12] Blood gas values of umbilical venous blood, which carries oxygenated blood to the fetus, reflect maternal acid-base status and placental function; values of umbilical arterial blood reflect the acid-base balance of the fetus, typically with lower pH and P_{O_2} and higher P_{CO_2} than umbilical venous blood.[13]

Isolated respiratory acidosis, caused by CO_2 accumulation usually occurs following short-lived decreases in uteroplacental perfusion, for example, associated with maternal hypotension, and seems to have little impact on clinical outcome.[11] More pronounced hypoxemia is associated with anaerobic glycolysis and development of a mixed respiratory and metabolic acidosis. With acute onset and insufficient time for equilibration with maternal blood, there is slower placental transfer of non-volatile acids such as lactic acid, so a pattern of high umbilical arterial base deficit and low umbilical venous base deficit is likely to occur. When both the umbilical arterial and umbilical venous base deficit are large, hypoxemia is likely to have been less acute, because the fetal acid load has had the opportunity to saturate placental buffering capacity.

Umbilical arterial pH is determined by metabolic and respiratory acid components. Differences in umbilical arterial and umbilical venous pH may also be revealing. When uteroplacental perfusion is diminished, both the umbilical artery and umbilical vein are impacted, with the pH difference being about 0.06. Poor fetal perfusion leads to a large difference between the umbilical arterial and venous pH (about 0.12).[14] Large differences between umbilical arterial and venous pH, P_{CO_2} and P_{O_2} tend to occur with cord compression. Small differences tend to be seen where there is reduced maternal perfusion of the placenta, for example, with abruptio placentae.[11]

Moderate or severe newborn complications are associated with a base deficit of 12 mmol/L or more.[15] Belai and colleagues[16] found that with umbilical arterial pH <7, a large difference between the umbilical arterial and venous values of P_{CO_2} was predictive of the risk of developing hypoxic-ischemic encephalopathy, and was a more sensitive indicator than the difference in P_{O_2}.

Anesthesia for Cesarean Delivery

The choice of anesthetic technique for cesarean delivery must be tailored to the urgency of surgery with consideration of anesthetic, obstetric, maternal and fetal factors. However, neuraxial anesthesia is preferred to general anesthesia in most cases as it avoids the risks of maternal difficult intubation and pulmonary aspiration, avoids the depressant effects of anesthetics on the fetus, allows the mother to be awake for her childbirth experience, is associated with lower blood loss, and provides superior post-operative pain control.[17] General anesthesia is associated with a higher risk of adverse events including anesthesia-related complications, surgical site infection, increased risk of deep venous thrombosis and pulmonary embolism, and accordingly, use of general anesthesia for cesarean delivery has substantially decreased.[18] A 2005 meta-analysis of neonatal acid-base data from patients receiving different types of anesthesia for cesarean delivery revealed greater neonatal acidosis associated with spinal versus general or epidural anesthesia.[19] Between spinal and general anesthesia (13 studies and 1272 subjects), the umbilical cord blood pH difference was −0.015 (95% CI -0.029 to −0.001) and the base deficit difference (seven studies and 695 subjects) was 1.109 (95% CI 0.434–1.784 mEq/L).[19] Although there may be multiple contributing factors, these findings are likely due to the rapid onset of sympathetic blockade associated with spinal anesthesia, leading to higher requirements for ephedrine, which in turn imposes metabolic effects on the fetus. They should not be interpreted as discouragement for the use of spinal anesthesia, but highlight the importance of aggressive blood pressure management and optimal vasopressor selection, which will be discussed below.

Neuraxial Anesthesia

Spinal anesthesia is the most popular neuraxial technique utilized for cesarean delivery in contemporary practice, used in 75% to 88% of elective cases in the US.[20] The technique provides rapid onset of dense motor and sensory blockade, and blockade of sympathetic preganglionic sites. Local anesthetic injected into the intrathecal space undergoes dilution in cerebrospinal fluid (CSF). Individual variation in lumbosacral CSF volume and distribution within the CSF, and individual variability in the anatomy of spinal nerve roots contribute to variability of response.[21] Therefore, with the single-shot technique, there is a challenge to choose an optimal dose that provides an adequate block, especially given that intraoperative pain is a major potential adverse outcome (and very important cause of litigation). Because of the variability of response, with single-shot spinal anesthesia, a dose is typically chosen that has a high probability of an adequate block but is a relative "overdose" in a large proportion of patients, hence the risk of hypotension is further increased.[22] The combined spinal-epidural technique is an alternative that allows selection of lower doses with less hypotension.

Sympathetic blockade is usually 2 segments higher than sensory blockade to pinprick at the recommended T4-T6 sensory level.[21] Sympatholysis decreases tonic sympathetic tone, resulting in peripheral vasodilation. The resulting decrease in blood pressure may be further compounded by blockade of cardioaccelerator nerves (T1 – T4), and reflex responses to decreased atrial and ventricular stretch with decreased cardiac filling.[21,23] Hypotension develops in over 70% of parturients,[24] accompanied by a compensatory baroreceptor-mediated rise in heart rate, stroke volume and cardiac output.[25] Uncorrected hypotension may lead to nausea and vomiting, decreased uteroplacental blood flow, fetal acidosis and in rare cases, cardiovascular collapse. In addition to reduced perfusion pressure, decreases in uteroplacental blood flow may be compounded by a reflex rise in endogenous vasoconstrictors, steal of blood to the lower limbs, and exogenous vasoconstrictor administration.[26]

Hypotension associated with epidural anesthesia tends to be less profound because of the slower onset of the sympathectomy and the ability to titrate the local anesthetic dose. Vena caval compression, which begins at the 20th week of gestation and is near complete at term, exacerbates hypotension by reducing the rate of venous return from the lower extremities.

OPTIMAL MATERNAL BLOOD PRESSURE

Evidence from the past 2 decades supports ideally maintaining maternal systolic arterial pressure near baseline with rapid correction of any decrease. Ngan Kee and colleagues[27] randomly assigned parturients receiving spinal anesthesia for cesarean delivery to receive a phenylephrine infusion targeted to maintain maternal systolic blood pressure at 100% (Group 100), 90% (Group 90) or 80% (Group 80) of baseline. Higher neonatal umbilical arterial pH and a lower incidence of nausea and vomiting was found when maternal blood pressure was targeted at 100% of baseline; the Group 100 umbilical arterial pH mean was 7.32 (95% CI 7.31–7.34) and the Group 80 mean was 7.30 (95% CI 7.31–7.34). Limiting the duration of episodes of hypotension is also supported by a report by Okudaira and Suzuki, who reported that women undergoing cesarean delivery with spinal anesthesia with ≥2 minutes of hypotension (defined as systolic blood pressure <100 mm Hg or <80% of baseline) had higher levels of oxygen free radicals in the fetoplacental circulation, evidenced by higher umbilical venous oxypurines and lipid peroxides than women who had <2 minutes of hypotension, despite no significant differences in umbilical arterial blood gases or pH.[28]

General Anesthesia

General anesthesia for cesarean delivery is appropriate for certain clinical situations, for example, where neuraxial anesthesia is contraindicated or refused by the patient, to facilitate ex utero intrapartum treatment (EXIT) procedures where uterine relaxation is beneficial, and for emergencies, where time may not permit performance of neuraxial anesthesia. Commonly used induction agents have little direct effect on uteroplacental blood flow, but may indirectly do so via their effects on maternal blood pressure.

Jouppila and colleagues[29] showed an average 35% decrease in intervillous blood flow at the time of induction of general anesthesia for cesarean delivery with thiopental and succinylcholine. The sympathetic response to laryngoscopy and tracheal intubation may also have a detrimental effect on uteroplacental perfusion.[30] Although there is no clear evidence that this is important in low-risk patients, the reduction in uteroplacental perfusion may be of importance for high-risk fetuses and has resulted in interest in the use of rapid-acting opioids to attenuate the response. Gin and colleagues[31] showed that alfentanil decreased the hemodynamic response and catecholamine surge following intubation. Multiple investigators have also demonstrated the effectiveness of remifentanil in blunting the response to intubation (ED_{95} 1.34 µg/kg),[32] however providers must be prepared to manage the transient neonatal respiratory depression that may occur in up to 50% of cases, depending on the dose given.[32,33]

Inhaled volatile anesthetics cause a dose-dependent decrease in systemic vascular resistance, and in high concentrations are associated with decreases in maternal cardiac output, blood pressure, and uterine blood flow.[34] The relaxation of the uterus in circumstances of increased tone, may be beneficial by increasing uterine blood flow.

During general anesthesia, it is generally advocated that hyperventilation be avoided because of concerns about reducing uteroplacental blood flow. Of further concern is that maternal respiratory alkalosis may cause a leftward shift in the oxyhemoglobin dissociation curve, which may reduce fetal oxygenation.[35] Investigators have reported an association between hypocapnia and fetal hypoxia and acidosis in animals and humans.[36] By impairing venous return, mechanical hyperventilation may indirectly reduce uterine blood flow.[37] Hypercapnia may indirectly reduce uterine blood flow by sympathetic activation.[38] Normocapnia (adjusted for pregnancy) should therefore be maintained (ie, $Paco_2$ 30–32 mm Hg [4.0–4.3 kPa]).

Vasopressors

Historically, strategies to prevent hypotension during neuraxial anesthesia for cesarean delivery focused on improving venous return with intravenous fluids, altering maternal position to decrease aortocaval compression, and leg wrapping or elevation. However, in recognition of the fact that the dominant cause of hypotension associated with sympathetic blockade is arteriolar vasodilation, with only modest venodilation,[39] contemporary practice now emphasizes the importance of the use of vasopressors agents as the most effective method for preventing and treating hypotension.[40]

Ephedrine was previously considered to be the first-line agent based on animal studies that indicated sparing of uterine artery vasoconstriction relative to systemic vessels and increased release of nitric oxide from uterine artery endothelium.[41] However, the increase in uterine vascular resistance associated with alpha-adrenergic receptor agonists may be more of an effect on myometrium, with vessels perfusing the placenta relatively spared.[42,43] Today, the bulk of available evidence supports the use of phenylephrine as the vasopressor of choice to treat spinal anesthesia-induced hypotension.[40]

PHENYLEPHRINE

Phenylephrine is a potent alpha-1 adrenergic receptor agonist with virtually no beta adrenergic effect at normal clinical doses. It is preferred to ephedrine because of its fast onset and short duration which facilitates administration via either boluses or infusion, its greater efficacy, lower placental transfer, and smaller propensity to depress fetal pH. Numerous high quality studies support the superiority of phenylephrine in maintaining maternal blood pressure, for preventing maternal nausea and vomiting and in producing less neonatal acidosis.[44–47]

The superior outcomes associated with phenylephrine with respect to neonatal acid base status contrast with animal studies which have suggested either no improvement or decreased uterine blood flow, and no difference in fetal acid-base status or lactate with phenylephrine compared with ephedrine.[48–50] The discrepancies are likely due to species differences in placenta morphology. Less placental transfer of ephedrine in sheep may occur because of the thicker synepitheliochorial placenta, which may represent a barrier to drug transfer, compared with the memomonochorial placenta of humans. Reassuringly, no increase in placental vascular resistance was demonstrated with phenylephrine 50 μg/min or ephedrine 4 mg/min infusions in women undergoing cesarean delivery with epidural anesthesia.[51]

A lingering concern related to use of phenylephrine is its propensity to cause a dose-related baroreceptor-mediated reflex decrease in heart rate with a concomitant decrease in cardiac output.[25,52] Generally, these changes appear to be well tolerated and thus their clinical significance is unknown. However, since most studies have been conducted in healthy subjects there is concern for potential harm in the setting of a compromised fetus who may not be able to compensate for any additional reductions in flow because of vasoconstriction or a decrease in maternal cardiac output.

To date, studies have not shown a difference in fetal acidosis with respect to ephedrine and phenylephrine for spinal anesthesia for non-elective delivery or in the setting of acute fetal compromise.[53,54] A randomized comparison of bolus phenylephrine and ephedrine for treating spinal anesthesia-induced hypotension among parturients (n = 133) with severe preeclampsia and fetal compromise undergoing cesarean delivery found no difference between groups with respect to mean base excess or clinical outcomes; the mean umbilical arterial base excess was −4.9 (SD 3.7) versus −6.0 (4.6) mmol/L for patients receiving ephedrine and phenylephrine respectively.[55] Ngan Kee and colleagues[53] conducted a double-blinded randomized trial among 204 parturients undergoing non-elective cesarean delivery with spinal anesthesia; patients were randomized to receive boluses of phenylephrine or ephedrine to treat hypotension. Clinical outcome, and umbilical arterial and venous pH and base excess were similar between groups, but in the ephedrine group, umbilical arterial lactate concentration was higher (median 2.6 [interquartile range 2.3–3.3] vs 2.4 [1.9–3.0] mmol/L, P = .016). Among protocol-compliant patients, umbilical arterial and venous Po_2 were lower in the phenylephrine group, but the oxygen content was similar between groups. The authors speculated this could indeed reflect a vasoconstrictive effect of phenylephrine leading to a reduction in uteroplacental flow and more efficient fetal extraction of oxygen. A meta-analysis by Heesen and colleagues[56] concluded there are insufficient data to make a recommendation in the setting of non-elective and high-risk patients. During non-elective cases the induction-to-delivery interval may be short, so exposure of the fetus to vasopressors is limited; it is also known that laboring patients have a reduced susceptibility to hypotension from spinal anesthesia so vasopressor requirement (exposure) is reduced.

EPHEDRINE

Ephedrine has indirect and weak direct adrenergic activity, which may explain the relatively slow onset and long duration. Its predominantly beta-adrenergic agonist effect, due to the indirect presynaptic release of norepinephrine, does not match the main physiologic disturbance of vasodilation which is produced by neuraxial blockade; ephedrine primarily produces an increase in cardiac output with relatively less vasoconstriction. The delayed onset and long duration of action of ephedrine make it more difficult to titrate to target blood pressure and the delayed pressor response is thought to contribute to the higher incidence of nausea and vomiting.[45]

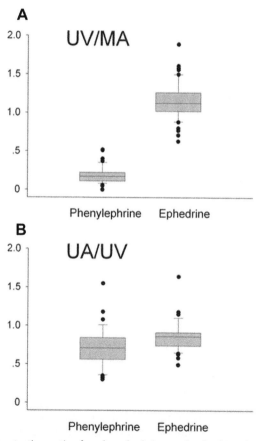

Fig. 1. Plasma concentration ratios for phenylephrine and ephedrine for parturients undergoing elective cesarean delivery with spinal anesthesia who randomly received either an infusion of phenylephrine (100 μg/mL) or ephedrine (8 mg/mL) titrated to maintain maternal systolic blood pressure near baseline. Data are shown for (*A*) umbilical venous to maternal arterial (UV/MA) and (*B*) umbilical arterial to umbilical venous (UA/UV) ratios. Box plots display the 25th, 50th, and 75th percentiles as horizontal lines on a bar, whiskers above and below the box indicate the 90th and 10th percentiles, and data beyond the 10th and 90th percentiles are displayed as individual points. Data were significantly different between groups ($P \leq .001$) for both concentration ratios. (*From:* Ngan Kee WD, Khaw KS, Tan PE, et al. Placental transfer and fetal metabolic effects of phenylephrine and ephedrine during spinal anesthesia for cesarean delivery. Anesthesiology. 2009;111(3):506-512; with permission.)

Although effective for managing maternal hypotension, ephedrine's higher lipid solubility results in higher transplacental transfer than phenylephrine (**Fig. 1**). Fetal sympathetic metabolism is stimulated in a dose-dependent manner, leading to neonatal acidemia; elevated umbilical arterial and venous concentrations of lactate, glucose, epinephrine and norepinephrine, and higher umbilical venous Pco_2 were reported by Ngan Kee and colleagues[47] Median umbilical vein/maternal arterial ratios were 1.13 for ephedrine and 0.17 for phenylephrine.[47] A systematic review by Veeser and colleagues[57] including 20 trials reported the risk ratio for true fetal acidosis to be 5.29 [95% CI 1.62–17.25] for ephedrine versus phenylephrine, $P = .006$.

Pharmacogenetics

Variations in maternal and fetal responses to adrenergic receptor agonists may relate in part to variations in genetic characteristics. Maternal haplotype of the beta2-adrenoceptor gene (ADRB2) influences ephedrine requirements. Glycine at position 16 and/or glutamate at position 27 was associated with 40% - 50% lower ephedrine requirement compared with other genotypes, among a US cohort of mixed ethnicity,[58] whereas in a Chinese cohort maternal ADRB2 genotype had no effect on ephedrine dose but neonatal homozygosity at codon 16 had a protective effect against the development of ephedrine-induced acidosis, with higher umbilical arterial pH and lower umbilical arterial lactate concentration.[59]

NOREPINEPHRINE

Norepinephrine (noradrenaline) is a catecholamine with potent alpha-1 adrenergic receptor agonist, and moderate beta adrenergic receptor agonist activity resulting in both direct positive chronotropic and reflex negative chronotropic effects; the net result is an approximately neutral effect on heart rate.[60] Comparative studies during spinal anesthesia for cesarean delivery have shown that, compared with phenylephrine, use of equipotent doses of norepinephrine is associated with less reflexive decreases in heart rate and cardiac output (**Fig. 2**).

The features of higher cardiac output, lower systemic vascular resistance and the lack of placental transfer[61] potentially may make norepinephrine more favorable for promoting uteroplacental perfusion than phenylephrine and has triggered interest in exploring its use as an alternative vasopressor for obstetric patients.[62,63] It has a fast onset and short duration of action, and has been demonstrated to be feasible for use as boluses and infusions, including prophylactic infusion.[62,64,65] The less pronounced effects of norepinephrine on heart rate compared with phenylephrine may reduce the need to administer anticholinergic drugs to treat bradycardia.

Norepinephrine is more available around the world than phenylephrine. However, clinicians may be more familiar with its use in the intensive care and cardiac anesthesia settings, and may be concerned about the risk of tissue injury from extravasation, which mandates the use of large-bore intravenous access and utilization of dilute norepinephrine solutions. Nevertheless, it should be noted that when norepinephrine is diluted to a concentration that is equipotent with commonly used phenylephrine solutions, the considerations and precautions should be the same for both agents.[66] Although some institutions that have limited experience with the use of peripherally administered vasopressors may currently have specific restrictions against peripheral use of norepinephrine,[67] there is no evidence that norepinephrine is associated with a higher risk of tissue ischemia compared with other vasopressors and the manufacturers do not stipulate administration via a central venous line.[68]

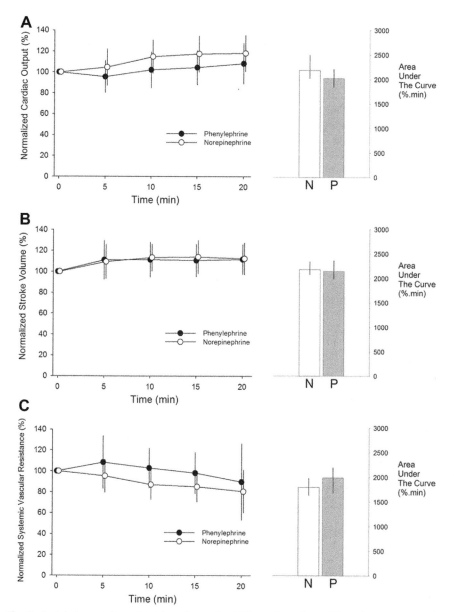

Fig. 2. Serial changes in maternal cardiac output (*A*), stroke volume (*B*), and systemic vascular resistance (*C*) among healthy patients undergoing cesarean delivery with spinal anesthesia who were randomized to have systolic blood pressure maintained with a computer-controlled infusion of norepinephrine 5 μg/mL or phenylephrine 100 μg/mL. On the left side of the panels, data are serial values for the first 20 minutes after the induction of spinal anesthesia normalized to percentage of baseline values. On the right side of the panels, bars show the area under the curve for the 2 groups. Comparison of the calculated values for area under the curve showed that cardiac output was greater over time (*P*<.001) and systemic vascular resistance was lower over time (*P*<.001) in the norepinephrine group compared with that in the phenylephrine group, but there was no difference in stroke volume (*P* = .44). Values are shown as median and interquartile range. N, norepinephrine; P, phenylephrine. (*From*: Ngan Kee WD, Lee SW, Ng FF, et al. Randomized double-blinded comparison of norepinephrine and phenylephrine for maintenance of blood pressure during spinal anesthesia for cesarean delivery. Anesthesiology. 2015;122(4):736-745; with permission.)

OTHER VASOPRESSORS

Other vasopressors may be effective for maintenance of maternal blood pressure at cesarean delivery, but have generally been less well-studied.

Metaraminol has direct and indirect adrenergic receptor agonist activity. It is a potent alpha-1 adrenergic receptor agonist and a weak beta adrenergic receptor agonist. A meta-analysis including 4 studies showed that, compared with ephedrine-treated patients, metaraminol was associated with higher mean umbilical arterial pH (standardized mean difference 0.82, 95% CI 0.01–1.62, $P = .05$).[69] McDonnell and colleagues,[70] in a randomized double-blinded comparison of metaraminol and phenylephrine found that metaraminol was at least non-inferior to phenylephrine for the primary outcome of umbilical arterial pH.

Mephenteramine is a mixed alpha and beta adrenergic receptor agonist with direct and indirect effects, used in many low- and middle-income countries. There is limited evidence regarding its transplacental transfer and effect on fetal metabolism but it has been shown to have comparative effectiveness to ephedrine and phenylephrine for treating maternal hypotension associated with spinal anesthesia during cesarean delivery.[71,72]

Methoxamine is an alpha-1 adrenergic receptor agonist reported to have efficacy for restoring maternal blood pressure, but the evidence is insufficient to support routine use in obstetric patients.[73] In Germany, a combination of cafedrine (covalently linked norephedrine and theophylline) and theoadrenaline (covalently linked noradrenaline and theophylline) in a 20:1 ratio is widely used to treat hypotension during cesarean delivery.[74] Administration of this drug combination leads to increased blood pressure primarily because of increased stroke volume and cardiac output, with unchanged systemic vascular resistance. Beta adrenergic receptor agonism (beta 1) is the predominant effect. The theoadrenaline component causes peripheral vasoconstriction via alpha adrenergic receptor agonist activity, which may compete with partial agonist activity of cafedrine's norephedrine component. The drug has not undergone extensive research. One retrospective study comparing a cohort who received the drug (n = 117) to a cohort not requiring pharmacologic treatment of hypotension (n = 56) found an onset of effect within 2 to 3 minutes and no detrimental effect on Apgar scores or umbilical arterial pH.[75]

5-HYDROXYTRYPTAMINE-3 RECEPTOR ANTAGONISTS

The Bezold-Jarisch reflex may be triggered during spinal anesthesia in response to decreased venous return and cardiac filling, resulting in bradycardia and vasodilation, which may exaggerate the severity of maternal hypotension. 5-Hydroxytryptamine-3 (5-HT3) receptors are among the chemoreceptors involved in mediating the reflex and blockade of 5-HT3 receptors has been shown to prevent the reflex in animal studies.[76] Among obstetric patients undergoing cesarean delivery with spinal anesthesia, 5-HT3 antagonists are moderately effective in decreasing the incidence of hypotension and bradycardia. A meta-analysis by Heesen and colleagues[77] reviewed trials involving obstetric patients and concluded that treatment with 5-HT3 blockers is effective in decreasing the incidence of hypotension; although no effect on the number of patients who received treatment for hypotension was found, the dose of vasopressor required was decreased. Seven of 8 trials studied ondansetron (dose range 2–12 mg); the relative risk for hypotension among treated patients was 0.70, 95% CI 0.49 to 0.99, $I^2 = 71\%$.

Intravenous Fluids

Intravenous fluid loading, in combination with vasopressor administration, is a key strategy for the prevention and treatment of spinal anesthesia-induced hypotension.

Several controversies including choice of fluid (crystalloid vs colloid), timing (pre-vs coload), and dose have led numerous investigators to pursue studies to determine the optimal approach. Intravenous fluids were previously given to maintain venous return and cardiac output; however, studies show that in most cases cardiac output actually increases after spinal anesthesia, which is contrary to the original rationale of using fluids. Studies have not consistently shown intravenous fluids to be effective and vasopressors are normally always required.

Timing of fluid administration

Because of rapid redistribution into the interstitial space,[78] crystalloid preloading (10 - 30 mL/kg Ringer's lactate) has been debunked as ineffective by multiple investigators[79]; a more effective approach is rapid administration at the time of intrathecal injection, known as "coloading" or "cohydration".[46,80]

Dyer and colleagues[81] randomly assigned women (n = 50) undergoing spinal anesthesia for elective cesarean delivery to receive either 20 mL/kg crystalloid preload or coload. More patients in the coload group did not require ephedrine before delivery (P = .047) and the coload group required a lower median dose of ephedrine (P = .03). Ngan Kee and colleagues[46] (n = 53) determined that a combination of prophylactic phenylephrine infusion 100 μg/min in addition to a rapid lactated Ringer's solution coload to a maximum of 2 L was an effective strategy for preventing hypotension during spinal anesthesia for cesarean delivery compared with patients receiving crystalloid at a minimal maintenance rate. One potential benefit of rapid cohydration might be simply to enhance distribution of the vasopressor.[46]

Crystalloids versus colloids

Colloid preloading effectively lowers the incidence and severity of hypotension as infused fluid remains intravascular for a longer period,[82] but routine use has been discouraged because of the risk of allergy, higher cost, and the effect on coagulation of first-generation hetastarch.[83] Furthermore, the degree of placental transfer and potential for adverse effects on the neonate have not been studied.

Because a colloid intravenous bolus remains longer in the intravascular space than crystalloid, no advantage has been found for administering a colloid coload versus preload.[84] McDonald and colleagues[85] randomized healthy term women scheduled for elective cesarean delivery with spinal anesthesia to receive either a 1-L coload of hetastarch or Hartmann's (lactated Ringer's) solution. The investigators reported no difference in the primary outcome, cardiac output, between groups and no difference in phenylephrine requirement. Most recently, Tawfik and colleagues[86] found no advantage to a combination of a 500 mL colloid preload and 500 mL crystalloid coload compared with a 1000 mL crystalloid coload to reduce ephedrine dose to treat spinal induced maternal hypotension during cesarean delivery.

Maternal Position and Aortocaval Compression During Cesarean Delivery

At the 20th week of gestation, the gravid uterus begins to compress the inferior vena cava in the supine position.[87] At term, both older dye injection studies and more recent magnetic resonance imaging (MRI) studies have demonstrated near-complete inferior vena cava occlusion in the supine position at term.[88,89] Physiologic compensation involves peripheral venoconstriction, which increases venous return via collateral channels which develop over the course of pregnancy. Holmes[90] classically demonstrated that 8.2% of women exhibited the "supine hypotensive syndrome" with a decrease in systolic blood pressure of greater than 30 mm Hg or decrease in systolic blood pressure to less than 80 mm Hg. Improvement in symptoms occurs with lateral positioning, performing manual displacement or with delivery.[87] Imaging studies have demonstrated significant relief of vena caval obstruction only occurs at 30° of lateral tilt.[89] Accordingly, lateral positioning of the patient is a key component of intrauterine resuscitation techniques in labor,[91] and both the Society of Obstetric Anesthesia and Perinatology (SOAP) and the American Heart Association (AHA) recommend manual lateral uterine displacement during cardiac arrest in pregnancy if the uterus is palpable or visible at the umbilicus.[92,93]

For decades, instituting 15° of left uterine displacement during cesarean delivery with the aid of wedges or tilting of the surgical table has been advocated to relieve aortocaval compression. The specification of a 15° angle appears to be arbitrary and was adopted following influential studies conducted in the 1970's – many of which were non-randomized, utilized varying anesthetic techniques, and avoided the use of vasopressors – that suggested that neonates of patients positioned with uterine displacement had less acidosis at birth.[94–97] 15° of tilt has since been shown not to produce significant relief of vena caval obstruction, in clinical practice the angle achieved is very variable and often overestimated, and surgeons may have difficulty operating in this position.[98]

The dogma of lateral tilt being essential in all patients undergoing cesarean delivery is being questioned because it is so infrequently achieved, and in contemporary practice maternal blood pressure may otherwise be maintained close to baseline with vasopressors and fluids. Recently, Lee and colleagues[99] randomized non-laboring, healthy women with uncomplicated pregnancies at term to be placed supine or with 15° of left tilt during spinal anesthesia for elective cesarean delivery. They found that when systolic blood pressure was maintained at baseline with a

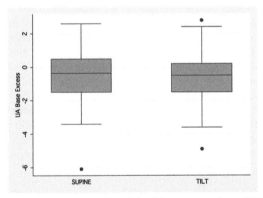

Fig. 3. Box plot of neonatal umbilical arterial (UA) base excess (mmol/L) by group. Subjects were healthy nonobese term parturients undergoing elective cesarean delivery with spinal anesthesia, who were randomly allocated to be in the supine horizontal position (SUPINE group) or in 15° of left lateral tilt (TILT group) until delivery. Maternal blood pressure was supported with a crystalloid coload and a prophylactic phenylephrine infusion, titrated to maintain maternal systolic blood pressure near baseline. Dots represent outlier values. (*From* Lee AJ, Landau R, Mattingly JL, et al. Left Lateral table tilt for elective cesarean delivery under spinal anesthesia has no effect on neonatal acid-base status: a randomized controlled trial. Anesthesiology. 2017;127(2):241-249; with permission.)

crystalloid coload and phenylephrine infusion there was no difference in umbilical arterial base excess in the supine group (mean −0.5 (SD ± 1.6) mmol/L) versus the tilted group (−0.6 (±1.5) mmol/L, P = .64) (**Fig. 3**).[99] Notably, however, the systolic blood pressure and cardiac output during the first 15 minutes post-spinal anesthesia were lower in the supine group. Despite no negative effect on neonatal acid-base status among healthy women in the supine position, it is unknown whether the difference in blood pressure and cardiac output would be clinically important in the setting of fetal compromise or impaired placental perfusion (eg, preeclampsia or intrauterine growth restriction).[100] A subset of patients will experience the supine hypotensive syndrome and some patients are at risk of exaggerated aortocaval compression (eg, multiple gestation, macrosomia or polyhydramnios), and these patients would very likely benefit from left uterine displacement. At this time there is no reliable screening tool to predict who these women will be. Although having women tilted or wedged during cesarean delivery may not be necessary in all cases, particularly if not preferred by the patient or surgeon, experts caution we should not necessarily abandon the practice; one suggested compromise is to maintain tilt for the period of preparation and draping, at least until the start of surgery.

Best Practices

What is the current practice for the use of vasoactive medications and maternal positioning during cesarean delivery?

Best practice, guideline, and care path objective
• Take active measures to prevent and treat hypotension during regional anesthesia for cesarean delivery.
• Administer fluids and medications with the aim of maintaining systolic blood pressure near baseline values until delivery.
• Apply left uterine displacement to mitigate the effects of inferior vena cava compression by the gravid uterus.

What changes in current practice are likely to improve outcomes?

• Utilization of a prophylactic infusion of phenylephrine started immediately after induction of spinal anesthesia.
• Measures to reduce maternal bradycardia during the administration of pure alpha-adrenergic agonists.

Major recommendations

• Administer intravenous fluid preload or coload.
• Prophylactically administer phenylephrine or other alpha adrenergic agonist via intravenous boluses or infusion.
• Restrict use of ephedrine to cases of hypotension and bradycardia in order to limit transplacental transfer and dose-dependent fetal metabolic effects.
• Provide left lateral uterine displacement until delivery although if not tolerated may be omitted in healthy, non-obese, elective cases if blood pressure is maintained with vasopressors.
• Avoid prolonged bradycardia by limiting vasopressor dose or using vasopressor with positive chronotropic properties (eg, norepinephrine).
• Monitor cardiac output non-invasively or indirectly using maternal heart rate as a surrogate.

Bibliographic Source(s): *Data from* Refs.[40,46,47,99]

REFERENCES

1. Thaler I, Manor D, Itskovitz J, et al. Changes in uterine blood flow during human pregnancy. Am J Obstet Gynecol 1990;162(1):121–5.
2. Wehrenberg WB, Chaichareon DP, Dierschke DJ, et al. Vascular dynamics of the reproductive tract in the female rhesus monkey: relative contributions of ovarian and uterine arteries. Biol Reprod 1977;17(1):148–53.
3. Palmer SK, Zamudio S, Coffin C, et al. Quantitative estimation of human uterine artery blood flow and pelvic blood flow redistribution in pregnancy. Obstet Gynecol 1992;80(6):1000–6.
4. Novy MJ, Thomas CL, Lees MH. Uterine contractility and regional blood flow responses to oxytocin and prostaglandin E2 in pregnant rhesus monkeys. Am J Obstet Gynecol 1975;122(4):419–33.
5. Burton GJ, Fowden AL. The placenta: a multifaceted, transient organ. Philos Trans R Soc Lond B Biol Sci 2015;370(1663):20140066.
6. Leiser R, Kaufmann P. Placental structure: in a comparative aspect. Exp Clin Endocrinol 1994;102(3):122–34.
7. Wilkening RB, Meschia G. Fetal oxygen uptake, oxygenation, and acid-base balance as a function of uterine blood flow. Am J Physiol 1983;244(6):H749–55.
8. Boyle JW, Lotgering FK, Longo LD. Acute embolization of the uteroplacental circulation: uterine blood flow and placental CO diffusing capacity. J Dev Physiol 1984;6(4):377–86.
9. Greiss FC Jr. Pressure-flow relationship in the gravid uterine vascular bed. Am J Obstet Gynecol 1966;96(1):41–7.
10. Greiss FC Jr, Still JG, Anderson SG. Effects of local anesthetic agents on the uterine vasculatures and myometrium. Am J Obstet Gynecol 1976;124(8):889–99.
11. Armstrong L, Stenson BJ. Use of umbilical cord blood gas analysis in the assessment of the newborn. Arch Dis Child Fetal Neonatal Ed 2007;92(6):F430–4.
12. Ngan Kee WD, Lee A. Multivariate analysis of factors associated with umbilical arterial pH and standard base excess after Caesarean section under spinal anaesthesia. Anaesthesia 2003;58(2):125–30.
13. Westgate J, Garibaldi JM, Greene KR. Umbilical cord blood gas analysis at delivery: a time for quality data. Br J Obstet Gynaecol 1994;101(12):1054–63.
14. Johnson JW, Richards DS, Wagaman RA. The case for routine umbilical blood acid-base studies at delivery. Am J Obstet Gynecol 1990;162(3):621–5.
15. Low JA, Panagiotopoulos C, Derrick EJ. Newborn complications after intrapartum asphyxia with metabolic acidosis in the term fetus. Am J Obstet Gynecol 1994;170(4):1081–7.
16. Belai Y, Goodwin TM, Durand M, et al. Umbilical arteriovenous PO2 and PCO2 differences and neonatal morbidity in term infants with severe acidosis. Am J Obstet Gynecol 1998;178(1 Pt 1):13–9.
17. Practice guidelines for obstetric anesthesia: an updated report by the American Society of Anesthesiologists Task Force on Obstetric Anesthesia and the Society for Obstetric Anesthesia and Perinatology. Anesthesiology 2016;124(2):270–300.
18. Guglielminotti J, Landau R, Li G. Adverse events and factors associated with potentially avoidable use of general anesthesia in cesarean deliveries. Anesthesiology 2019;130(6):912–22.

19. Reynolds F, Seed PT. Anaesthesia for Caesarean section and neonatal acid-base status: a meta-analysis. Anaesthesia 2005;60(7):636–53.
20. Traynor AJ, Aragon M, Ghosh D, et al. Obstetric anesthesia workforce survey: a 30-year update. Anesth Analg 2016;122(6):1939–46.
21. Liu SS, McDonald SB. Current issues in spinal anesthesia. Anesthesiology 2001; 94(5):888–906.
22. Ginosar Y. Mini-dose single-shot spinal anesthesia for cesarean delivery: for whom the bell-shaped curve tolls. Int J Obstet Anesth 2012;21(3):207–11.
23. Crystal GJ, Salem MR. The Bainbridge and the "reverse" Bainbridge reflexes: history, physiology, and clinical relevance. Anesth Analg 2012;114(3):520–32.
24. Ngan Kee WD, Khaw KS, Lee BB, et al. A dose-response study of prophylactic intravenous ephedrine for the prevention of hypotension during spinal anesthesia for cesarean delivery. Anesth Analg 2000;90(6):1390–5.
25. Dyer RA, Reed AR, van Dyk D, et al. Hemodynamic effects of ephedrine, phenylephrine, and the coadministration of phenylephrine with oxytocin during spinal anesthesia for elective cesarean delivery. Anesthesiology 2009;111(4):753–65.
26. Baumann H, Alon E, Atanassoff P, et al. Effect of epidural anesthesia for cesarean delivery on maternal femoral arterial and venous, uteroplacental, and umbilical blood flow velocities and waveforms. Obstet Gynecol 1990;75(2):194–8.
27. Ngan Kee WD, Khaw KS, Ng FF. Comparison of phenylephrine infusion regimens for maintaining maternal blood pressure during spinal anaesthesia for Caesarean section. Br J Anaesth 2004;92(4):469–74.
28. Okudaira S, Suzuki S. Influence of spinal hypotension on fetal oxidative status during elective cesarean section in uncomplicated pregnancies. Arch Gynecol Obstet 2005;271(4):292–5.
29. Jouppila P, Kuikka J, Jouppila R, et al. Effect of induction of general anesthesia for cesarean section on intervillous blood flow. Acta Obstet Gynecol Scand 1979;58(3):249–53.
30. Shnider SM, Wright RG, Levinson G, et al. Uterine blood flow and plasma norepinephrine changes during maternal stress in the pregnant Ewe. Anesthesiology 1979;50(6):524–7.
31. Gin T, Ngan-Kee WD, Siu YK, et al. Alfentanil given immediately before the induction of anesthesia for elective cesarean delivery. Anesth Analg 2000;90(5): 1167–72.
32. Yoo KY, Kang DH, Jeong H, et al. A dose-response study of remifentanil for attenuation of the hypertensive response to laryngoscopy and tracheal intubation in severely preeclamptic women undergoing caesarean delivery under general anaesthesia. Int J Obstet Anesth 2013;22(1):10–8.
33. Van de Velde M. The use of remifentanil during general anesthesia for caesarean section. Curr Opin Anaesthesiol 2016;29(3):257–60.
34. Okutomi T, Whittington RA, Stein DJ, et al. Comparison of the effects of sevoflurane and isoflurane anesthesia on the maternal-fetal unit in sheep. J Anesth 2009;23(3):392–8.
35. Levinson G, Shnider SM, DeLorimier AA, et al. Effects of maternal hyperventilation on uterine blood flow and fetal oxygenation and acid-base status. Anesthesiology 1974;40(4):340–7.
36. Peng AT, Blancato LS, Motoyama EK. Effect of maternal hypocapnia v. eucapnia on the foetus during Caesarean section. Br J Anaesth 1972;44(11):1173–8.
37. Levinson G, Shnider SM, Gildea JE, et al. Maternal and foetal cardiovascular and acid-base changes during ketamine anaesthesia in pregnant ewes. Br J Anaesth 1973;45(11):1111–5.

38. Makowski EL, Hertz RH, Meschia G. Effects of acute maternal hypoxia and hyperoxia on the blood flow to the pregnant uterus. Am J Obstet Gynecol 1973; 115(5):624–31.

39. Rabow S, Olofsson P. Pulse wave analysis by digital photoplethysmography to record maternal hemodynamic effects of spinal anesthesia, delivery of the baby, and intravenous oxytocin during cesarean section. J Matern Fetal Neonatal Med 2017;30(7):759–66.

40. Kinsella SM, Carvalho B, Dyer RA, et al. International consensus statement on the management of hypotension with vasopressors during caesarean section under spinal anaesthesia. Anaesthesia 2018;73(1):71–92.

41. Li P, Tong C, Eisenach JC. Pregnancy and ephedrine increase the release of nitric oxide in ovine uterine arteries. Anesth Analg 1996;82(2):288–93.

42. Rosenfeld CR, West J. Circulatory response to systemic infusion of norepinephrine in the pregnant Ewe. Am J Obstet Gynecol 1977;127(4):376–83.

43. Greiss FC Jr. Differential reactivity of the myoendometrial and placental vasculatures: adrenergic responses. Am J Obstet Gynecol 1972;112(1):20–30.

44. Mercier FJ, Riley ET, Frederickson WL, et al. Phenylephrine added to prophylactic ephedrine infusion during spinal anesthesia for elective cesarean section. Anesthesiology 2001;95(3):668–74.

45. Cooper DW, Carpenter M, Mowbray P, et al. Fetal and maternal effects of phenylephrine and ephedrine during spinal anesthesia for cesarean delivery. Anesthesiology 2002;97(6):1582–90.

46. Ngan Kee WD, Khaw KS, Ng FF. Prevention of hypotension during spinal anesthesia for cesarean delivery: an effective technique using combination phenylephrine infusion and crystalloid cohydration. Anesthesiology 2005;103(4): 744–50.

47. Ngan Kee WD, Khaw KS, Tan PE, et al. Placental transfer and fetal metabolic effects of phenylephrine and ephedrine during spinal anesthesia for cesarean delivery. Anesthesiology 2009;111(3):506–12.

48. Ralston DH, Shnider SM, DeLorimier AA. Effects of equipotent ephedrine, metaraminol, mephentermine, and methoxamine on uterine blood flow in the pregnant Ewe. Anesthesiology 1974;40(4):354–70.

49. Erkinaro T, Makikallio K, Kavasmaa T, et al. Effects of ephedrine and phenylephrine on uterine and placental circulations and fetal outcome following fetal hypoxaemia and epidural-induced hypotension in a sheep model. Br J Anaesth 2004;93(6):825–32.

50. Erkinaro T, Kavasmaa T, Pakkila M, et al. Ephedrine and phenylephrine for the treatment of maternal hypotension in a chronic sheep model of increased placental vascular resistance. Br J Anaesth 2006;96(2):231–7.

51. Guo R, Xue Q, Qian Y, et al. The effects of ephedrine and phenylephrine on placental vascular resistance during cesarean section under epidural anesthesia. Cell Biochem Biophys 2015;73(3):687–93.

52. Stewart A, Fernando R, McDonald S, et al. The dose-dependent effects of phenylephrine for elective cesarean delivery under spinal anesthesia. Anesth Analg 2010;111(5):1230–7.

53. Ngan Kee WD, Khaw KS, Lau TK, et al. Randomised double-blinded comparison of phenylephrine vs ephedrine for maintaining blood pressure during spinal anaesthesia for non-elective Caesarean section*. Anaesthesia 2008;63(12): 1319–26.

54. Jain K, Makkar JK, Subramani Vp S, et al. A randomized trial comparing prophylactic phenylephrine and ephedrine infusion during spinal anesthesia for

emergency cesarean delivery in cases of acute fetal compromise. J Clin Anesth 2016;34:208–15.

55. Dyer RA, Emmanuel A, Adams SC, et al. A randomised comparison of bolus phenylephrine and ephedrine for the management of spinal hypotension in patients with severe preeclampsia and fetal compromise. Int J Obstet Anesth 2018;33:23–31.

56. Heesen M, Rijs K, Hilber N, et al. Ephedrine versus phenylephrine as a vasopressor for spinal anaesthesia-induced hypotension in parturients undergoing high-risk caesarean section: meta-analysis, meta-regression and trial sequential analysis. Int J Obstet Anesth 2019;37:16–28.

57. Veeser M, Hofmann T, Roth R, et al. Vasopressors for the management of hypotension after spinal anesthesia for elective caesarean section. Systematic review and cumulative meta-analysis. Acta Anaesthesiol Scand 2012;56(7):810–6.

58. Smiley RM, Blouin JL, Negron M, et al. β_2-adrenoceptor genotype affects vasopressor requirements during spinal anesthesia for cesarean delivery. Anesthesiology 2006;104(4):644–50.

59. Landau R, Liu SK, Blouin JL, et al. The effect of maternal and fetal beta2-adrenoceptor and nitric oxide synthase genotype on vasopressor requirement and fetal acid-base status during spinal anesthesia for cesarean delivery. Anesth Analg 2011;112(6):1432–7.

60. Ferguson-Myrthil N. Vasopressor use in adult patients. Cardiol Rev 2012;20(3):153–8.

61. Puolakka J, Kauppila A, Tuimala R, et al. The effect of parturition on umbilical blood plasma levels of norepinephrine. Obstet Gynecol 1983;61(1):19–21.

62. Ngan Kee WD, Lee SW, Ng FF, et al. Randomized double-blinded comparison of norepinephrine and phenylephrine for maintenance of blood pressure during spinal anesthesia for cesarean delivery. Anesthesiology 2015;122(4):736–45.

63. Carvalho B, Dyer RA. Norepinephrine for spinal hypotension during cesarean delivery: another paradigm shift? Anesthesiology 2015;122(4):728–30.

64. Onwochei DN, Ngan Kee WD, Fung L, et al. Norepinephrine intermittent intravenous boluses to prevent hypotension during spinal anesthesia for cesarean delivery: a sequential allocation dose-finding study. Anesth Analg 2017;125(1):212–8.

65. Ngan Kee WD, Lee SWY, Ng FF, et al. Prophylactic norepinephrine infusion for preventing hypotension during spinal anesthesia for cesarean delivery. Anesth Analg 2018;126(6):1989–94.

66. Ngan Kee WD. A random-allocation graded dose-response study of norepinephrine and phenylephrine for treating hypotension during spinal anesthesia for cesarean delivery. Anesthesiology 2017;127(6):934–41.

67. Smiley RM. More perfect? Int J Obstet Anesth 2017;29:1–4.

68. Medlej K, Kazzi AA, El Hajj Chehade A, et al. Complications from administration of vasopressors through peripheral venous catheters: an observational study. J Emerg Med 2018;54(1):47–53.

69. Chao E, Sun HL, Huang SW, et al. Metaraminol use during spinal anaesthesia for caesarean section: a meta-analysis of randomised controlled trials. Int J Obstet Anesth 2019;39:42–50.

70. McDonnell NJ, Paech MJ, Muchatuta NA, et al. A randomised double-blind trial of phenylephrine and metaraminol infusions for prevention of hypotension during spinal and combined spinal-epidural anaesthesia for elective caesarean section. Anaesthesia 2017;72(5):609–17.

71. Kansal A, Mohta M, Sethi AK, et al. Randomised trial of intravenous infusion of ephedrine or mephentermine for management of hypotension during spinal anaesthesia for Caesarean section. Anaesthesia 2005;60(1):28–34.
72. Mohta M, Janani SS, Sethi AK, et al. Comparison of phenylephrine hydrochloride and mephentermine sulphate for prevention of post spinal hypotension. Anaesthesia 2010;65(12):1200–5.
73. Luo XJ, Zheng M, Tian G, et al. Comparison of the treatment effects of methoxamine and combining methoxamine with atropine infusion to maintain blood pressure during spinal anesthesia for cesarean delivery: a double blind randomized trial. Eur Rev Med Pharmacol Sci 2016;20(3):561–7.
74. Bein B, Christ T, Eberhart LH. Cafedrine/Theodrenaline (20:1) is an established alternative for the management of arterial hypotension in Germany-a review based on a systematic literature search. Front Pharmacol 2017;8:68.
75. Clemens KE, Quednau I, Heller AR, et al. Impact of cafedrine/theodrenaline (Akrinor(R)) on therapy of maternal hypotension during spinal anesthesia for Cesarean delivery: a retrospective study. Minerva Ginecol 2010;62(6):515–24.
76. Yamano M, Ito H, Kamato T, et al. Characteristics of inhibitory effects of serotonin (5-HT)3-receptor antagonists, YM060 and YM114 (KAE-393), on the von Bezold-Jarisch reflex induced by 2-Methyl-5-HT, veratridine and electrical stimulation of vagus nerves in anesthetized rats. Jpn J Pharmacol 1995;69(4):351–6.
77. Heesen M, Klimek M, Hoeks SE, et al. Prevention of spinal anesthesia-induced hypotension during cesarean delivery by 5-hydroxytryptamine-3 receptor antagonists: a systematic review and meta-analysis and meta-regression. Anesth Analg 2016;123(4):977–88.
78. Ewaldsson CA, Hahn RG. Volume kinetics of Ringer's solution during induction of spinal and general anaesthesia. Br J Anaesth 2001;87(3):406–14.
79. Rout CC, Rocke DA, Levin J, et al. A reevaluation of the role of crystalloid preload in the prevention of hypotension associated with spinal anesthesia for elective cesarean section. Anesthesiology 1993;79(2):262–9.
80. Banerjee A, Stocche RM, Angle P, et al. Preload or coload for spinal anesthesia for elective Cesarean delivery: a meta-analysis. Can J Anaesth 2010;57(1):24–31.
81. Dyer RA, Farina Z, Joubert IA, et al. Crystalloid preload versus rapid crystalloid administration after induction of spinal anaesthesia (coload) for elective caesarean section. Anaesth Intensive Care 2004;32(3):351–7.
82. Ueyama H, He YL, Tanigami H, et al. Effects of crystalloid and colloid preload on blood volume in the parturient undergoing spinal anesthesia for elective Cesarean section. Anesthesiology 1999;91(6):1571–6.
83. Mercier FJ. Fluid loading for cesarean delivery under spinal anesthesia: have we studied all the options? Anesth Analg 2011;113(4):677–80.
84. Teoh WH, Sia AT. Colloid preload versus coload for spinal anesthesia for cesarean delivery: the effects on maternal cardiac output. Anesth Analg 2009;108(5):1592–8.
85. McDonald S, Fernando R, Ashpole K, et al. Maternal cardiac output changes after crystalloid or colloid coload following spinal anesthesia for elective cesarean delivery: a randomized controlled trial. Anesth Analg 2011;113(4):803–10.
86. Tawfik MM, Tarbay AI, Elaidy AM, et al. Combined colloid preload and crystalloid coload versus crystalloid coload during spinal anesthesia for cesarean delivery: a randomized controlled trial. Anesth Analg 2019;128(2):304–12.
87. Lee AJ, Landau R. Aortocaval compression syndrome: time to revisit certain dogmas. Anesth Analg 2017;125(6):1975–85.

88. Scott DB, Kerr MG. Inferior vena caval pressure in late pregnancy. J Obstet Gynaecol Br Commonw 1963;70:1044–9.
89. Higuchi H, Takagi S, Zhang K, et al. Effect of lateral tilt angle on the volume of the abdominal aorta and inferior vena cava in pregnant and nonpregnant women determined by magnetic resonance imaging. Anesthesiology 2015; 122(2):286–93.
90. Holmes F. Incidence of the supine hypotensive syndrome in late pregnancy. A clinical study in 500 subjects. J Obstet Gynaecol Br Emp 1960;67:254–8.
91. Simpson KR, James DC. Efficacy of intrauterine resuscitation techniques in improving fetal oxygen status during labor. Obstet Gynecol 2005;105(6): 1362–8.
92. Lipman S, Cohen S, Einav S, et al. The Society for Obstetric Anesthesia and Perinatology consensus statement on the management of cardiac arrest in pregnancy. Anesth Analg 2014;118(5):1003–16.
93. Jeejeebhoy FM, Zelop CM, Lipman S, et al. Cardiac arrest in pregnancy: a scientific statement from the American Heart Association. Circulation 2015; 132(18):1747–73.
94. Ansari I, Wallace G, Clemetson CA, et al. Tilt caesarean section. J Obstet Gynaecol Br Commonw 1970;77(8):713–21.
95. Crawford JS, Burton M, Davies P. Time and lateral tilt at Caesarean section. Br J Anaesth 1972;44(5):477–84.
96. Clemetson CA, Hassan R, Mallikarjuneswara VR, et al. Tilt-bend cesarean section. Obstet Gynecol 1973;42(2):290–8.
97. Downing JW, Coleman AJ, Mahomedy MC, et al. Lateral table tilt for Caesarean section. Anaesthesia 1974;29(6):696–703.
98. Aust H, Koehler S, Kuehnert M, et al. Guideline-recommended 15° left lateral table tilt during cesarean section in regional anesthesia - practical aspects. An observational study. J Clin Anesth 2016;32:47–53.
99. Lee AJ, Landau R, Mattingly JL, et al. Left lateral table tilt for elective cesarean delivery under spinal anesthesia has no effect on neonatal acid-base status: a randomized controlled trial. Anesthesiology 2017;127(2):241–9.
100. Farber MK, Bateman BT. Phenylephrine infusion: driving a wedge in our practice of left uterine displacement? Anesthesiology 2017;127(2):212–4.

Anesthesia for Urgent Cesarean Section

Nicole L. Fernandes, MBChB, DA (SA), FCA (SA), Robert A. Dyer, MBChB, FCA (SA), PhD*

KEYWORDS

- Anesthesia • Urgent • Emergency • Cesarean • Fetal compromise

KEY POINTS

- The management of maternal comorbidities and the compromised fetus at urgent cesarean section (CS) requires precise teamwork and communication, where the anesthesiologist has a central role.
- Urgency of CS is best described as a continuum of risk. The decision-to-delivery interval (DDI) is an important audit tool in safe maternal management and neonatal outcomes.
- Although general anesthesia (GA) shortens the DDI, the risk to the mother and fetus is higher.
- Regional anesthesia (RA) is safely performed in the emergency setting, provided no contraindications exist, without compromising neonatal outcomes.
- Anesthesia for urgent CS always requires an individualized approach, taking into consideration specific high-risk clinical scenarios.

INTRODUCTION

Over the past 30 years, the rate of delivery by cesarean section (CS) has steadily increased, in high-, middle-, and low-income countries. Many countries have exceeded the optimal cesarean delivery rate of 10% to 15% as proposed by the World Health Organization in 1985.[1] Data from Africa show that although cesarean delivery is on the increase, it is still well less than the recommended 15%, and the World Health Organization global survey on maternal and perinatal health in Africa reports an operative delivery rate of only 8.8%. This is likely caused by a lack of access to appropriate surgical interventions, as evidenced by only 73% of facilities participating in the survey offered cesarean delivery.[2] It is well established that maternal mortality is higher in areas where the overall rate of delivery by CS is lower than recommended standards.

The authors have nothing to disclose.
Department of Anaesthesia and Perioperative Medicine, University of Cape Town, Groote Schuur Hospital, D23 Groote Schuur Hospital, Anzio Road, Observatory, Cape Town 7925, South Africa
* Corresponding author.
E-mail address: Robert.dyer@uct.ac.za

In terms of perioperative maternal mortality, Gebhardt and colleagues[3] reported that in South Africa specific areas of concern were hemorrhage during or after CS; hypertensive disorders of pregnancy; puerperal sepsis; and importantly, anesthesia-related deaths. This phenomenon is probably caused by a lack of skills, and inexperienced staff. This is also true in the overall African context, where obstetric hemorrhage and anesthesia expertise have recently been identified as major challenges.[4]

Considering the multiple maternal comorbidities and often compromised fetal biophysical profile, particularly in limited-resource environments, it is of the utmost importance that the anesthesia practitioner is familiar with the management of urgent and emergency anesthesia. A knowledge of the classification of urgency of caesarean delivery, and the diagnosis and management of maternal comorbidities indicating urgent operative delivery, and fetal compromise, is not only the ambit of the obstetrician, but requires precise teamwork and communication.[5] This narrative review discusses how anesthesiologist may influence maternal and neonatal outcome, by choosing the most appropriate method of anesthesia for maternal safety, and achieving timeous delivery to reduce fetal morbidity. Novel issues are addressed, related to anesthesia training for emergency delivery.

URGENCY OF CESAREAN SECTION

The most widely adopted classification system of urgency of CS is the four-point classification described by Lucas and colleagues[6] in 2000. This was subsequently endorsed for use by the Royal College of Obstetricians and Gynecologists (RCOG) and the National Institute for Health and Care Excellence in 2004. **Table 1** describes the categories of urgency in detail, which are best regarded as a continuum of risk.[7] To date, no more comprehensive classification of the urgency of CS has been described.

THE IMPORTANCE OF THE DECISION-TO-DELIVERY INTERVAL

Considerable early literature suggests that much of the damage to the fetal brain that precipitates hypoxic ischemic encephalopathy and cerebral palsy is antepartum, and often beyond the control of the obstetrician and anesthesiologist. However, a landmark paper on MRI and post mortem in 351 infants with neonatal encephalopathy and/or early seizures, has shown evidence for acute injury in 80% of infants.[8] This highlights the importance of timely responses to intrapartum hypoxia.

The decision-to-delivery interval (DDI) is the time taken from recognition of an abnormality on fetal heart tracing using cardiotocography and decision to proceed with operative delivery, to the time of delivery of the fetus. International guidelines from the American College of Obstetricians and Gynecologists and RCOG agree on maximum DDI of 30 minutes in urgent cases.[9,10] The RCOG further expands on their guidelines, stating that category 1 patients should have a DDI no longer than 30 minutes, but delivery in category 2 and 3 CS is safely achieved within 75 minutes of decision-making.[10] However, the National Institute for Health and Care Excellence Guidelines emphasize that these times are for audit standards only, and not a strict judgment of practice in individual cases. There may be conflicting concerns regarding the safe management of mother and baby; expediting delivery with a view to improve neonatal outcomes may compromise thoroughness and care in maternal management. The ideal DDI in clinical practice is unknown, with the suggested time intervals in the current literature all based on observational data. It is difficult to draw firm conclusions on neonatal outcome based on the DDI alone. Although some authors report improved outcomes if delivery is completed within 30 minutes,[11] others have found no difference, until DDI exceeds 75 minutes, by which time a significantly lower 5-minute

Table 1
Categories of urgency for cesarean section

Category	Definition	Indications
1	Immediate threat to life of mother or fetus	Placental abruption, uterine rupture, active bleeding, severe fetal distress, and cord prolapse
2	Maternal or fetal compromise that is not immediately life threatening	Breech presentation, previous CS, and nonreassuring fetal status
3	No maternal or fetal compromise, but needs early delivery	Low amniotic fluid index, previous CS, not in labor
4	At a time to suit the mother and the maternity team	

Adapted from Lucas DN, Yentis SM, Kinsella SM et al. Urgency of caesarean section: a new classification. J R Soc Med. 2000;93 (7): 346 – 50; with permission.

Apgar score is noted, and the chance of maternal admission to a high-care setting is 50% higher.[12]

Factors influencing the DDI vary greatly between obstetric units. A recent randomized trial in a middle-income country comparing vasopressors for spinal hypotension during category 1 to 3 CS in patients with preeclampsia and fetal compromise reported DDI as a secondary outcome. Patients with fetal bradycardia were excluded. DDI was 62 minutes and 70 minutes, respectively, in the two groups of patients.[13] The long mean DDI in this study likely reflects a high-pressure, overburdened system in an underresourced environment.

Obesity has been found to contribute to a longer DDI in category 1 CS, probably because of the more challenging nature of the surgical procedure in this population group. In this study, the contribution of epidural top-up to the reduction of the DDI was also examined, compared with the administration of combined spinal-epidural (CSE) anesthesia. The epidural top-up, when initiated on the labor ward at the time of decision making, was associated with a shorter DDI in all body mass index groups.[14]

An Australian audit of anesthesia for emergency CS reported the time to carry out general anesthesia (GA), epidural top-up, and spinal anesthesia (SA) as 17, 19, and 27 minutes, respectively.[15] A single-center study that compared DDI when GA, SA, or epidural top-up were used, found a similar interval with the two regional anesthesia (RA) options. SA was performed with a combination of bupivacaine, fentanyl, and morphine, whereas epidural top-up was achieved with a combination of ropivacaine and fentanyl. Neonatal outcomes were comparable between the two groups.[16]

Many obstetric units emphasize the importance of decreasing the DDI so as to achieve the 30-minute rule. A high-output obstetrics unit in Tel Aviv instituted a protocol to decrease the DDI over a 54-month period in their institution. They found that simply protocolizing actions following the decision to perform a CS for a nonreassuring fetal heart trace resulted in a shorter DDI and improved early neonatal outcomes. The protocol focused on improving communication between all members of the perioperative team, and practical interventions, such as quick transfer to theater, and emptying the urinary bladder while the abdomen of the patient was being prepared for surgery. The proposed protocol did, however, favor the provision of GA, which may not be the accepted practice in other units worldwide.[17]

A recent review has highlighted the heterogeneity of indications for CS in studies examining the association between DDI and neonatal outcomes.[7] The authors suggest that better evidence could arise from focusing on one indication for CS involving an irreversible cause of neonatal morbidity, such as uterine rupture, where poor outcomes have recently been demonstrated with DDIs greater than 18 minutes.[18] In the setting of placental abruption, an even shorter DDI is necessary to prevent adverse outcomes, with a rapid deterioration of fetal acid base status at approximately 10 minutes.[19]

METHOD OF ANESTHESIA
Risk Versus Benefit

The goals of obstetric anesthesia are to ensure maternal safety and comfort, and the delivery of a healthy infant. When performing purely elective CS, and even in most urgent operative deliveries, RA (spinal, epidural, or CSE) is the preferred and most widely accepted method. This avoids failed tracheal intubation and hypoxemia, and maternal awareness, when CS is performed under GA, and allows for early maternal bonding with her baby, and improved analgesia.

The incidence of failed tracheal intubation in the obstetric population has remained stable over the past 40 years at approximately 1 in 390, with maternal deaths mostly caused by pulmonary aspiration and/or hypoxic brain injury.[20] The recent NAP 5 audit showed that the obstetric population is at high risk for awareness under GA for CS. Risk factors included difficult airway management, obesity, limited time between induction of anesthesia and initiation of surgery, and the high incidence of urgent procedures performed outside normal clinical hours.[21]

Apart from the previously mentioned maternal risks as a result of GA for CS, there are multiple reports of risk to the neonate associated with GA.[22–24] Time to readiness for initiation of operative delivery has been shown to be shorter for GA when compared with SA.[25] A large Australian study showed that, despite more rapid delivery of the neonate, when adjusted for confounding factors, neonates born by category 1 CS under GA were significantly more likely to have a 5-minute Apgar score less than 7, to require respiratory support, and to be admitted to a neonatal intensive care unit, when compared with those delivered under SA.[24] These findings are supported by Edipoglu and colleagues[22] who found that the 1-minute Apgar score was significantly lower in neonates born by CS performed under GA. These authors report RA to be associated with shorter hospital stays, less maternal morbidity, and higher umbilical blood pH values in the neonate. A study by Hein and colleagues[16] found that the DDI for GA was considerably shorter than for SA and epidural top-up, but Apgar scores of less than 7 at 5 minutes were more frequent in GA-exposed neonates. It is, however, likely that poor neonatal outcomes in category 1 GA for CS are in part because of a higher degree of compromise in utero.

Overall, the choice of GA versus RA is governed by maternal comorbidities, urgency, and available equipment and expertise, in the context of obstetric anesthesia practice in the particular country and unit. A decision-analysis study, based on multiple high-quality systematic reviews, has recently evaluated three anesthesia options for the management of parturients with a predicted difficult laryngoscopy at preoperative assessment, in women requiring a category 1 CS for fetal compromise.[25] Options for anesthetic management were rapid sequence induction with videolaryngoscopy, awake fiberoptic intubation, or SA. Krom and colleagues[26] found that the rate of failure using videolaryngoscopy as a first-line intubation technique was extremely low, at 21 per 100,000. The mean time for induction of GA was 100 seconds, as compared with an SA time of 6.3 minutes, and 9 minutes for awake fiberoptic intubation. One can appreciate that the last option may be impracticable in low-resource environments, particularly when neonatal outcome is critically dependent on the time to delivery, such as is the case when there is severe fetal bradycardia.

RECENT ADVANCES
The Airway Algorithm

In recent times the difficult airway algorithm in obstetrics has undergone several improvements to reduce failed intubation.[27] These include early facemask ventilation and placement of a second-generation supraglottic airway (SGA), availability of a videolaryngoscope, release of cricoid pressure if laryngoscopy is difficult, and limiting intubation attempts to two. In addition, the importance of appropriate positioning of the parturient before tracheal intubation, and the potential utility of transnasal humidified rapid insufflation ventilatory exchange, has been recognized.

It is widely accepted that videolaryngoscopy improves the view obtained at laryngoscopy in the nonobstetric population[28] and is an integral tool in the management of initial failed intubation attempts.[29] The Difficult Airway Society, in conjunction with the Obstetric Anaesthetists' Association of the United Kingdom, have developed a set of guidelines for the safe management of the airway in obstetrics. They recommend that a videolaryngoscope be available in the operating room for all obstetric GA cases.[27] The obstetric airway is known to be inherently more difficult than in the general surgical population, and this is often further complicated by such conditions as maternal obesity and preeclampsia.

In obese parturients the ramped position, with the external auditory meatus and sternal notch aligned, has been shown to significantly improve the view at laryngoscopy.[30] In a recent survey, 57% of participants used the ramped position for all women undergoing a rapid sequence induction for CS.[31]

Tan and colleagues[32] recently evaluated the use of high-flow humidified oxygen as an alternative to standard preoxygenation for CS. They found 3 minutes of preoxygenation via high-flow humidified canulae to be inadequate to attain the recommended end-tidal oxygen concentration of greater than 90% before induction. Transnasal humidified rapid insufflation ventilatory exchange has not been widely adopted in obstetric practice as yet, despite its promising results in the nonobstetric literature.[31] The main benefit may be prolongation of time to desaturation after administration of muscle relaxant and ensuing apnea.

Oxygen Supplementation

Oxygen supplementation at CS has been widely studied. A concern is that hyperoxia may lead to the formation of harmful oxygen free radical species. It has, however, been shown that in the setting of urgent RA for CS for fetal compromise supplemental oxygen should be provided, while concurrently using other strategies to improve fetal oxygen delivery. There is no evidence to show increased lipid peroxidation in this population.[33,34] GA for CS is associated with free radical generation, but this is not related to the inspired oxygen concentration.[35]

Postoperative Analgesia

The method of postcesarean analgesia is dependent on the anesthesia technique adopted for urgent CS. RA allows for the safe use of 50 to 100 μg spinal or 3 mg epidural morphine. Transversus abdominis plane blocks are effective in the patient receiving GA, but confer no additional benefit over spinal morphine.[36] A recent advance is the introduction of the ultrasound-guided quadratus lumborum block.[37] Urgent CS does not preclude effective postcesarean analgesia.

URGENT REGIONAL ANESTHESIA

In the recent survey by Kinsella and coworkers[38] on anesthesia practice for category 1 CS, many units performed SA if a labor epidural catheter had not been placed. The number of attempts at insertion was limited to two, with a maximum time for insertion of 5 minutes. To decrease the time spent performing SA, while avoiding the risks of GA, the concept of the rapid sequence SA (RSSA) has been developed, which aims to perform SA with only the essential equipment and limit the number of attempts at insertion. Kinsella and colleagues[39] suggest only one attempt at SA, and encourage the notion of the rapid adoption of the next option, as after a limited number of attempts at tracheal intubation (**Box 1**). The addition of opioids to the spinal injectate is also an area for consideration. Standard practice in the United Kingdom is to use diamorphine as an adjunct to SA. This is, however, not readily available as a low-dose preparation and requires dilution before injection, which is time-consuming. Therefore, the opioid of choice in the performance of RSSA is fentanyl, 50 μg/mL.

In a recent series of 25 patients who required category 1 CS and received RSSA, 22 had severe fetal compromise as assessed by an abnormal fetal heart tracing, and the remaining three presented with cord prolapse.[39] The DDI was 22.5 minutes, and the median time from spinal injection until readiness for surgery, as assessed by the sensory level, was 4 minutes. The authors cautioned against the practice of RSSA by novice anesthesia providers. It is important to assess at the outset whether SA may be difficult to achieve, in which case GA may be preferred. Concerns were that three women reported pain on initiation of surgery requiring conversion to GA, and the abandonment of strict asepsis raises questions regarding safety. For these reasons RSSA is not uniformly supported at this point.[40]

Further RA options are CSE, and top-up of an existing labor epidural catheter for anesthesia purposes. CSE has been found to be more time-consuming than either SA or epidural anesthesia alone in the elective and emergency setting.[41]

Many protocols exist for the extension of labor epidural analgesia for emergency CS. Meta-analysis shows that the fastest onset of surgical anesthesia is achieved with the administration of 2% lignocaine with epinephrine and fentanyl. The use of ropivacaine, 0.75%, results in the lowest requirement for intraoperative supplementation of the epidural block. Bupivacaine and levobupivacaine, 0.5%, were found to be the least favorable with respect to speed of onset and quality of block.[42] All included

---

Box 1
Components of rapid sequence spinal anesthesia

- Other staff members to secure intravenous access and apply monitoring; spinal dose not to be injected before intravenous cannula is secured
- Preoxygenate during attempt, for more rapid conversion to GA
- Adopt "no-touch" technique (gloves only, no gown necessary). Skin prepared with a single wipe of 0.5% chlorhexidine solution
- Consider omitting intrathecal opioid if this adds unnecessary delay
- If no opioid, consider increased dose of hyperbaric bupivacaine, 0.5%, up to 3 mL
- Surgery is commenced when sensory block is higher than the T10 level, and ascending
- All equipment prepared and staff ready to convert to GA

Data from Dongare PA, Nataraj MS. Anaesthetic management of obstetric emergencies. Indian J Anaesth. 2018;62(9):704-709.

studies in the meta-analysis using a lignocaine top-up with or without fentanyl had a median onset time of 15 minutes. Despite being common practice, this is not a well-studied area of obstetric anesthesia, and the meta-analysis is difficult to interpret because of the heterogeneity of practice protocols, in the administration and assessment of the level of epidural blockade.

SPECIFIC CLINICAL CONDITIONS: URGENT SPINAL ANESTHESIA
Preeclampsia

After early fears concerning intravascular volume depletion and theoretic risks of hypotension, research in the past 25 years has confirmed the safety of SA in preeclampsia in the absence of contraindications to RA. SA is associated with mild afterload reduction, and a lower vasopressor requirement than in healthy patients.[43] In the only randomised trial comparing GA and SA in patients with preeclampsia and a non-reassuring fetal heart trace, fetal base deficit was higher in the SA group.[44] However, ephedrine, which is associated with more fetal acid-base disturbance, was used more often in the SA group. Modern practice ensuring tight control of blood pressure using phenylephrine might eliminate this difference.

A recent observational study reported favorable outcomes after SA for CS in severe preeclampsia, as evidenced by a lower requirement for maternal critical care support and better neonatal outcomes.[45] These results are, however, difficult to interpret. The patients managed under GA in this cohort were more likely to require blood pressure control with labetalol before induction, possibly indicating more severe disease. The mean gestational age was also lower in the parturients who received GA and the most frequent indication for GA was cited as severe fetal compromise. A further large study, involving a cohort of more than 300,000 women, found that GA for CS in preeclampsia was associated with a greater than two-fold increase in the risk of stroke when compared with SA. This was, however, not a randomized trial, and despite attempts by the authors to correct for confounders, it is likely that the results reflect that patients receiving GA had more severe disease.[46]

Cardiac Disease

Most peripartum cardiac comorbidities (congenital or acquired) may be safely managed under carefully conducted RA, with GA reserved for specific, individualized indications. Wherever possible, a multidisciplinary team in a specialized unit should manage such patients throughout pregnancy. Ideally, patients with advanced cardiac lesions should have carefully planned elective caesarean delivery, including serial echocardiography assessments. However, sudden deterioration of maternal or fetal condition may precipitate urgent CS, and GA may be necessary if the patient is anticoagulated, or if mechanical ventilation, complex cardiac interventions, or extracorporeal membrane oxygenation are required. A thorough understanding of risk categories and pathophysiology are required, as outlined in a recent extensive review.[47]

Premature Delivery

The EPIPAGE studies examined neurodevelopmental outcomes in preterm babies in nine hospitals in France in 1997. A secondary analysis found that in infants of less than 33 weeks gestation, SA was associated with a higher mortality than GA (12.2% vs 10%). However, the data are from a nonrandomized study with many confounding variables, including anesthesia technique and vasopressor use.[48]

Choice of Vasopressor for Urgent Cesarean Section

Spinal hypotension is a common management challenge during CS, and is a major concern for maternal safety and comfort, and neonatal outcome. The most commonly used agents in clinical practice are the mixed α and β agonist ephedrine and the α agonist phenylephrine. Recent research has confirmed that in healthy parturients ephedrine results in significant neonatal acidosis, when compared with phenylephrine.[49] This is likely caused by stimulation of fetal β-adrenergic receptors resulting in an increased metabolic rate.

There are limited data in the setting of urgent delivery. In 2008, Ngan Kee and colleagues[50] conducted a randomized controlled trial evaluating the effects of ephedrine versus phenylephrine in SA for urgent CS. They reported no difference in markers of neonatal acidemia; however, only a small proportion of the deliveries were performed because of fetal compromise. A smaller study, including only patients with severe fetal compromise, showed similar rates of neonatal acidemia in the study groups, but significantly more nausea and vomiting in the ephedrine group, which compromised maternal comfort.[51]

The choice of vasopressor is based on fetal and maternal considerations. A recent randomized trial found the choice vasopressor does not influence fetal acid-base status in cesarean delivery for a nonreassuring fetal heart tracing in preeclampsia,[13] and concluded that the management should be based on maternal hemodynamic responses. In a further randomized trial on SA for urgent cesarean delivery for a maternal indication in preeclampsia, phenylephrine, 50 μg, has been shown to be more effective than ephedrine, 15 mg, in restoring systemic vascular resistance. Phenylephrine is therefore preferred in the management of most cases of spinal hypotension in women with preeclampsia, in the absence of systolic heart failure.

URGENT GENERAL ANESTHESIA

There are instances where SA is ineffective, or contraindicated. Failed SA requires conversion to GA in urgent cases. Primary indications for GA may be maternal, fetal, or combined. The commonest maternal indications include severe hemorrhage, thrombocytopenia and/or coagulopathy, and cardiorespiratory compromise. Abnormal placentation, which often gives rise to urgent CS, was previously considered a relative contraindication to SA. However, CS has for the past 25 years been safely performed under SA in select groups of this population.[52] The patient presenting with hemorrhage requires context-sensitive management. Some well-equipped units with immediate access to advanced obstetric interventions may offer such patients RA, but for most parturients in whom severe hemorrhage is anticipated, GA is likely to be a safer option.[53]

A survey carried out in the United Kingdom[38] found that 54% of category 1 CS were performed under GA. The authors noted that in larger units there was a trend toward lower rates of GA. The most frequently cited reason for the choice of GA in category 1 CS was that it was the default option in such cases. Some units had specific indications for the choice of GA ahead of RA, including cord prolapse, placental abruption, uterine rupture, and fetal bradycardia.

The choice of induction agent for emergency CS seems to have no significant effect on neonatal outcomes. Recent work has shown that Apgar scores are no different in neonates born to mothers induced with propofol when compared with thiopental. This was despite a longer time to delivery noted in the thiopental group.[54] The choice of induction agent should be based on the clinical situation, maternal hemodynamics, and experience of the anesthesia provider with the agent.

SAFETY CONCERNS IN THE PRACTICE OF GENERAL ANESTHESIA
Resources and Training

A concern in low- and middle-income countries is the lack of resources (human and infrastructural) to provide safe GA to women requiring cesarean delivery. A program for the training of nonphysician practitioners in the provision of GA for CS has been rolled out across Kenya. The ESM-Ketamine program consists of training of appropriate practitioners, including nurse midwives, to safely administer anesthesia with a prepackaged GA toolbox. This includes ketamine as the induction agent and a range of airway management devices. An audit of the service found no serious adverse events, with no deaths being attributed to anesthesia-related complications; however, this was a small cohort of 109 patients and larger series are awaited to establish patient safety.[55]

Even in high- and middle-income countries, high rates of SA performed for CS has led to a lack of skills, especially among junior trainees, in the safe provision of GA for CS. Anesthesia training is continuously evolving. Simulation has become an integral part of anesthesia trainee curricula worldwide. It has been shown in meta-analysis that simulation training improves clinical skills and knowledge in the short and long term.[56] Work from two American training institutions[57,58] has evaluated the usefulness of simulation training among trainees on their obstetric anesthesia rotation. Ortner and colleagues[58] specifically evaluated the performance of trainees when performing GA for emergency CS. They found that the institution of a structured simulation learning program led to retention of these skills for 8 months post-training. The level of expertise attained was found to be at that of an attending obstetric anesthetist.

Training programs, such as the Safer Anesthesia from Education obstetrics and pediatrics, and the Essential Steps in the Management of Obstetric Emergencies course aim to ensure sound obstetric anesthesia care through the provision of factual knowledge, while emphasizing the acquisition of clinical and nontechnical skills.[59]

The Use of a Supraglottic Airway During Emergency Cesarean Section

The Difficult Airway Society advocates the use of an SGA as a rescue device in the event of failed intubation in obstetrics.[27] Many studies have explored the use of SGA as a first-line airway device in GA for CS without severe fetal compromise.[60–62] All of the current work has been performed with second-generation SGAs, based on the concept that higher sealing pressures and a gastric suction port is protective against the higher risk of pulmonary aspiration in parturients. No adverse events, airway or otherwise, have been reported by any of the authors. This work is, however, all observational in nature and remains controversial, not having been widely adopted into current accepted clinical practice, particularly in limited-resource environments.

A single, retrospective observational study has been conducted evaluating the use of an SGA for emergency cesarean delivery.[63] The supreme LMA, also a second-generation device, was used in all patients. Outcomes measured were adverse events related to the device, maternal mortality, and neonatal outcomes. The authors reported successful use in 1039 deliveries, with no maternal laryngospasm, bronchospasm, regurgitation, aspiration, or death reported. Neonatal outcomes were similar to those in other studies conducted on outcomes in GA for CS, with a 5-minute Apgar score of 7 to 10 in most cases. However, most patients had a normal body mass index, and no details were supplied of patients with recent oral intake or symptoms of gastroesophageal reflux, in whom there would surely have been a low threshold for tracheal intubation. No randomized controlled trials exist to support the routine use of an SGA for urgent GA for CS, other than in the emergency failed intubation scenario. The overwhelming body of clinical opinion would be that rapid sequence induction with endotracheal intubation remains the safest management option in emergency GA for CS.

SPECIFIC CLINICAL CONDITIONS: URGENT GENERAL ANESTHESIA
Preeclampsia and Eclampsia

Preeclampsia remains a major perioperative medical challenge, particularly in lower- and middle-income countries, often involving maternal and fetal indications for GA, most commonly HELLP syndrome, hemorrhage, and cardiorespiratory failure. Anesthesiologists are best placed to assess severity of cardiopulmonary involvement,[64,65] resuscitation, perform anesthesia for urgent delivery, and assist in critical care management.

Key issues surrounding urgent operative delivery under GA are:

- Fluid management (usually a restrictive policy, but acute intravascular volume changes are best guided by arterial line placement and transthoracic echocardiography, and seldom central venous or pulmonary artery catheter placement),[66]
- Availability of a videolaryngoscope,
- Obtundation of hypertensive response to intubation,[67,68] and
- Avoidance of nondepolarizing muscle relaxants in patients receiving magnesium sulfate.

The eclamptic patient requires an individualized approach. A South African series[69] found no difference in maternal and neonatal outcomes in women with stable eclampsia who received epidural anesthesia or SA compared with GA for cesarean delivery. This suggests that patients with eclampsia whose seizures have terminated and show no signs of raised intracranial pressure are safely managed with RA. Patients presenting with ongoing, uncontrolled seizures are best managed with GA. Propofol and thiopentone are considered acceptable induction agents because they support favorable neurophysiologic conditions. Mechanical ventilation should be continued after cesarean delivery in patients who have not recovered neurologically, using a sedative with some anticonvulsant activity. An infusion of propofol supplemented with a short-acting opiate is an acceptable alternative to benzodiazepine infusions, which are associated in the nonobstetric setting with more drug accumulation and a potentially longer period of mechanical ventilation. Sedation should be carefully titrated to maintain adequate cerebral perfusion pressure, in view of cerebral edema and raised intracranial pressure.

SUMMARY

Access to urgent caesarean delivery, with adequate surgery and anesthesia skills, is essential for maternal and fetal safety worldwide. Categorization of urgency of CS has generated an important audit tool, namely the 30-minute DDI. Focused studies suggest that a considerably shorter DDI is required in cases of irreversible fetal hypoxia. Some form of decision analysis is required in every case, to estimate the risks and benefits to mother and fetus of GA versus RA. RA for CS has become highly sophisticated, including the rapid performance of SA with tight vasopressor control of maternal hemodynamics, epidural anesthesia, and CSE anesthesia. Indications for GA include maternal anticoagulation, hemorrhage, unstable cardiac disease, complicated preeclampsia, and fetal bradycardia with imminent fetal demise. Physician and nonphysician education, in the clinical and simulation scenarios, is crucial, so that RA is safely practiced, and GA is safely performed if specifically indicated, or should RA fail.

Best Practices

What is the current practice for anesthesia for urgent CS?

CS should be classified by urgency and subsequently performed within prescribed time limits

The DDI is an important audit tool

For category 1 CS, this interval should be less than 30 minutes

RA is safe and effective in urgent CS, unless specific contraindications exist

Specific clinical scenarios (hemorrhage, hypertensive disorders, cardiac disease, obesity, the difficult airway, and severe fetal compromise) require an individualized approach to anesthesia

What changes in current practice are likely to improve outcome?

Access to skilled surgery and anesthesia for CS should be prioritized

Ongoing and improving training, including simulation, is integral to the provision of safe anesthesia for urgent CS

Adherence to the latest difficult airway algorithm may improve outcomes after GA

Major recommendations

RA for CS is favored in the absence of contraindications

All clinicians practicing obstetric anesthesia should understand the indications for and contraindications to RA and GA for CS

Adequate training in both methods is crucial, and continuously updated

There are limited randomized controlled trials on which to base clinical practice

Best references for the previous recommendations.[6,7,15,21,22]

REFERENCES

1. Betran AP, Torloni MR, Zhang J, et al. What is the optimal rate of caesarean section at population level? A systematic review of ecologic studies. Reprod Health 2015;12(7):57.
2. Shah A, Fawole B, M'Imunya JM, et al. Cesarean delivery outcomes from the WHO global survey on maternal and perinatal health in Africa. Int J Gynecol Obstet 2009;107(3):191–7.
3. Gebhardt GS, Fawcus S, Moodley J, et al. Maternal death and caesarean section in South Africa: results from the 2011-2013 saving mothers report of the National Committee for Confidential Enquiries into maternal deaths. S Afr Med J 2015; 105(4):287–91.
4. Bishop D, Dyer RA, Maswime S, et al. Maternal and neonatal outcomes after caesarean delivery in the African Surgical Outcomes Study: a 7-day prospective observational cohort study. Lancet Glob Health 2019;7:e513–22.
5. Moaveni DM, Birnbach DJ, Ranasinghe JS, et al. Fetal assessment for anesthesiologists: are you evaluating the other patient? Anesth Analg 2013;116(6): 1278–92.
6. Lucas DN, Yentis SM, Kinsella SM, et al. Urgency of caesarean section: a new classification. J R Soc Med 2000;93(7):346–50.
7. Tomlinson JH. Lucas DN. Decision-to-delivery interval: is 30 min the magic time? What is the evidence? Does it work? Best Pract Res Clin Anaesthesiol 2017;31(1): 49–56.

8. Cowan F, Rutherford M, Groenendaal F, et al. Origin and timing of brain lesions in term infants with neonatal encephalopathy. Lancet 2003;361(9359):736–42.

9. ACOG. Practice bulletin no. 116: management of intrapartum fetal heart rate tracings. Obstet Gynecol 2010;116(5):1232–40.

10. RCOG. Classification of urgency of caesarean section: a continuum of risk. Good Pract 2010;11(11):1–4.

11. Hillemanns P, Strauss A, Hasbargen U, et al. Crash emergency cesarean section: decision-to-delivery interval under 30 min and its effect on Apgar and umbilical artery pH. Arch Gynecol Obstet 2005;273(3):161–5.

12. Thomas J, Paranjothy S, James D. National cross sectional survey to determine whether the decision to delivery interval is critical in emergency caesarean section. BMJ 2004;328(7441):665.

13. Dyer RA, Emmanuel A, Adams SC, et al. A randomised comparison of bolus phenylephrine and ephedrine for the management of spinal hypotension in patients with severe preeclampsia and fetal compromise. Int J Obstet Anesth 2018;33:23–31.

14. Väänänen AJ, Kainu JP, Eriksson H, et al. Does obesity complicate regional anesthesia and result in longer decision to delivery time for emergency cesarean section? Acta Anaesthesiol Scand 2017;61(6):609–18.

15. Popham P, Buettner A, Mendola M. Anaesthesia for emergency caesarean section, 2000-2004, at the Royal Women's Hospital, Melbourne. Anaesth Intensive Care 2007;35(1):74–9.

16. Hein A, Thalen D, Eriksson Y, et al. The decision to delivery interval in emergency caesarean sections: impact of anaesthetic technique and work shift. F1000Res 2017;6:1977.

17. Weiner E, Bar J, Fainstein N, et al. The effect of a program to shorten the decision-to-delivery interval for emergent cesarean section on maternal and neonatal outcome. Am J Obstet Gynecol 2014;210(3):224.

18. Holmgren C, Scott JR, Porter TF, et al. Uterine rupture with attempted vaginal birth after cesarean delivery: decision-to-delivery time and neonatal outcome. Obstet Gynecol 2012;119(4):725–31.

19. Kayani SI, Walkinshaw SA, Preston C. Pregnancy outcome in severe placental abruption. BJOG 2003;110(7):679–83.

20. Kinsella SM, Winton AL, Mushambi MC, et al. Failed tracheal intubation during obstetric general anaesthesia: a literature review. Int J Obstet Anesth 2015; 24(4):356–74.

21. Pandit JJ, Andrade J, Bogod DG, et al. 5th National Audit Project (NAP5) on accidental awareness during general anaesthesia: summary of main findings and risk factors. Br J Anaesth 2014;113(4):549–59.

22. Edipoglu IS, Celik F, Marangoz EC, et al. Effect of anaesthetic technique on neonatal morbidity in emergency caesarean section for foetal distress. PLoS One 2018;13(11):e0207388.

23. Algert CS, Bowen JR, Giles WB, et al. Regional block versus general anaesthesia for caesarean section and neonatal outcomes: a population-based study. BMC Med 2009;7:20.

24. Beckmann M, Calderbank S. Mode of anaesthetic for category 1 caesarean sections and neonatal outcomes. Aust N Z J Obstet Gynaecol 2012;52(4):316–20.

25. Mccahon RA, Catling S. Time required for surgical readiness in emergency caesarean section: spinal compared with general anaesthesia. Int J Obstet Anesth 2003;12(3):178–82.

26. Krom AJ, Cohen Y, Miller JP, et al. Choice of anaesthesia for category-1 caesarean section in women with anticipated difficult tracheal intubation: the use of decision analysis. Anaesthesia 2017;72:156–71.

27. Mushambi MC, Kinsella SM, Popat M, et al. Obstetric Anaesthetists' Association and Difficult Airway Society guidelines for the management of difficult and failed tracheal intubation in obstetrics. Anaesthesia 2015;70(11):1286–306.

28. Healy DW, Maties O, Hovord D, et al. A systematic review of the role of video-laryngoscopy in successful orotracheal intubation. BMC Anesthesiol 2012; 12:32.

29. Frerk C, Mitchell VS, McNarry AF, et al. Difficult Airway Society 2015 guidelines for management of unanticipated difficult intubation in adults. Br J Anaesth 2015; 115(6):827–48.

30. Soens MA, Birnbach DJ, Ranasinghe JS, et al. Obstetric anesthesia for the obese and morbidly obese patient: an ounce of prevention is worth more than a pound of treatment. Acta Anaesthesiol Scand 2008;52(1):6–19.

31. Desai N, Wicker J, Sajayan A, et al. A survey of practice of rapid sequence induction for caesarean section in England. Int J Obstet Anesth 2018;36:3–10.

32. Tan PCF, Millay OJ, Leeton L, et al. High-flow humidified nasal preoxygenation in pregnant women: a prospective observational study. Br J Anaesth 2018;122(1): 86–91.

33. Meyersfeld N, Ngan-Kee WD, Segal S, et al. Oxygen at caesarean section: too much of a good thing? South Afr J Anaesth Analg 2014;20(5):4–6.

34. Khaw KS, Wang CC, Ngan Kee WD, et al. Supplementary oxygen for emergency caesarean section under regional anaesthesia. Br J Anaesth 2009;102(1):90–6.

35. Khaw KS, Ngan Kee WD, Chu CY, et al. Effects of different inspired oxygen fractions on lipid peroxidation during general anaesthesia for elective caesarean section. Br J Anaesth 2010;105(3):355–60.

36. Champaneria R, Shah L, Wilson MJ, et al. Clinical effectiveness of transversus abdominis plane (TAP) blocks for pain relief after caesarean section: a meta-analysis. Int J Obstet Anesth 2016;28:45–60.

37. Krohg A, Ullensvang K, Rosseland LA, et al. The analgesic effect of ultrasound-guided quadratus lumborum block after cesarean delivery: a randomized clinical trial. Anesth Analg 2018;126(2):559–65.

38. Kinsella SM, Walton B, Sashidharan R, et al. Category-1 caesarean section: a survey of anaesthetic and peri-operative management in the UK. Anaesthesia 2010; 65(4):362–8.

39. Kinsella SM, Girgirah K, Scrutton MJL. Rapid sequence spinal anaesthesia for category-1 urgency caesarean section: a case series. Anaesthesia 2010;65(7): 664–9.

40. Hurford DM, De Zoysa N. Rapid sequence spinal anaesthesia: a survey of current use. Anaesthesia 2012;67(11):1284–5.

41. Gonzales Fiol A, Meng ML, Danhakl V, et al. A study of factors influencing surgical cesarean delivery times in an academic tertiary center. Int J Obstet Anesth 2018; 34:50–5.

42. Hillyard SG, Bate TE, Corcoran TB, et al. Extending epidural analgesia for emergency caesarean section: a meta-analysis. Br J Anaesth 2011;107(5):668–78.

43. Dyer RA, Piercy JL, Reed AR, et al. Hemodynamic changes associated with spinal anesthesia for cesarean delivery in severe preeclampsia. Anesthesiology 2008;108(5):802–11.

44. Dyer RA, Els I, Farbas J, et al. Prospective , randomized trial comparing general with spinal anesthesia for cesarean delivery in preeclamptic patients with a non-reassuring fetal heart trace. Anesthesiology 2003;3:561–9.

45. Chattopadhyay S, Das A, Pahari S. Fetomaternal outcome in severe preeclamptic women undergoing emergency cesarean section under either general or spinal anesthesia. J Pregnancy 2014;2014:325098.

46. Huang CJ, Fan YC, Tsai PS. Differential impacts of modes of anaesthesia on the risk of stroke among preeclamptic women who undergo caesarean delivery: a population-based study. Br J Anaesth 2010;105(6):818–26.

47. Arendt KW, Lindley KJ. Obstetric anesthesia management of the patient with cardiac disease. Int J Obstet Anesth 2019;37:73–85.

48. Laudenbach V, Mercier FJ, Rozé JC, et al. Anaesthesia mode for caesarean section and mortality in very preterm infants: an epidemiologic study in the EPIPAGE cohort. Int J Obstet Anesth 2009;18(2):142–9.

49. Veeser M, Hofmann T, Roth R, et al. Vasopressors for the management of hypotension after spinal anesthesia for elective caesarean section. Systematic review and cumulative meta-analysis. Acta Anaesthesiol Scand 2012;56(7):810–6.

50. Ngan Kee WD, Khaw KS, Lau TK, et al. Randomised double-blinded comparison of phenylephrine vs ephedrine for maintaining blood pressure during spinal anaesthesia for non-elective caesarean section. Anaesthesia 2008;63(12): 1319–26.

51. Jain K, Makkar JK, Subramani Vp S, et al. A randomized trial comparing prophylactic phenylephrine and ephedrine infusion during spinal anesthesia for emergency cesarean delivery. J Clin Anesth 2016;34:208–15.

52. Parekh N, Husaini SW, Russell IF. Caesarean section for placenta praevia: a retrospective study of anaesthetic management. Br J Anaesth 2000;84(6):725–30.

53. Beilin Y. Maternal hemorrhage: regional versus general anesthesia. Anesth Analg 2018;127(4):805–7.

54. Tumukunde J, Lomangisi DD, Davidson O, et al. Effects of propofol versus thiopental on Apgar scores in newborns and peri-operative outcomes of women undergoing emergency cesarean section: a randomized clinical trial. BMC Anaesthesiol 2015;15:63.

55. Burke TF, Nelson BD, Kandler T, et al. International Journal of Gynecology and Obstetrics Evaluation of a ketamine-based anesthesia package for use in emergency cesarean delivery or emergency laparotomy when no anesthetist is available. Int J Gynecol Obstet 2018;135(3):295–8.

56. Lorello GR, Cook DA, Johnson RL, et al. Simulation-based training in anaesthesiology: a systematic review and meta-analysis. Br J Anaesth 2014;112(2):231–45.

57. Scavone BM, Toledo P, Higgins N, et al. A randomized controlled trial of the impact of simulation-based training on resident performance during a simulated obstetric anesthesia emergency. Simul Healthc 2010;5(6):320–4.

58. Ortner CM, Richebé P, Bollag LA, et al. Repeated simulation-based training for performing general anesthesia for emergency cesarean delivery: long-term retention and recurring mistakes. Int J Obstet Anesth 2014;23(4):341–7.

59. Vasco M, Pandya S, Van Dyk D, et al. Maternal critical care in resource-limited settings. Narrative review. Int J Obstet Anesth 2019;37:86–95.

60. Han TH, Brimacombe J, Lee EJ, et al. The laryngeal mask airway is effective (and probably safe) in selected healthy parturients for elective cesarean section: a prospective study of 1067 cases. Can J Anaesth 2001;48(11):1117–21.

61. Yao WY, Li SY, Sng BL, et al. The LMA Supreme in 700 parturients undergoing cesarean delivery: an observational study. Can J Anaesth 2012;59(7):648–54.

62. Li SY, Yao WY, Yuan YJ, et al. Supreme laryngeal mask airway use in general anesthesia for category 2 and 3 cesarean delivery: a prospective cohort study. BMC Anesthesiol 2017;17:169.

63. Fang X, Xiao Q, Xie Q, et al. General anesthesia with the use of SUPREME laryngeal mask airway for emergency cesarean delivery: a retrospective analysis of 1039 parturients. Sci Rep 2018;8(1):13098.

64. Hofmeyr R, Matjila M, Dyer R. Preeclampsia in 2017: obstetric and anaesthesia management. Best Pract Res Clin Anaesthesiol 2017;31(1):125–38.

65. Ortner CM, Krishnamoorthy V, Neethling E, et al. Point-of-care ultrasound abnormalities in late-onset severe preeclampsia: prevalence and association with serum albumin and brain natriuretic peptide. Anesth Analg 2019;128(6):1208–16.

66. Pretorius T, Van Rensburg G, Dyer RA, et al. The influence of fluid management on outcomes in preeclampsia: a systematic review and meta-analysis. Int J Obstet Anesth 2018;34:85–95.

67. Pant M, Fong R, Scavone B. Prevention of peri-induction hypertension in preeclamptic patients: a focused review. Anesth Analg 2014;119(6):1350–6.

68. James MF, Dyer RA. Prevention of peri-induction hypertension in pre-eclamptic patients. Anesth Analg 2015;121(6):1678–9.

69. Moodley J, Jjuuko G, Rout C. Epidural compared with general anaesthesia for caesarean delivery in conscious women with eclampsia. Br J Obstet Gynaecol 2001;108(4):378–82.

Anesthesia for Fetal Surgery and Fetal Procedures

Laurence E. Ring, MD[a],*, Yehuda Ginosar, BSc, MBBS[b,c]

KEYWORDS

- Fetal anesthesia • Fetal surgery • Congenital defects

KEY POINTS

- Before providing a fetal anesthetic, significant consideration must be given to the ethics of fetal surgery, specifically what qualifies a fetus as a "fetal patient."
- Fetal surgeries may be performed during a periviable period of the late second to early third trimester, through either minimally invasive or open approaches.
- Fetal surgeries may also be performed at the time of cesarean delivery using the ex utero intrapartum treatment procedure.
- Knowledge of physiologic changes of pregnancy, uteroplacental perfusion, and fetal physiology is crucial in providing a safe and effective anesthetic.
- The surgical approach and gestational age of the fetus are key factors used in the determination of specific aspects of the anesthetic approach.

INTRODUCTION

The past 20 years have seen advances in surgical technique and technology that have allowed surgeons and obstetricians to push the boundaries of interventional therapies available to fetuses with congenital and developmental abnormalities. Here we define fetal anesthesia as the anesthetic delivered at the time of fetal surgery; that is, the anesthetic provided to the pregnant mother, or the anesthesia administered directly to the fetus, or both. Sitting at the nexus of obstetric and pediatric anesthesia, anesthesiologists providing fetal anesthesia must be well-acquainted with general concepts of the physiologic changes of pregnancy, placental physiology, and fetal

Disclosures: None.
Financial Support: None.
[a] Columbia University Medical Center, 630 West 168th Street PH-5, New York, NY 10032, USA;
[b] Mother and Child Anesthesia Unit, Department of Anesthesiology, Critical Care, and Pain Medicine, Hebrew University – Hadassah School of Medicine, Anesthesia Research Institute, The Wohl Institute for Translational Medicine, Hadassah Hebrew University Medical Center, Ein Karem Campus, POB 12000, Jerusalem 91120, Israel; [c] Division of Obstetric Anesthesiology, Washington University School of Medicine, Barnes Jewish Hospital, 660 South Euclid - Campus Box 8054, St Louis, MO 63110-1093, USA
* Corresponding author.
E-mail address: Ler20@cumc.columbia.edu

0095-5108/19/© 2019 Elsevier Inc. All rights reserved.

anatomy and neurodevelopment, as well as any concerns specific to the fetal surgical procedures. This review focuses on the types of and indications for fetal surgeries currently being performed, the unique maternal and fetal aspects of physiology that impact a fetal anesthetic, and finally, the actual provision of the fetal anesthetic.

THE ETHICS OF FETAL SURGERY

Before considering any of the specifics of fetal surgeries and fetal anesthesia, it is imperative that the ethics surrounding these procedures be first considered. The very idea of fetal surgery, especially on a previable fetus, is an ethical quagmire. For anesthesiologists, especially, the question of establishing fetal patient-hood, and the rigor it demands, is crucial. In a much cited ethical argument, Chervenak and McCoullough[1] describe the previable fetus as a "cipher," a zero. It has no possibility of existing outside of the uterus, they argue, and hence no independent moral status. They further argue that what establishes moral status for the fetus is the idea that the fetus, later as a child and eventually as an adult will achieve independent moral status. Hence viability, or the gestational age at which scientific and technologic advance may support the life of a neonate ex utero, establishes the fetus as a fetal patient. Likewise, a pregnant woman's autonomy and commitment to not terminating her pregnancy, thereby eventually bringing her fetus to term (and presumably to birth, childhood, etc) imbues the fetus with moral status.[1] Put another way, the "dependent moral status of the fetus" depends on "whether it is reliably expected later to achieve the relatively unambiguous moral status of becoming a child and, still later, the more unambiguous moral status of becoming a person."[2]

The rationale for moral status is important, because it provides a framework for addressing the personal risk that a pregnant woman must understand before consenting to fetal surgery and anesthesia. Every fetal surgery necessarily involves some risk to the pregnant woman. A recent meta-analysis found a maternal severe complication rate (hemorrhage, hysterectomy, sepsis, or maternal cardiac arrest, among others) of almost 5% in open fetal surgeries and about 1.5% in fetoscopic surgeries.[3] Furthermore, the patient's expectations and the measurement of success or failure of a fetal surgery should be carefully defined during the consent process. Depending on the primary fetal abnormality and outcome of the intervention, a fetus may:

1. Suffer significant injury owing to the surgical intervention, in some cases converting a viable pregnancy in to a nonviable one.
2. Fail to respond to the surgical intervention, neither worsening nor improving outcomes.
3. Have a "successful" intervention, avoiding in utero demise or early neonatal death, but nevertheless being born with severe morbidity and a devastating life trajectory. In some cases, this may be considered as a worse outcome, with a more profound impact on the family and on society.
4. Have a successful intervention, but still require neonatal surgical intervention.
5. Have a successful intervention with either no morbidity or acceptable morbidity and a good future life trajectory.

Because many fetal procedures remain in experimental or early clinical stages, all participating surgical and anesthesia staff must be meticulous in their collection and presentation of current data on the risks, benefits, and alternatives. New fetal care programs should consider getting local institutional review board approval for fetal surgeries and should ensure that their procedures follow basic beneficence-based obligations to both the mother and fetus.

Ultimately, the decision to perform fetal surgery should be made by the mother, based on the best available evidence. Caregivers should endeavor to guarantee that the consent process is thorough, dispassionate, and nondirective, and that it presents alternatives to fetal surgery including termination or postdelivery surgical intervention, where appropriate.

The decision process is inevitably a personal one for the mother (and her partner) and is often affected by their own prior traditional, religious, or even political beliefs, and these concerns are perfectly reasonable and legitimate. It is, however, important also to appreciate that previously held beliefs for theoretic scenarios may be revised or even abandoned by patients when these scenarios become real and personal. Staff should be able to shield patients from pressure brought on them from advocates of these beliefs, even when these are close family members. Ultimately, these complex and difficult decisions are the maternal patient's decision, and hers alone.

TYPES OF FETAL SURGERY

Fetal surgeries can be divided into 2 main categories: (1) surgeries to the fetus or placenta in which imminent delivery is not planned (usually occurring in the late second trimester) and (2) surgeries to the fetus at or around term where immediately after the surgery is completed, delivery is planned (summarized in **Table 1**).

With some crossover, fetal surgeries in which imminent delivery is not planned can be subdivided into 2 approaches: minimally invasive and open procedures. Generally, minimally invasive procedures present less maternal risk, but direct fetal risk or risk of preterm labor is not necessarily lower than in open procedures. Minimally invasive procedures fall into either percutaneous needle or endoscopic (fetoscopic) approaches. Although some of these procedures are variations of open surgeries, many minimally invasive procedures were developed de novo and have no open correlate.

Minimally Invasive, Ultrasound-Guided Midgestation Fetal Surgeries

During needle-based procedures, high-fidelity ultrasound examination is used to identify the placental location and fetal structures. Then, using real-time ultrasound guidance, a needle is advanced, percutaneously, through the uterine wall, into the intrauterine space, and ultimately to the structure of interest. A wide range of therapies may be provided directly through the needle, or through a specialized catheter extended through the needle. This approach can be used to access the umbilical vein for fetal blood sampling or transfusion of packed red blood cells in a fetus with hydrops or anemia.

The ultrasound-guided needle technique may also be used to treat prenatally diagnosed plural effusions and congenital cystic adenomatoid malformations. Left untreated, some of these malformations can become large enough to cause mediastinal compression and lung hypoplasia. In cases in which hydrops develops, the prognosis without fetal intervention can be very poor, with at least 1 study reporting a greater than 95% mortality rate.[4] In the largest study of its kind, Peranteau and colleagues[5] reported significantly improved outcomes after ultrasound guided placement of fetal thoracoamniotic shunts in high-risk fetuses, with survival at birth of 68%.

A similar approach of amniotic shunt has been described in the fetal treatment of lower urinary tract obstruction (LUTO). LUTO may be caused by posterior urethral valves (most common), urethral stricture or prune belly syndrome. Resultant oligohydramnios or anhydramnios can lead to lung hypoplasia.[6] The PLUTO study examined the effect of ultrasound-guided placement of a fetal vesicoamniotic shunt versus no fetal treatment with disappointing results. The study found improved 28-day survival

Table 1
Summary of currently preformed fetal surgeries

Indication	Surgery	Approach
Midgestational procedures		
Congenital cystic adenomatoid malformations	Thoracoamniotic shunting	Minimally invasive, ultrasound guided
Lower urinary tract obstruction	Vesicoaminotic shunting	Minimally invasive, ultrasound guided
	Valve ablation (posterior urethral valves)	Fetal cystoscopic
Twin reversed arterial perfusion	Radiofrequency ablation of umbilical cord	Minimally invasive, ultrasound guided
Aortic valve stenosis, pulmonic valve stenosis or hypoplastic left heart syndrome	Balloon valvuloplastyor septoplasty	Minimally invasive, ultrasound guided
Twin–twin transfusion syndrome	Laser ablation of placental anastomosis	Minimally invasive, fetoscopic
Amniotic band syndrome	Ligation of amniotic bands	Minimally invasive, fetoscopic
Congenital diaphragmatic hernia	FETO	Minimally invasive, fetoscopic
Myelomeningocele	Patching of neural tube defect	Most centers currently perform this surgery open; fetoscopic surgery is currently used in several centers.
Sacrococcygeal teratoma	Resection of tumor	Open
Procedures performed at term		
EXIT	Airway management (eg, tracheostomy, intubation, FETO removal, cystic hygroma removal); other surgical procedures have been described.	Open, with planned immediate delivery after the EXIT surgery.

Abbreviation: FETO, fetal endoscopic tracheal occlusion.

in the shunt group, but renal function at 1 and 2 years was poor in both groups. The authors suggest that, at the time of diagnosis of LUTO, damage to the fetal kidneys may already be too significant to be overcome with a shunt.[7] When the cause of LUTO is found to be posterior urethral valves, an endoscopic (fetal cystoscopic) approach has been used to provide treatment. Outcomes for this combination of etiology and treatment have been promising, with an increase in perinatal survival (odds ratio, 20.51[8]) and normal renal function in 75% of those who survive.[9]

Certain complicated monochorionic twin gestations can present an opportunity for highly effective ultrasound-guided fetal surgery. Twin reversed arterial perfusion sequence is a rare abnormality of monochorionic twins that describes a syndrome in which there is 1 normal fetus (pump twin) and 1 dysmorphic fetus with an absent heart, which is incompatible with life. The acardiac fetus receives perfusion from the pump twin, which puts the pump twin at risk for high -output cardiac failure, polyhydramnios, hydrops, and death.[10] In a retrospective review of 10 years of practice and 98 treated twin pairs, ultrasound-guided radiofrequency ablation of the acardiac fetus's umbilical cord was found to result in 80% survival rate of the pump twin, compared with a historical reference of greater than 50% mortality of the pump twin in untreated twin pairs.[11]

Remarkably, the ultrasound-guided percutaneous needle approach can be used to treat certain critical congenital heart malformations. Reserved for only the most severe cases of aortic or pulmonic valve stenosis, or hypoplastic left heart syndrome with a highly restrictive atrial septum, a needle can be used to guide the placement of a balloon catheter through the fetal chest wall, through the fetal myocardium, dilating a restrictive aortic valve, pulmonic valve, or foramen ovale, respectively. In a retrospective study examining outcomes in fetuses who underwent fetal aortic valvuloplasty, Freud Lindsay and colleagues[12] reported biventricular function at birth in more than 30% of neonates who had been treated. Although almost all of these patients required postnatal surgical intervention, there was still a survival benefit seen in the valvuloplasty group over a group of patients with hypoplastic left heart syndrome who did not undergo fetal therapy.

Minimally Invasive, Midgestation Fetoscopic Procedures

Twin–twin transfusion syndrome is a rare, severe complication of monochorionic twin pregnancies that results from an intertwin imbalance of blood flow through placental anastomoses. This syndrome results in 1 fetus experiencing complications of hypovolemia and anemia (oligouria, oligohydramnios, and significant growth restriction) while the other experiences complications of hypervolemia and polycythemia (polyuria, polyhydramnios, hydrops, and cardiac failure). Without treatment, twin–twin transfusion syndrome can result in mortality rates of up to 90%.[13] Laser ablation of the placental anastomoses can reduce mortality to less than 20%. Under fetoscopic vision of the placenta, the proceduralist is able to identify, and with a laser disrupt, blood vessels that transverse the separating membrane of the placenta, obliterating the circulatory connection between the 2 fetuses. Laser ablation for twin–twin transfusion syndrome has proven even more successful that the alternate approach of amnioreduction, with fewer neurologic complications seen in the laser ablation group at 6 months and 6 years of age.[14]

Amniotic band syndrome is a rare condition in which strands of the amniotic sac tangle and constrict fetal parts, which could result in significant deformity. A fetoscopic approach has been described in releasing the bands, especially when they are entangling extremities. For appropriately selected candidates (abnormal but present Doppler flow within the affected extremity), release of the band can result in normal functionality of that extremity at birth.[15] Premature preterm rupture of membranes is very common after the procedure, and the tradeoff of risk for preterm delivery for improvement of a nonlethal deformity must be considered.

Congenital diaphragmatic hernia (CDH) was one of the first fetal malformations to be treated with fetal surgery. The diaphragmatic defect is readily repaired after delivery, but the major complication of CDH is persistent pulmonary hypoplasia owing to inadequate fetal lung inflation in utero. Although the fetus does not breathe in utero, the fetal lungs are inflated with fluid. The pressure exerted by abdominal organs such as the stomach and liver inside the fetal thorax leads to collapse of the developing fetal lung. Theoretically, if the abdominal contents that had herniated into the thorax were to be pushed into the abdomen and the diaphragm repaired early enough in gestation, the developing fetal lung would have significantly more time to develop normally. Historically, an open approach was used to repair CDH, but the results were disappointing. A different approach has been used over the past 20 years that relies on the idea that developing fetal lungs exposed to long periods of upper airway obstruction become hypertrophic.[16] In the early third trimester in an affected fetus, through endoscopic visualization, fetal surgeons are able to advance a balloon occlusive device through the fetal mouth, into the fetal trachea. The balloon is then inflated and left in place for a period of weeks to months (fetal endoscopic tracheal occlusion [FETO]; **Fig. 1**). The occlusive device is generally removed during a second fetoscopic procedure at 32 to 34 weeks of gestation, or occasionally by planned operative delivery (ex utero intrapartum treatment [EXIT] procedure, see Open, Late Gestation Fetal Surgery with Planned Delivery). There is a serious potential risk to the fetus if there is unplanned delivery with the FETO device still located in the trachea, because neonatal breathing will be impossible. Immediate balloon puncture and deflation in an asphyxiating neonate is a highly stressful procedure with a high likelihood of neonatal asphyxia and death. In a 2016 meta-analysis, Al-Maary and colleagues[17] analyzed 5 studies to determine the effectiveness of the FETO procedure versus standard postnatal treatment in fetuses with severe CDH and found the procedure favored survival by an odds ratio more than 13.

Open Midgestation Fetal Surgeries

Fetal repair of myelomenigocele (MMC) is perhaps the most robustly studied major fetal surgery, although controversy exists with regard to the surgical approach. MMC is a congenital defect in which the meninges and spinal cord or nerve roots protrude through a defect of a vertebral arch or arches and the overlying skin. Although folic acid supplementation has deceased the prevalence of MMC, it still has a prevalence of about 1 in 5000 births in the United States.[18] The standard treatment of MMC has been postdelivery closure of the defect at birth. This approach has frequently lead to permanent and significant neurologic defects, as well as high rates ventriculomegaly necessitating a ventriculoperitoneal shunt.[19]

The Management of Myelomeningocele (MoM) study[20] has been a breakthrough in the treatment of myelomeningocele specifically and fetal surgery in general. The 2011 article compared fetal repair of MMC with postnatal repair and found a 50% decrease in the need for ventriculoperitoneal shunt in the fetally repaired group and overall better neurologic and functional scores in the fetally repaired group. A 30-month outcomes analysis of the cohort confirmed improved mental and motor function,

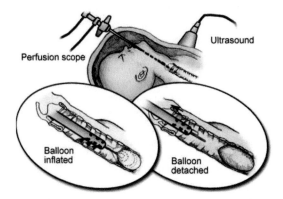

Fig. 1. Fetal endotracheal occlusion (FETO) procedure, using a catheter-based detachable balloon that is inserted through a fetoscope directly into the fetal trachea. (Image reproduced with permission from Medscape Drugs & Diseases (https://emedicine.medscape.com/), Fetal Surgery for Congenital Diaphragmatic Hernia, 2017, available at: https://emedicine.medscape.com/article/2109500-overview.)

including ambulation and self-care scores in the fetally treated group.[21] The cases reported in the MoMs trial were done as open procedures. To achieve access to the fetal back, surgeons made a Pfannenstiel incision, positioned the fetus within the uterus so that the lesion was in an easily accessed location, and then made a hysterotomy about 6 to 8 cm in length. An open technique, while providing better surgical exposure than a minimally invasive technique, also carries with it a greater risk of maternal complications, including maternal hemorrhage, sepsis, and the ultimate need to deliver the affected fetus, and any subsequent pregnancies, by Cesarean section.

With these maternal concerns in mind, groups have also pursued a fetoscopic approach to fetal MMC repair.[22] In these cases, a camera and laparoscopic instruments are inserted percutaneously through the uterus, most of the amniotic fluid is drained, and the uterus is insufflated with carbon dioxide. This approach (and a related hybrid approach of maternal open incision but uterine insufflation and laparoscopic repair[23]) should probably be viewed as more experimental than the open approach at this time. Although the success of the repair is reported to be encouraging, obstetric complications, including premature preterm rupture of membranes and preterm labor and delivery, do seem to be more common in the laparoscopic approach. Unlike with the open approach, women who undergo a fetoscopic approach to MMC repair may safely deliver the affected fetus (and any other subsequent pregnancies) vaginally.[24] This factor is important when considering that many women opting for fetal surgery are religiously traditional and reject the option of termination of pregnancy; they also may desire future pregnancies. The impact of fetal surgery on subsequent pregnancies may be an issue of great importance.

Sacrococcygeal teratoma, with a prevalence of 1 in 40,000 live births, represents the most common tumor of the newborn. These tumors are uniformly attached to the coccyx and may extend inside the abdomen and pelvis, or, more commonly, may exist largely outside of the pelvis. The mortality rate associated with these tumors has been reported to be as high as 50%.[25] Largely external tumors have been reported as amenable to resection via an open approach. Although the chance of mortality from this sort of fetal surgery is high, fetal surgery does likely increase survival rate, especially in cases of large tumor load.[26]

Open, Late Gestation Fetal Surgery with Planned Delivery

The EXIT procedure is the broad term used to describe a fetal procedure done when the fetus is in the process of being delivered. During the procedure, the fetus maintains its fetal circulation and oxygenation is from the umbilical cord via continued perfusion of the placenta. Rare indications for the EXIT approach have been for the resection of large lung or pleural tumors,[27] but the EXIT approach is much more commonly used when there is concern that the fetal airway will not be patent at the time of birth, including cases of congenital high airway obstruction, cystic hygroma, cervical teratoma, and of course following fetal tracheal occlusion for CDH. In these cases, the head and neck of the fetus is delivered as in a typical Cesarean section, but rather than deliver the remainder of the fetus, the fetal surgical and/or airway team begins work immediately. Securing the airway may involve something as simple as the placement of an endotracheal tube by direct laryngoscopy, or may be more complicated, necessitating advanced airway devices or tracheostomy. Depending on the primary fetal malformation, after confirmation of a secure airway, the remainder of the fetus is delivered with ultimate management with neonatal surgery, or fetal circulation may be maintained and other surgical interventions (extracorporeal membrane oxygenation, mediastinal tumor resection) performed. EXIT replaced the earlier operation on placental support procedure, where the fetus was completely delivered, the cord was not clamped, and the fetus was placed at the same vertical level as the uterus (either on a side table or on the patient's legs). During the period of placental perfusion to the fetus simple surgical procedures could be performed. However, the duration of placental support on operation on placental support was typically several minutes only, while the duration of placental support on EXIT may approach 2 hours.

Critical features of EXIT include

a. not delivering the fetus except for the fetal head, neck, and 1 hand (for intravenous access and pulse oximetry), the remainder stays in the uterus as reductions in uterine volume lead to uterine contractions and impaired fetal perfusion;
b. augmenting the intrauterine volume by warm amnioinfusion;
c. profound tocolysis with general anesthesia including volatile anesthetics, and augmented by nitroglycerine if needed;
d. provision for maternal hemorrhage with blood replacement and volume resuscitation; and
e. fetal monitoring using echocardiography to assess heart rate, contractility, and ventricular filling. Fetal bradycardia may reflect maternal hemodynamic instability, elevated uterine tone, placental separation, kinking of the umbilical cord, or fetal hemorrhage.

UNIQUE PHYSIOLOGIC CONCERNS IN THE PREGNANT AND FETAL PATIENTS
Physiologic Changes of Pregnancy

Owing to the primary topic of this article, it is not the intent for this to be an exhaustive analysis of the physiologic changes of pregnancy, but rather to discuss important highlights of maternal changes that must be considered when providing anesthesia for fetal surgery.

By the middle of the second trimester of pregnancy, likely in response to progesterone-mediated decreases in systemic vascular resistance (25%–30%), a pregnant woman's cardiac output will have increased about 40% from baseline. Plasma volume will have increased by almost 50%, resting heart rate will have increased to about 100 beats per minute, stroke volume will have increased by about 25%, and autonomic nervous system tone will have increased from prepregnancy levels. These changes have direct structural implications on the maternal heart, remodeling the cardiac myocytes, and increasing left and right ventricular wall mass and thickness, as well as leading to dilation of all chambers.[28] These changes have critical anesthetic implications, specifically in the realm of maintenance of maternal blood pressure. Because of the increased sympathetic tone seen in pregnant patients, anesthetic interventions that cause a sympathectomy (neuraxial blocks) or that directly vasodilate (volatile inhaled agents, some intravenous induction agents) can lead to a surprising degree of hypotension. It is thus critical that directly vasoconstricting agents (usually phenylephrine and ephedrine) be immediately available for any pregnant patient undergoing anesthesia.

Pregnancy-related changes to the respiratory system are also significant considerations during fetal surgery. An increase in the metabolic demand by both the pregnant woman and the fetus increases oxygen consumption and carbon dioxide production by as much as 60% at term. Owing to the increasing size of the gravid uterus, the diaphragm is displaced upward and the chest becomes more barrel shaped, leading to decreased in functional residual capacity.[29] Together, these changes can lead to rapid oxygen desaturation during the apneic period after the induction of general anesthesia. This condition makes adequate preinduction preoxygenation critical in these patients. Optimizing patient positioning and the ready availability of a multitude of intubation tools will assist in securing the airway quickly and efficiently as soon as unconsciousness is confirmed. Changes in the pregnant patient's upper airway can often work against this goal, however. Upper airway edema and tissue friability can make endotracheal intubation difficult in some pregnant patients, making preoperative airway assessment and the preparation of backup airway devices that much more crucial.

Although nonlaboring pregnant woman have normal gastric emptying,[30] and hence an empty stomach after the typical preoperative fasting time, pregnant patients may still be at increased risk for regurgitation and aspiration of stomach contents during the induction of general anesthesia. For this reason, rapid sequence induction (quick administration of induction and paralytic agent, cricoid pressure, and avoidance of bag-mask ventilation) is generally practiced for the induction of mid-second trimester and later pregnant patients. Likewise, owing to concerns of loss of airway reflexes and risk of aspiration, moderate to deep sedation is generally not practiced in patients later than the mid-second trimester. Exceptions may be made after prolonged periods of fasting and confirmation of gastric residual volume by ultrasound examination.

Pregnancy has been shown to increase a patient's sensitivity to anesthetic agents, including agents which induce and maintain general anesthesia as well as local anesthetics. Functionally, this translates into a reduced minimum alveolar concentration of inhaled anesthetics during general anesthesia, and reduced doses of neuraxial local anesthetics needed to achieve adequate anesthetic level during spinal or epidural anesthesia.

The Uterus and Placenta

Functional aspects of the uterus and placenta must be well-understood and considered during a fetal surgery.

The developing fetus completely depends on the developing uterine–placental interface for the exchange of oxygen, nutrients, and metabolites. This dependence necessarily means that maintaining maternal uterine blood flow is crucial to a fetus's well-being. Without a mechanism of autoregulation of blood flow, uterine blood flow depends on maternal cardiac output and blood pressure to maintain adequate perfusion. As noted, many anesthetic interventions can reduce maternal blood pressure, so the anesthesiologist must be prepared to (1) frequently and fastidiously monitor blood pressure and (2) administer vasopressor agents to treat hypotension. This caution is especially important in situations where continuous fetal heart rate monitoring (as an indicator of fetal well-being) is not possible.

Maternal pain, through the elaboration of catecholamines, can also negatively affect uterine blood flow and should be avoided as much as possible during fetal surgeries. Likewise, uterine contractions decrease uterine blood flow. Uterine irritability and contractions are nearly a universal result of uterine manipulation during fetal surgery and should be avoided or treated using uterine smooth muscle relaxing or tocolytic agents, which most commonly include high-dose inhaled volatile agents, magnesium, nitroglycerin, indomethacin, and terbutaline. Of course, many of these agents, especially at high doses, have the effect of peripheral vasodilation or reduction of cardiac contractility, leading to maternal hypotension, underscoring the need for careful monitoring and treatment of blood pressure.

Transfer of maternally dosed medications must be a consideration during fetal anesthesia. **Table 2** summarizes the maternal–fetal transfer of some of the most commonly administered anesthetic agents.

Table 2
Commonly used pharmaceutical agents during fetal anesthesia and their ability to cross the placenta

Drug Class	Examples	Crosses Placenta?	Notes
Opioids	Morphine, fentanyl, remifentanil	Yes	All cross readily, remifentanil quickly metabolized in fetus
Induction agents	Propofol	Yes	Crosses quickly, rapidly metabolized by fetus
Inhalational agents	Sevoflurane, desflurane	Yes	Prolonged maternal dosing increases fetal concentration (context-sensitive half-life)
Neuromuscular blocking agents	Rocuronium, vecuronium, succinylcholine	No	
Local anesthetics	Lidocaine, bupivacaine	Yes	Ion trapping may occur in fetus[a]
Quaternary ammonium anticholinergic	Glycopyrrolate	No	Ionized; large molecule
Acetylcholinesterase inhibitor	Neostigmine	Yes	Pair with anticholinergic such as atropine for reversal of neuromuscular blockade
Benzodiazepines	Midazolam	Yes	Crosses readily; ion trapping may occur in fetus[a]

[a] Phenomenon by which weak bases are not ionized in neutral pH (maternal circulation) but become ionized in acidic environment (fetal circulation, especially if fetus is in distress). In this case, these drugs may diffuse from the maternal to the fetal circulation, and then become 'trapped' there, leading to disproportionately high fetal drug concentration. The clinical significance is uncertain, but will depend on the drug and dose used.

Fetal Concerns in Fetal Anesthesia

The major fetal-related goals of any anesthetic for fetal surgery are (1) minimizing any long-term effects of the anesthetic, (2) mitigation of the fetal response to noxious stimuli, (3) fetal immobilization, and (4) maintenance of fetal hemodynamics and hemodynamic rescue, if needed. Any of these aspects may become more or less important depending on the scope of the fetal surgery.

Ideas about minimizing long-term fetal effects of the fetal anesthetic refers to ideas about the teratogenicity of agents used during the anesthetic, as well as the neurotoxicity of any of the agents used. Luckily, commonly used anesthetic drugs (opioids, volatile agents, induction agents, neuromuscular blockers, and benzodiazepines) do not seem to have teratogenic effects on the developing fetus, especially at the gestational ages that would be clinically relevant for fetal surgeries (midgestation and later). Over the past 15 years there has been significant focus on the possible neuroapoptotic effects of commonly used anesthetic agents on children, as well as fetuses. Although there have been several large-scale, high-quality studies looking at neurodevelopmental outcome in children exposed to anesthetic agents finding negligible or no difference between exposed and nonexposed groups,[31,32] there have been no comparable human studies exploring the neurodevelopmental effect of anesthesia on the developing fetus.

The idea of whether a fetus can feel pain is controversial and has been influenced not just by scientific findings, but also by closely held political, cultural, and religious opinions. Lee and colleagues[33] provide an excellent fact-based review of the topic, including a critical discussion of the very definition of pain itself. Sympathetic response or withdrawal reflex to noxious stimuli is not sufficient to demonstrate perception of pain, because these responses can exist without higher cortical function. Pain perception requires conscious recognition of a noxious stimulus, and the thalamocortical pathways implicated in these functions are unlikely to be functional before 29 weeks of gestation.

Even if the fetus is not feeling pain, the existence of autonomic or withdrawal responses to noxious stimuli requires the use of analgesic agents to blunt or mitigate them. As mentioned, opioids do cross the uteroplacental barrier. Alternatively, opioids (usually fentanyl) can be administered directly to the fetus via an ultrasound-guided transuterine intramuscular injection. Opioid treatment of the fetus should decrease overall fetal motor responsiveness, but it will not cease all fetal movements. If absolute fetal immobility is required, direct intramuscular or intravascular dosing of a nondepolarizing neuromuscular blocker (pancuronium, vecuronium, or rocuronium) to the fetus should be provided. Because fentanyl may cause bradycardia, especially if coadministered with vecuronium, atropine is generally coadministered with these direct intramuscular fetal injections in the fetal cocktail.

Maintenance of the fetal cardiovascular system is of utmost importance when providing a fetal anesthetic. As noted, the primary driver of fetal oxygenation is adequate uteroplacental perfusion, but direct effects of anesthetic agents on the fetal circulatory system can also negatively affect fetal well-being. As in the neonate, cardiac output in the fetus is highly dependent on fetal heart rate, and fetal bradycardia can rapidly lead to fetal acidosis leading to a vicious cycle of worsening fetal bradycardia. High doses of volatile anesthetics (as can sometimes be used for uterine relaxation) can act as myocardial depressants, reducing ventricular function or even heart rate directly.[34] Simple interventions like maternal repositioning or increased maternal Fio_2 delivery may sometimes resolve the bradycardia, but the intraoperative team must be prepared to treat bradycardia with fetally administered drugs like atropine and/or epinephrine.

ANESTHESIA FOR FETAL SURGERY

The anesthetic approach to fetal surgery can be grouped into 3 categories: anesthesia for minimally invasive fetal surgery, anesthesia for open fetal surgery, and anesthesia for EXIT procedure; the anesthetic approach and goals vary based on the type of procedure planned (**Table 3**).

Anesthesia for Minimally Invasive Fetal Surgery

Anesthesia for minimally invasive fetal surgical procedures with minimal uterine manipulation (laser ablation for twin–twin transfusion syndrome, radiofrequency ablation procedures, shunting procedures), can be quite simple, and might consist of mild maternal intravenous sedation and/or neuraxial (usually epidural or combined spinal epidural) anesthesia paired with local anesthesia to the skin site of the needle or trocar. Certain cases may require fetal immobilization (particularly in procedures with fetal stimulation, such as FETO), which can be achieved through maternal administration of a remifentanil infusion, or via direct fetal administration of agents, typically administered as an ultrasound-guided intramuscular injection of a fetal cocktail of fentanyl, a neuromuscular blocker, and atropine into a fetal leg. There is rarely a need for significant intraoperative uterine relaxation, although doses of tocolytic drugs may be given before or after these cases as prophylaxis against preterm labor.

	Open Fetal Surgery	Fetoscopic Surgery	EXIT Procedure	Cesarean Delivery
Table 3 **Anesthetic goals differ based on surgical plan and gestational age of fetus (and these contrast with the typical anesthesia goals in cesarean delivery)**				
Preferred anesthesia	General	General or regional	General	Regional
Direct fetal anesthesia	Desirable	Desirable	Desirable	Undesirable
Uterine relaxation	Desirable	Desirable	Desirable[a]	Undesirable
Amnioinfusion	Yes	Depends on surgery	Yes	No
Postoperative tocolysis	Yes	Yes	No	No
Anesthesia personnel	One team	One team	Two teams (pediatric as well as obstetric)	One team

[a] Until completion of EXIT and delivery, after which uterine contraction is desirable.

During most minimally invasive fetal surgeries, the fetal heart rate is monitored, either by Doppler or visually using ultrasound examination, frequently or on a near continuous basis. A thorough discussion between the operating team and the patient, as well as among members of the operating room team to plan what actions will be taken in the event of a fetal emergency. As discussed, multiple doses of fetal atropine and epinephrine (dosed based on estimated fetal weight, either intramuscularly, intravenous, or intracardiac) should be part of the plan, and predrawn sterile doses should be provided to the surgical team before the start of the case. A crucial question is whether, in a case of prolonged fetal bradycardia, the fetus should be delivered. The idea of viability is important here, and not just viability based on gestational age. For example, a fetus at 26 weeks of gestation, but with severe intrauterine growth restriction and severe aortic stenosis may be thought to be nonviable if it were to be delivered.

The anesthetic approach to minimally invasive (fetoscopic) MMC repair differs from other minimally invasive procedures, because significantly more anesthetic involvement is required. Maternal patients usually undergo general anesthesia for these cases. Anesthesia is typically maintained with inhaled anesthetics (which also contribute to uterine relaxation) as well as a remifentanil infusion. A combination approach with lower doses of an inhaled anesthetic as well as a propofol infusion has also been described.[35] An arterial line is generally placed after the induction of general anesthesia. Additional uterine relaxants, including magnesium and/or nitroglycerin may be used, per clinical indication. The fetus is dosed directly with a fetal cocktail, as discussed elsewhere in this article. The most unique part of this surgery, and perhaps the riskiest, occurs when a majority of the amniotic fluid is drained and the uterus is insufflated with carbon dioxide. Uptake of carbon dioxide into the maternal and fetal circulation should be expected and hyperventilation of the pregnant patient could be required to maintain normocarbia. Vexingly, during the time of pneumouterus (which could last more than an hour), ultrasound or Doppler monitoring of the fetal heart rate will not be possible. Occasional visual checks for pulsatility in the umbilical cord or placental vessels may be an adequate substitute.

Anesthesia for Open Fetal Surgery

For open fetal surgeries, preoperative consideration should be given to a postoperative multimodal approach to pain management. Although open fetal surgery is usually done under general anesthesia with an endotracheal tube, preoperative placement of a lumbar epidural catheter is recommended for later use in the postoperative period. Epidural analgesia (usually with a combination of an opioid and a local anesthetic) is thought to be superior to parenteral or orally delivered analgesics, owing to the ability of the epidurally delivered drugs to block (not just modulate) pain transmission and sympathetic outflow. This may have a positive effect in avoiding postoperative catecholamine mediated uterine irritability and preterm labor.[36]

After induction of general anesthesia, an arterial line should be placed. Because there will be a need for significant uterine relaxation during the case, and many of the uterine relaxing agents have the side effect of peripheral vasodilation and hypotension, especially at a high dose (volatile agents, nitroglycerin, magnesium), the placement of a central venous catheter for potential administration of high-dose, potent vasopressors should be considered. Special considerations in these cases should be given to fluid administration and maintenance of core body temperature. Owing to the combination of the pregnant state, as well as the dosing of tocolytic medications, these patients are prone to intraoperative and postoperative pulmonary edema. Fluid administration, hence, should be judicious, and urine output, as a sign of volume status, should be closely monitored. Heat loss from both the maternal and fetal patients can be significant. A forced air warmer and fluid warmer should be used. Because hemorrhage is a significant risk, cross-matched blood should be immediately available for both the maternal and fetal patient.

During the case, a fetal cocktail is given. At the time of hysterotomy, some centers drain and reserve some of the amniotic fluid (for replacement into the intra-amniotic space at the conclusion of the procedure). Fetal parts will partially occlude the hysterotomy, decreasing the continued loss of amniotic fluid, but there will still be a steady and continuous loss, prompting concerns for intrauterine hypotension, uterine irritability, and uteroplacental separation. To address these concerns, an amnioinfusion should be initiated with a warmed isotonic solution being provided through a pump (large volumes >10 L may be needed, depending on the duration of the surgery).

The conclusion of the surgery is managed as any other general anesthetic. Inhaled anesthetic gases are weaned to off and any residual neuromuscular blockade in the pregnant patient is reversed. The mother should be dosed with a dilute local anesthetic through the epidural catheter before emergence to minimize pain. The mother should not be extubated until she meets the following criteria: adequate unassisted ventilation, stable vital signs, can follow simple commands, and demonstrates muscle strength. Magnesium infusion, as well as other tocolytics, may be continued well into the postoperative period.

Anesthesia for the Ex Utero Intrapartum Treatment Procedure

Initial anesthesia management for the EXIT procedure is similar to the management seen in open fetal surgeries—the maternal patient receives general anesthesia (although there are reports of the use of regional anesthesia for EXIT procedure[37]), an arterial line, and consideration for placing a central venous line, because bleeding and hypotension requiring significant vasopressor support is a possibility. Uterine relaxant agents used should be short acting; desflurane is the volatile anesthetic of choice owing to its rapid onset and offset, and nitroglycerin is commonly used. After hysterotomy, the fetal head and neck are delivered, the fetus is dosed with an opioid and a neuromuscular blocker, and a definitive airway is placed and confirmed with the use of a fiberoptic bronchoscope. In some cases, the placement of the airway is the end goal of the procedure, in which case ventilation of the fetus is begun and the surgeons complete the delivery and neonatal separation. In cases where there are further planned procedures although the fetus remains on placental support (mass resection, extracorporeal membrane oxygenation), the lungs are not ventilated until those procedures are completed. After neonatal separation, the anesthesiologist must focus on the uterus contracting and regaining its tone. The volatile anesthetic should be discontinued and the patient should be switched to propofol infusion for maintenance of anesthesia. Uterotonics (oxytocin, methylergonvine) should be administered.

Unlike in midgestation surgeries, fetal viability defines the EXIT procedure, which means delivery of the fetus after either a successful or unsuccessful procedure. Neonatal intensive care and pediatric surgical teams should be immediately available should the fetal patient need to be delivered emergently, before the completion of the planned procedure.

SUMMARY

Pushed by advances in imagining, technology, and technique, fetal surgery and fetal anesthesia are developing at an accelerated pace, with several high-quality studies demonstrating that specific fetal procedures can improve neonatal outcomes when compared with expectant and neonatal management.

REFERENCES

1. Chervenak FA, McCullough LB. Ethics of maternal–fetal surgery. Semin Fetal Neonatal Med 2007;12(6):426–31.
2. Bliton MJ. Ethics: "life before birth" and moral complexity in maternal-fetal surgery for spina bifida. Clin Perinatol 2003;30(3):449–64.
3. Sacco A, Van der Veeken L, Bagshaw E, et al. Maternal complications following open and fetoscopic fetal surgery: a systematic review and meta-analysis. Prenatal Diagn 2019;39(4):251–68.
4. Grethel EJ, Wagner AJ, Clifton MS, et al. Fetal intervention for mass lesions and hydrops improves outcome: a 15-year experience. J Pediatr Surg 2007;42(1): 117–23.
5. Peranteau WH, Scott Adzick N, Boelig MM, et al. Thoracoamniotic shunts for the management of fetal lung lesions and pleural effusions: a single-institution review and predictors of survival in 75 cases. J Pediatr Surg 2015;50(2):301–5.
6. Farrugia M-K. Fetal bladder outlet obstruction: embryopathology, in utero intervention and outcome. J Pediatr Urol 2016;12(5):296–303.
7. Morris RK, Malin GL, Quinlan-Jones E, et al. Percutaneous vesicoamniotic shunting versus conservative management for fetal lower urinary tract obstruction (PLUTO): a randomised trial. Lancet 2013;382(9903):1496–506.
8. Kilby MD, Morris RK. Fetal therapy for the treatment of congenital bladder neck obstruction. Nat Rev Urol 2014;11:412.
9. Sananes N, Cruz-Martinez R, Favre R, et al. Two-year outcomes after diagnostic and therapeutic fetal cystoscopy for lower urinary tract obstruction. Prenatal Diagn 2016;36(4):297–303.

10. Ghartey K, Miller RS, Simpson LL. 163 - twin reversed arterial perfusion sequence. In: Copel JA, D'Alton ME, Feltovich H, et al, editors. Obstetric imaging: fetal diagnosis and care. 2nd edition. Elsevier; 2018. p. 659–63.e1.

11. Lee H, Bebbington M, Crombleholme TM. The North American Fetal Therapy Network Registry data on outcomes of radiofrequency ablation for twin-reversed arterial perfusion sequence. Fetal Diagn Ther 2013;33(4):224–9.

12. Freud Lindsay R, McElhinney Doff B, Marshall Audrey C, et al. Fetal aortic valvuloplasty for evolving hypoplastic left heart syndrome. Circulation 2014;130(8): 638–45.

13. Johnson A. Diagnosis and management of twin-twin transfusion syndrome. Clin Obstetrics Gynecol 2015;58(3):611–31.

14. Roberts D, Neilson JP, Kilby M, et al. Interventions for the treatment of twin-twin transfusion syndrome. Cochrane Database Syst Rev 2008;(1). CD002073. Available at: http://europepmc.org/abstract/MED/18254001. Accessed September 24, 2019.

15. Hüsler MR, Wilson RD, Horii SC, et al. When is fetoscopic release of amniotic bands indicated? Review of outcome of cases treated in utero and selection criteria for fetal surgery. Prenatal Diagn 2009;29(5):457–63.

16. Hedrick MH, Ferro MM, Filly RA, et al. Congenital high airway obstruction syndrome (CHAOS): a potential for perinatal intervention. J Pediatr Surg 1994; 29(2):271–4.

17. Al-Maary J, Eastwood MP, Russo FM, et al. Fetal tracheal occlusion for severe pulmonary hypoplasia in isolated congenital diaphragmatic hernia: a systematic review and meta-analysis of survival. Ann Surg 2016;264(6):929–33.

18. Racial/ethnic differences in the birth prevalence of spina bifida - United States, 1995-2005. MMWR Morbidity Mortality Weekly Rep 2009;57(53):1409–13.

19. Sileo FG, Pateisky P, Curado J, et al. Long-term neuroimaging and neurological outcome of fetal spina bifida aperta after postnatal surgical repair. Ultrasound Obstetrics Gynecol 2019;53(3):309–13.

20. Adzick NS, Thom EA, Spong CY, et al. A randomized trial of prenatal versus postnatal repair of myelomeningocele. N Engl J Med 2011;364(11):993–1004.

21. Farmer DL, Thom EA, Brock JW III, et al. The Management of Myelomeningocele Study: full cohort 30-month pediatric outcomes. Am J Obstetrics Gynecol 2018; 218(2):256.e1-13.

22. Pedreira DAL, Zanon N, Nishikuni K, et al. Endoscopic surgery for the antenatal treatment of myelomeningocele: the CECAM trial. Am J Obstetrics Gynecol 2016; 214(1):111.e1-11.

23. Belfort MA, Whitehead WE, Shamshirsaz AA, et al. Fetoscopic repair of meningomyelocele. Obstetrics Gynecol 2015;126(4):881–4.

24. Joyeux L, Engels AC, Russo FM, et al. Fetoscopic versus open repair for spina bifida aperta: a systematic review of outcomes. Fetal Diagn Ther 2016;39(3): 161–71.

25. Holterman A-X, Filiatrault D, Lallier M, et al. The natural history of sacrococcygeal teratomas diagnosed through routine obstetric sonogram: a single institution experience. J Pediatr Surg 1998;33(6):899–903.

26. Hirose S, Farmer DL. Fetal surgery for sacrococcygeal teratoma. Clin Perinatol 2003;30(3):493–506.

27. Adzick NS. Management of fetal lung lesions. Clin Perinatol 2003;30(3):481–92.

28. Sanghavi M, Rutherford John D. Cardiovascular physiology of pregnancy. Circulation 2014;130(12):1003–8.

29. Wise RA, Polito AJ, Krishnan V. Respiratory physiologic changes in pregnancy. Immunol Allergy Clin North America 2006;26(1):1–12.
30. Wong CA, Loffredi M, Ganchiff JN, et al. Gastric emptying of water in term pregnancy. Anesthesiology 2002;96(6):1395–400.
31. Davidson AJ, Disma N, de Graaff JC, et al. Neurodevelopmental outcome at 2 years of age after general anaesthesia and awake-regional anaesthesia in infancy (GAS): an international multicentre, randomised controlled trial. Lancet 2016;387(10015):239–50.
32. Sun LS, Li G, Miller TLK, et al. Association between a single general anesthesia exposure before age 36 months and neurocognitive outcomes in later childhood. JAMA 2016;315(21):2312–20.
33. Lee SJ, Ralston HJP, Drey EA, et al. Fetal Pain a systematic multidisciplinary review of the evidence. JAMA 2005;294(8):947–54.
34. Rychik J, Cohen D, Tran KM, et al. The role of echocardiography in the intraoperative management of the fetus undergoing myelomeningocele repair. Fetal Diagn Ther 2015;37(3):172–8.
35. Boat A, Mahmoud M, Michelfelder EC, et al. Supplementing desflurane with intravenous anesthesia reduces fetal cardiac dysfunction during open fetal surgery. Pediatr Anesth 2010;20(8):748–56.
36. Brusseau R, Mizrahi-Arnaud A. Fetal anesthesia and pain management for intrauterine therapy. Clin Perinatology 2013;40(3):429–42.
37. George RB, Melnick AH, Rose EC, et al. Case series: combined spinal epidural anesthesia for Cesarean delivery and ex utero intrapartum treatment procedure. Can J Anesth 2007;54(3):218.

Neonatal Abstinence Syndrome
Review of Epidemiology, Care Models, and Current Understanding of Outcomes

Kathryn Dee Lizcano MacMillan, MD, MPH[a,b,*]

KEYWORDS

- Neonatal abstinence syndrome (NAS)
- Neonatal opioid withdrawal syndrome (NOWS) • Opioid exposed newborn (OEN)
- Prenatal substance exposure • Eat sleep console (ESC) • Pharmacotherapy
- Length of stay (LOS) • Developmental outcomes

KEY POINTS

- Multiple individual and demographic factors contribute to neonatal abstinence syndrome severity and clinical course.
- Emerging evidence supports the importance of parental roles in care.
- Studies support evolving care models to focus on nonpharmacologic treatment and family-centered care.
- Long-term outcomes from neonatal abstinence syndrome are poorly understood and must be considered in context of multiple individual, familial, and societal factors.

BACKGROUND

Neonatal abstinence syndrome (NAS) includes an array of symptoms impacting opioid-exposed newborns (OEN) owing to postnatal withdrawal from in utero substance exposure. More recently, the term neonatal opioid withdrawal syndrome has emerged to specify prenatal opioid exposure, but NAS remains the dominant term in the literature. NAS symptoms generally occur in the first 24 hours of life for short-acting opioid exposure and within 72 to 96 hours of life for long-acting

Disclosure Statement: The author has nothing to disclose.
[a] Division of Neonatology and Newborn Medicine, Massachusetts General Hospital for Children, Good Samaritan Medical Center, 55 Fruit Street, Founders 5-530, Boston, MA 02114, USA;
[b] Division of Pediatric Hospital Medicine, Massachusetts General Hospital for Children, Good Samaritan Medical Center, 55 Fruit Street, Founders 5-530, Boston, MA 02114, USA
* Division of Neonatology and Newborn Medicine, Massachusetts General Hospital for Children and Good Samaritan Medical Center, 55 Fruit Street, Founders 5-530, Boston, MA 02114.
E-mail address: kdmacmillan@mgh.harvard.edu
twitter: @KateMacMD (K.D.L.M.)

Clin Perinatol 46 (2019) 817–832
https://doi.org/10.1016/j.clp.2019.08.012
0095-5108/19/© 2019 Elsevier Inc. All rights reserved.

perinatology.theclinics.com

opioid exposure. The most frequently reported symptoms include tremors, restlessness, hyperactive reflexes, regurgitation, increased tone, high-pitched cry, frantic suck, and difficulty sleeping.[1-3] OEN have lengthy hospital stays, higher costs, and in some settings, separation from their mothers, during the newborn hospitalization.[4-7] NAS can impact an infant's ability to grow and thrive and contribute to caregiver distress.[8,9] Emerging evidence supports the importance of environment of care and parental engagement in NAS care, mitigating symptoms, improving outcomes, and supporting families.[10-12] This review summarizes current evidence on epidemiology and predictive factors, evolving assessment and treatment models, and the current understanding of postdischarge considerations and long-term outcomes.

EPIDEMIOLOGY AND PREDICTIVE FACTORS

With the expansion of the opioid epidemic in the United States, prenatal exposure to both illicit and prescribed opioids and subsequent incidence of NAS has also increased dramatically.[4,13-16] A recent study based on the National Inpatient Sample, a representative sample of US hospital discharges, found that from 2000 to 2014, incidence of NAS in the United States has increased 5-fold, from 1.5 to 8.0 per 1000 hospital births.[4] In the United States, NAS has disproportionately impacted rural and public health insurance–dependent populations, with both rates of NAS and associated hospital costs growing at a faster pace compared with urban and privately insured peers. Rural families impacted by NAS are more likely than their urban peers to have a lower family income and be dependent on health insurance.[16] Those insured by Medicaid are more likely to have longer hospital stays and to require transfer to other hospitals for NAS management,[4] potentially creating new burdens and barriers for families. A recent single-site, prospective cohort study found that maternal food insecurity is correlated with an increased likelihood for the need for pharmacologic treatment of NAS in their infants. This association was independent of maternal depression or type of opioid agonist medication-assisted treatment (MAT) prescribed to mothers.[17]

NAS risk seems to be associated with several demographic factors. Based on national data compiled by the Agency for Healthcare Research and Quality, NAS rates are higher among non-Hispanic white infants, with more than 10 per 1000 births compared with fewer than 3 per 1000 births among infants of other races/ethnicities in the United Stgates.[18] In a retrospective cohort study of infants enrolled in Medicaid in Tennessee, male sex was associated with increased likelihood of NAS requiring pharmacologic treatment, independent of multiple maternal factors including age, race, and education, anxiety, or depression; in utero exposures to selective serotonin reuptake inhibitors or cigarettes; opioid type or dosing; and infant birth weight or small for gestation age.[19] However, prior studies have shown conflicting results regarding whether there was an effect of gender on symptom severity or likelihood to need treatment independent of maternal and neonatal factors.[20-22]

Coexposure to other psychotropic medication, including selective serotonin reuptake inhibitors, benzodiazepines, and other illicit substances increases the risk of significant withdrawal symptoms.[2,7,23] Genetic and epigenetic factors also seem to influence the clinical course of NAS. Studies have identified variation in genotype and epigenetic markers related to mu-opioid receptors, modulators of pain sensitivity, dopamine metabolism, and stress pathways as important to variation NAS symptom severity, response to opioid medications in the neonatal period, and clinical outcomes such as hospital length of stay (LOS).[24-26] Ongoing exploration of genetic and epigenetic markers may further elucidate individual variation in response to pharmacotherapy and development of clinical prediction models.

VARIATION IN INPATIENT CARE

There is wide variability in the inpatient care and costs for NAS.[5,27–29] Standardizing hospital policies and care processes for NAS is recommended by the American Academy of Pediatrics and has been shown to improve hospital care and outcomes.[2,15] A survey of policies and practices in hospitals participating in the Better Outcomes Through Research For Newborns (BORN) network in 2015 found that the majority of responding hospitals had NAS management protocols. Of these, 72% addressed pharmacologic treatment, although only 58% addressed nonpharmacologic supportive care. Observation periods for OENs varied: for short-acting opioids, 57% observed for 2 to 3 days and 30% for 5 or more days. For long-acting opioids 71% observed for 4 to 5 days, 8% observed for 7 or more days, and 19% observed for only 2 to 3 days. A majority of hospitals observed for NAS in level 1 nurseries, but of these most (87%) transferred to neonatal intensive care unit (NICU) settings when starting pharmacotherapy.[27] Similarly, a study of infants with NAS discharged from children's hospitals in the Pediatric Health Information System found 93% of newborns receiving pharmacotherapy were admitted to the NICU, although individual hospital rates varied from 0% to 100%. Rates of pharmacotherapy were high overall, with 70% of newborns with NAS treated pharmacologically and pharmacotherapy rates by hospital ranging from 13% to 90%. Consistent with findings in earlier studies, pharmacotherapy was linked to a more than 2-fold increase in LOS (22.0 vs 10.9 days) and total hospital costs ($44,720 vs $20,708) compared with newborns with NAS not treated pharmacologically.[28]

CHOICE OF PHARMACOLOGIC AGENT

When pharmacotherapy for NAS is indicated, an opioid agonist is often selected as first line. In the BORN network survey, morphine was the most common first-line pharmacologic agent used by participating hospitals, followed by methadone.[27] A review of NAS hospitalizations in the Pediatric Health Information System records also found morphine to be the most common pharmacotherapy choice for NAS, received by 90% of pharmacologically treated newborns, whereas 13% received methadone. Phenobarbital was the adjunctive agent of choice, with 20% of treated newborns receiving both morphine and phenobarbital.[28]

A large retrospective review using 2011 to 2015 data from the Pediatrix Clinical Data Warehouse compared outcomes among newborns treated with either morphine or methadone in the first week of life. The majority (85%) received morphine; however, those who received methadone as first-line pharmacotherapy had a 22% decrease in average hospital LOS, spent less time in the NICU, and were less likely to require an adjunctive agent.[30] A recent multicenter, randomized, controlled trial comparing methadone with morphine in NAS patients pharmacologically treated in 2014 to 2017 found a 14% decrease in mean hospital LOS and a 16% decrease in opioid treatment days in the methadone group.[31] Earlier smaller studies comparing morphine and methadone have shown conflicting results. A single-center, randomized trial found newborns with NAS treated with methadone rather than morphine had fewer opioid treatment days,[32] and a retrospective cohort study found fewer opioid treatment days to be associated with morphine compared with methadone.[33] Buprenorphine has also been proposed as an alternative opioid agonist therapy for NAS and several small studies have found a shorter duration of treatment and shorter hospital LOS with buprenorphine compared with either methadone or morphine.[34–36] Overall, these findings seem to favor longer acting opioid agonists over shorter acting agents.

A second pharmacologic agent is often added when a newborn with NAS has symptoms that are difficult to control with opioid agonist treatment or is having difficulty weaning their dose. A second agent may be particularly useful in cases of prenatal polypharmacy, including exposure to selective serotonin reuptake inhibitors and benzodiazepines in addition to opioids.[37–40] Phenobarbital is most frequently used[27,28]; however, concerns have been raised about impact on the developing brain with potential impact on behavioral and cognitive outcomes.[41–43] Studies have showed mixed benefits of clonidine as an alternative second agent. A single-center, prospective, nonblinded, block randomized trial found that adjunctive treatment with phenobarbital rather than clonidine led to a lesser average number of days of morphine treatment, but no difference in total morphine dose and longer total pharmacologic treatment duration, with phenobarbital continued for a mean of 3.8 months after discharge. There was no significant difference in adverse events or treatment failures.[38] Conversely, a retrospective study of adjunctive treatment with clonidine versus phenobarbital found the clonidine group had 8.5 days shorter mean opioid treatment duration.[39]

PHARMACOTHERAPY DOSING

Structured protocols for pharmacotherapy initiation and weaning have been associated with improved NAS outcomes.[15,44] Conventionally, once pharmacotherapy is initiated, it is titrated until symptoms are considered captured below the treatment threshold and then weaned off slowly, typically by 10% of the peak dose once or twice daily when symptoms remain below the threshold; the infant is discharged only after a period of observation off pharmacotherapy.[2,3,6] This practice contributes to lengthy hospital stays and there is no evidence base to support the necessity of slow weans or prolonged pharmacotherapy courses.[15,44] Alternative dosing approaches are emerging in the literature.[6,40,45–52] One single-center retrospective cohort report found a decreased LOS and decreased cumulative morphine using a structured weight-based weaning protocol compared with a symptom-based weaning protocol.[45] Multiple studies comparing outpatient weaning of opioid pharmacotherapy versus inpatient weaning have demonstrated shorted hospital LOS and decreased hospital costs without increased hospital readmission. However, there were mixed findings regarding the total duration of opioid treatment[46–51] and 1 study found increased postdischarge emergency department use in the outpatient treatment group.[48] Several institutions have moved to using single as-needed doses of morphine or methadone as opposed to the typical titration and weaning course as part of larger quality improvement initiatives.[6,52] One published report demonstrated that, when combined with optimized nonpharmacologic treatment as the first line of NAS care, the number of doses and cumulative amount of opioid therapy can be substantially and safely decreased.[52]

EVOLVING CARE MODELS

MAT, typically with the opioid agonists methadone or buprenorphine, is the currently recommended management for opioid use disorders in pregnancy to prevent risks associated with withdrawal during pregnancy in mothers. This has contributed to overall increased rates of NAS and altered the landscape of prenatal opioid exposure, with more infants exposed prenatally to daily opioid-mediated treatment.[3,4,53–55] This has impacted the family structures, home environments, and resources of infants with NAS, with a greater proportion of birth mothers actively in recovery and often better equipped to participate in their newborn's care both in the hospital and at home. There is an evolving frameshift in the literature around NAS care, with a greater emphasis on the mother–child dyad and family-centered care. The most recent American Academy of Pediatrics Clinical Report on Neonatal Drug Withdrawal states that, "the goals of therapy are to ensure that the infant achieves adequate sleep and nutrition to establish a consistent pattern of weight gain and begins to integrate into a social environment" and recognizes nonpharmacologic care as the first line in NAS treatment, including optimizing the environment of the infant, minimizing overstimulation and hunger, and providing a variety of soothing supports.[2] Suggested nonpharmacologic interventions may include soothing techniques that mimic the womb such as swaddling, holding and swaying motions, skin-to-skin contact, providing a low-stimulation environment, careful attention to feeding cues, on-demand feeding and provision of sufficient calories, encouraging mother–infant bonding, and creating supportive environments for families.[6,8,11,56,57]

NONPHARMACOLOGIC CARE

At many institutions, OENs are monitored in a NICU where infants are separated from their mothers. In some institutions, this separation occurs only once pharmacotherapy is initiated for those who need it, whereas in others, this practice is in place during observation for withdrawal symptoms.[27–29] However, the NICU environment may not be an ideal setting for these withdrawing newborns, who may already have difficulty with state regulation and may be especially sensitive to the noise, bright lights, and high activity levels in NICU.[8,58] Rooming-in environments, where mother and child stay together 24 hours a day unless separation is indicated for medical or safety reasons, is the World Health Organization recommended standard of care for newborns.[59] Rooming-in may be an important factor in optimizing nonpharmacologic care for the OEN. It has been shown in multiple single-center studies,[52,60–64] as well as a recent systematic review and meta-analysis,[12] to improve NAS hospitalization outcomes, decrease rates of pharmacotherapy, and shorten hospital LOS, without any reported increase in adverse events. A policy of separation of mothers from their infants during NAS hospitalization may interfere with bonding and contribute to maternal perceptions of stigma.[8,9,65] Additionally, a recent study demonstrated a positive correlation between amount of time mothers spend at the infants' bedside and improved NAS outcomes.[10]

FEEDING OPTIMIZATION AND BREASTFEEDING

Breastfeeding in mother–infant dyads with prescribed methadone or buprenorphine use is generally considered safe and beneficial to bonding and NAS symptoms management; however, there is wide variability in both breastfeeding rates, policies, and practices around breastfeeding in this population.[3,40,66–69] Among participating hospitals in the BORN network, 1 study found that 70% of hospitals had some policy or guideline in place regarding breastfeeding or feeding expressed breast milk to newborns being observed or treated for NAS. The criteria for breastfeeding eligibility was variable, with 50% requiring negative drug screening at delivery and 40% requiring enrollment in a substance use disorder treatment program.[27] Mothers may also face significant psychosocial and economic barriers to breastfeeding while receiving MAT.[69,70] Studies have shown lower rates of breastfeeding among infants with NAS than comparison groups. However, among eligible mother–infant dyads, rates of breastfeeding may be improved with integrated models of care for the mother and the infant.[66,68] Multiple studies have now linked breastfeeding with improved NAS hospital outcomes, including decreased hospital LOS and decreased pharmacotherapy.[66,71–74] Although these findings have not controlled for rooming-in, increased holding or other associated nonpharmacologic care, the potential benefit of increased maternal presence and engagement seems clear.

Standardizing nonpharmacologic and pharmacologic treatment holds promise for improving hospital care and experiences and can be implemented successfully on larger scales. One multicenter collaborative through the Vermont Oxford Network QI demonstrated improved outcomes, including decreased LOS and decreased pharmacotherapy, in participating hospitals through the adoption of a toolkit that addressed standardization of NAS identification, assessment, and management; standardization of processes for reporting and measuring NAS rates and outcomes; and focusing on creating environments that better supported the mother–child dyad, including instruction in trauma-informed care.[15]

ASSESSMENT MODELS

The Finnegan Neonatal Abstinence Scoring System (FNASS) and its variants have been the dominant models for assessment and management of NAS since it was first published in 1975.[1,27,75] Of hospitals participating in the BORN network, 92% reported using a version of the Finnegan Scale, with 70% using the Modified Finnegan Scale and 22% the Original Finnegan Scale.[27]

The FNASS has considerable limitations, including a lengthy symptom catalog, some of which have unclear clinical significance, and the assessment of which requires disturbing the infant and potentially exacerbating observed symptoms.[75] One analysis of the FNASS found poor internal psychometric properties and internal consistency guiding peak scores and pharmacotherapy initiation.[76] There is a lack of evidence supporting commonly used cut-offs guiding management, with most institutional FNASS based protocols starting or increasing pharmacologic treatment after an infant has received 3 scores of 8 or greater or 2 scores of 12 or greater.[6] This approach has never been validated and it is unclear how to differentiate fluctuations in FNASS score related to withdrawal versus variation in typical infant behaviors.[6,75,77] A study of infants without in utero substance exposure found that, although the FNASS scores were rarely greater than 7 in the first 3 days of life, scores increased with age and by 5 to 6 weeks of age, the 95th percentile cut-off score was as high as 8 with significant variations between day and night.[78]

Largely in response to these limitations, the Eat, Sleep, Console (ESC) approach was developed by Grossman and colleagues[52,75,77] as a foundation for functional clinical assessments of NAS guiding management. Infants are assessed based on their ability to successfully breastfeed or take a sufficient volume of expressed breastmilk or formula at each feed, sleep without interruption for at least 1 hour, and be consoled by caregivers within 10 minutes when fussing. If the infant is unable to meet these goals, multidisciplinary team huddles are called to optimize nonpharmacologic care first and consider pharmacologic management. This approach allows for frequent clinical assessments without disturbing the infant outside of routine care and encourages in-time responses that prioritize nonpharmacologic care. The investigators at Yale concurrently continued FNASS scoring and were able to compare outcomes with ESC management versus predicted outcomes using the Finnegan approach for a subset of OENs. The reported proportion of infants treated with morphine using the ESC approach was 12% compared with an estimated 62% predicted using the FNASS approach and average LOS for using the ESC tool was 5.9 days compared with an estimated average 16 days using FNASS.[77] Other institutions are adopting the ESC approach, largely as part of quality improvement initiatives and report substantial decreases in LOS and need for pharmacotherapy when used in combination with other measures supporting nonpharmacologic care.[75,79,80]

READMISSION AND HEALTH CARE USE

After the initial birth hospitalization, children with history of NAS have more frequent interactions with the health care system outside of routine health maintenance visits in the future. A longitudinal retrospective cohort study using data from the New York State Inpatient Database from 2006 to 2009 showed infants with a history of NAS had higher 30-day and 1-year readmission rates than infants born at term without NAS; readmission rates were similar to those of late preterm infants.[81] Conversely, a study using Pediatric Health Information System data found that term newborns with NAS had lower readmission rates than those without NAS at both 30 and 90 days compared with newborns without NAS, with no difference in hospital mortality.[28] An Australian population-based study linking hospital, birth, and death records found increased rates of hospitalization throughout childhood, persisting into adolescence. In childhood, NAS history was a predictor of admission for maltreatment and mental and behavioral disorders.[82] A retrospective longitudinal cohort study using linked claims data including inpatient, emergency department, and outpatient care found that children ages 1 to 8 years with a history of NAS had a significantly greater number of claims per year with nearly double mean annualized costs for all health services. Although costs and claims were steady or decreasing for other children after age 3, they progressively increased for children with a history of NAS. Additionally, well-child and preventive visits accounted for a significantly smaller proportion of encounter codes for children with NAS.[83] This finding reflects increased vulnerability among children with NAS and their families, not only increased health needs, but likely also social and economic needs impacting the way they navigate the health care system.

GROWTH AND NUTRITION

Infants with NAS are at risk for failure to thrive. Prenatal opioid exposure is associated with small for gestational age size at birth; in the neonatal period, this population often experiences poor feeding coordination and hyperphagia owing to increased metabolic needs.[1-3] Careful monitoring of feeding and growth is an important aspect of NAS care. Caloric fortification of formula and breastmilk may be initiated when there are signs of excessive early weight loss or failure to gain weight.[2,3] Survey of the BORN network found that one-third of responding hospitals provided caloric enhancement to all infants observed or treated for NAS.[27] A recent single-center study randomized newborns with prenatal methadone exposure to receive either standard (20 kcal/oz) or fortified (24 kcal/oz) formula and found similar days to weight nadir and percent maximum early weight loss, but a longitudinal analysis revealed a higher percent weight gained per day in the higher calorie group at 21 days, suggesting a potential benefit for early caloric fortification.[84]

Specific, longer term nutritional needs of this population remain uncertain. A retrospective of 70 term, singleton infants with NAS and controls matched for gestational age, birth weight, gender and insurance type at a tertiary center with level IV NICU followed growth over the first 400 days of life found both groups had similar growth curves. Interestingly, wider 10th and 90th percentile growth curves were seen for infants with NAS, although this finding did not attain statistical significance.[85] These findings may suggest a varied course in which some babies with NAS continue to struggle with growth after discharge, whereas others may be overfed in response to either hyperphagia, misinterpretation of feeding cues, or efforts to soothe fussy but fed infants. A further exploration of growth and feeding patterns in infancy and childhood for this population is needed.

BRAIN DEVELOPMENT

Several studies have demonstrated changes in the human brain in response to opioid exposure in adult humans, altering gray matter volume[86,87] as well changes in brain and cerebellar size and content in animal studies.[88–92] More recently, studies have demonstrated similar alteration in newborns with NAS.

A recent large prospective study of late preterm and term newborns found that those newborns with prenatal opioid exposure requiring pharmacologic treatment for NAS were more likely to have small head circumference (at or below both 3rd and 10th percentile curves) than controls without prenatal opioid or illicit substance exposure matched on gestational age, mode of delivery, race and maternal parity. The majority of mothers in the sample were receiving MAT and the relative reduction in head circumference seems to be independent of other substance coexposures.[93] Notably, those newborns with NAS not requiring pharmacologic treatment were excluded from results and there may other factors at play in the relationship between brain growth and withdrawal symptoms. Several earlier, smaller studies using MRIs of the brain have also found decreases in infant head circumference and whole brain volume and findings, suggesting that certain brain regions, including the basal ganglia, thalamus, and white matter tracts, may be particularly affected by prenatal opioid exposure.[94–97] These findings of altered brain volume and morphology seem to persist in childhood through school age,[97–100] but the functional significance of these findings as well as causal relationships with other prenatal and childhood stressors remain unclear.

COGNITIVE AND BEHAVIORAL OUTCOMES

Several studies have demonstrated an association of NAS with cognitive and developmental delay in preschool and grade school aged children.[101–107] In a recent study linking Tennessee Medicaid and Birth Certificate data with Tennessee State Department of Education special education data for those born between 2008 and 2011, ages 3 to 8 at the time of sampling, children with a history of NAS were more likely to have a referral made for evaluation of an educational disability, to meet criteria for either developmental delay or speech and language impairment, and also to receive services or therapies for these diagnoses than peers without history of NAS matched by age, gender, ethnicity, and Medicaid enrollment status.[103]

An Australian study linking health data and educational testing data from the National Assessment Program: Literacy and Numeracy examinations found that children with a history of NAS had significantly lower mean composite test scores and were more likely not to meet minimum standards at grades 3, 5, and 7 than peers matched for gender, gestational age at birth, and socioeconomic status. Older maternal age and higher level of maternal education seemed to be protective against failure to meet educational standards.[104]

Prenatal opioid exposure has also been linked to increased rates of attention deficit hyperactivity disorder, behavioral problems, and executive function issues.[108–113]

However, there are multiple factors that may impact these findings. In studies of children with prenatal heroin exposure, outcomes including findings of increased attention deficit hyperactivity disorder, inattention and aggressions, and lower performance on measures of intelligence were mitigated by home environment, adoption, and socioeconomic status.[102,109,114]

In a study of mother–child pairs with prenatal MAT, either methadone or buprenorphine, those in the MAT group had lower scores in measures of both cognitive development and mother–child interactions, but higher quality mother–child interactions positively impacted narrative memory and vocabulary scores across groups.[107] Additionally, recently published results from the MOTHER trial showed no difference in developmental outcomes between infants of mothers prenatally prescribed methadone and buprenorphine exposure and that children from both subsets were following normal tracks for physical growth and cognitive and language development. Mother–child pairs in this sample generally scored well in a measure of home environment.[115]

Early intervention services may be beneficial in mitigating the observed, likely multifactorial, impact of NAS on developmental, cognitive, and behavioral outcomes; this area deserves further exploration.[106,116,117] Despite being eligible, many children do not go on to receive early intervention services. A recent retrospective cohort study found less than one-half of infants with NAS eligible for early intervention services at time of discharge were subsequently enrolled. Those discharged home with a biological parent were more likely to be referred and those with longer hospital stays more likely to enroll, highlighting potential gaps in outpatient care for those discharged early or into nonparental care.[116]

SUMMARY AND FUTURE DIRECTIONS

Most studies of NAS outcomes have focused on linear causal relationships; however, as recently highlighted by Kaltenbach and colleagues,[115] there likely is no single cause to findings of longer term developmental and educational differences in children with prenatal opioid exposure, necessitating a shift in conceptual framework. The functional outcomes for this population likely reflect a complex interplay of genetic and epigenetic factors, prenatal and childhood stressors, and mitigating factors. More recent successful interventions in this population have addressed environmental and social factors and shifted focus to the mother–child dyad. It is worth noting that a majority of substance exposed infants have some involvement of child welfare services and many infants with NAS do not go home in the custody of their biological mothers.[15,118] Support is essential for these infants and their caregivers during the birth hospitalization, discharge to home, and early childhood. Future research on long-term outcomes is needed with careful planning to account for environmental factors and recognition of the role of family and community dynamics, in addition to individual variables, to understand causal relationships and better direct potential interventions at both the individual and policy levels.

REFERENCES

1. Finnegan LP, Connaughton JF, Kron RE, et al. Neonatal abstinence syndrome: assessment and management. Addict Dis 1975;2(1–2):141–58.

2. Hudak ML, Tan RC, Frattarelli DAC, et al. Neonatal drug withdrawal. Pediatrics 2012;129(2):e540–60.

3. Kocherlakota P. Neonatal abstinence syndrome. Pediatrics 2014;134(2):e547.

4. Winkelman T, Villapiano N, Kozhimannil K, et al. Incidence and costs of neonatal abstinence syndrome among infants with Medicaid: 2004–2014. Pediatrics 2018;141(4):1.

5. Patrick SW, Kaplan HC, Passarella M, et al. Variation in treatment of neonatal abstinence syndrome in US Children's Hospitals, 2004–2011. J Perinatol 2014;34(11):867–72.

6. Grossman M, Berkwitt A. Neonatal abstinence syndrome. Semin Perinatol 2019; 43(3):173–86.

7. Jones HE, Fielder A. Neonatal abstinence syndrome: historical perspective, current focus, future directions. Prev Med 2015;80:12–7.

8. Velez M, Jansson LM. The opioid dependent mother and newborn dyad: nonpharmacologic care. J Addict Med 2008;2(3):113.

9. Cleveland LM, Bonugli R. Experiences of mothers of infants with neonatal abstinence syndrome in the neonatal intensive care unit. J Obstet Gynecol Neonatal Nurs 2014;43(3):318–29.

10. Howard MB, Schiff DM, Penwill N, et al. Impact of parental presence at infants' bedside on neonatal abstinence syndrome. Hosp Pediatr 2017;7(2):63–9.

11. Atwood EC, Sollender G, Hsu E, et al. A qualitative study of family experience with hospitalization for neonatal abstinence syndrome. Hosp Pediatr 2016; 6(10):626–32.

12. MacMillan KDL, Rendon CP, Verma K, et al. Association of rooming-in with outcomes for neonatal abstinence syndrome: a systematic review and meta-analysis. JAMA Pediatr 2018;172(4):345–51.

13. Patrick SW, Davis MM, Lehmann C, et al. Increasing incidence and geographic distribution of neonatal abstinence syndrome: United States 2009 to 2012. J Perinatol 2015;35(8):650.

14. Ko JY, Patrick SW, Tong VT, et al. Incidence of neonatal abstinence syndrome—28 states, 1999–2013. MMWR Morb Mortal Wkly Rep 2016;65:799–802.

15. Patrick SW, Schumacher RE, Horbar JD, et al. Improving care for neonatal abstinence syndrome. Pediatrics 2016;137(5) [pii:e20153835].

16. Villapiano NL, Winkelman TN, Kozhimannil KB, et al. Rural and urban differences in neonatal abstinence syndrome and maternal opioid use, 2004 to 2013. JAMA Pediatr 2017;171(2):194–6.

17. Rose-Jacobs R, Trevino-Talbot M, Lloyd-Travaglini C, et al. Could prenatal food insecurity influence neonatal abstinence syndrome severity? Addiction 2019; 114(2):337–43.

18. Neonatal abstinence syndrome rates per 1,000 births by race/ethnicity, 2015 (Q1-Q3). Secondary neonatal abstinence syndrome rates per 1,000 births by race/ethnicity, 2015 (Q1-Q3). 2018. Available at: https://www.ahrq.gov/data/infographics/neonatal-abstinence-syndrome.html.

19. Charles MK, Cooper WO, Jansson LM, et al. Male sex associated with increased risk of neonatal abstinence syndrome. Hosp Pediatr 2017;7(6):328–34.

20. Unger A, Jagsch R, Bäwert A, et al. Are male neonates more vulnerable to neonatal abstinence syndrome than female neonates? Gend Med 2011;8(6): 355–64.

21. Jansson LM, DiPietro JA, Elko A, et al. Infant autonomic functioning and neonatal abstinence syndrome. Drug Alcohol Depend 2010;109(1–3):198–204.

22. Holbrook A, Kaltenbach K. Gender and NAS: does sex matter? Drug Alcohol Depend 2010;112(1–2):156–9.

23. Huybrechts KF, Bateman BT, Desai RJ, et al. Risk of neonatal drug withdrawal after intrauterine co-exposure to opioids and psychotropic medications: cohort study. BMJ 2017;358:j3326.

24. Wachman EM, Farrer LA. The genetics and epigenetics of neonatal abstinence syndrome. Semin Fetal Neonatal Med 2019;24(2):105–10.

25. Wachman EM, Hayes MJ, Sherva R, et al. Association of maternal and infant variants in PNOC and COMT genes with neonatal abstinence syndrome severity. Am J Addict 2017;26(1):42–9.

26. Wachman EM, Hayes MJ, Brown MS, et al. Association of OPRM1 and COMT single-nucleotide polymorphisms with hospital length of stay and treatment of neonatal abstinence syndrome. JAMA 2013;309(17):1821–7.

27. Bogen DL, Whalen BL, Kair LR, et al. Wide variation found in care of opioid-exposed newborns. Acad Pediatr 2017;17(4):374–80.

28. Milliren CE, Gupta M, Graham DA, et al. Hospital variation in neonatal abstinence syndrome incidence, treatment modalities, resource use, and costs across pediatric hospitals in the United States, 2013 to 2016. Hosp Pediatr 2018;8(1):15–20.

29. Filteau J, Coo H, Dow K. Trends in incidence of neonatal abstinence syndrome in Canada and associated healthcare resource utilization. Drug Alcohol Depend 2018;185:313.

30. Tolia VN, Murthy K, Bennett MM, et al. Morphine vs methadone treatment for infants with neonatal abstinence syndrome. J Pediatr 2018;203:185–9.

31. Davis JM, Shenberger J, Terrin N, et al. Comparison of safety and efficacy of methadone vs morphine for treatment of neonatal abstinence syndrome: a randomized clinical trial. JAMA Pediatr 2018;172(8):741–8.

32. Brown JD, Goodin AJ, Talbert JC. Rural and Appalachian disparities in neonatal abstinence syndrome incidence and access to opioid abuse treatment. J Rural Health 2018;34(1):6–13.

33. Young ME, Hager SJ, Spurlock D Jr. Retrospective chart review comparing morphine and methadone in neonates treated for neonatal abstinence syndrome. Am J Health Syst Pharm 2015;72(23_Supplement_3):S162–7.

34. Hall ES, Rice WR, Folger AT, et al. Comparison of neonatal abstinence syndrome treatment with sublingual buprenorphine versus conventional opioids. Am J Perinatol 2018;35(04):405–12.

35. Hall ES, Isemann BT, Wexelblatt SL, et al. A cohort comparison of buprenorphine versus methadone treatment for neonatal abstinence syndrome. J Pediatr 2016;170:39–44.e1.

36. Kraft WK, Adeniyi-Jones SC, Chervoneva I, et al. Buprenorphine for the treatment of the neonatal abstinence syndrome. N Engl J Med 2017;376(24):2341–8.

37. Coyle MG, Ferguson A, Lagasse L, et al. Diluted tincture of opium (DTO) and phenobarbital versus DTO alone for neonatal opiate withdrawal in term infants. J Pediatr 2002;140(5):561–4.

38. Surran B, Visintainer P, Chamberlain S, et al. Efficacy of clonidine versus phenobarbital in reducing neonatal morphine sulfate therapy days for neonatal abstinence syndrome. A prospective randomized clinical trial. J Perinatol 2013; 33(12):954.

39. Devlin LA, Lau T, Radmacher PG. Decreasing total medication exposure and length of stay while completing withdrawal for neonatal abstinence syndrome during the neonatal hospital stay. Front Pediatr 2017;5:216.

40. Wachman EM, Schiff DM, Silverstein M. Neonatal abstinence syndrome: advances in diagnosis and treatment neonatal abstinence syndrome: a review. JAMA 2018;319(13):1362–74.

41. Meador KJ, Baker G, Cohen MJ, et al. Cognitive/behavioral teratogenetic effects of antiepileptic drugs. Epilepsy Behav 2007;11(3):292–302.

42. Chen J, Cai F, Cao J, et al. Long-term antiepileptic drug administration during early life inhibits hippocampal neurogenesis in the developing brain. J Neurosci Res 2009;87(13):2898–907.

43. Reinisch JM, Sanders SA, Mortensen EL, et al. In Utero exposure to phenobarbital and intelligence deficits in adult men. JAMA 1995;274(19):1518–25.

44. Hall ES, Wexelblatt SL, Crowley M, et al. Implementation of a neonatal abstinence syndrome weaning protocol: a multicenter cohort study. Pediatrics 2015;136(4):e803.

45. Chisamore B, Labana S, Blitz S, et al. A comparison of morphine delivery in neonatal opioid withdrawal. Subst Abuse 2016;10(1):49–54.

46. Lee J, Hulman S, Musci M Jr, et al. Neonatal abstinence syndrome: influence of a combined inpatient/outpatient methadone treatment regimen on the average length of stay of a Medicaid NICU population. Popul Health Manag 2015; 18(5):392–7.

47. Backes CH, Backes CR, Gardner D, et al. Neonatal abstinence syndrome: transitioning methadone-treated infants from an inpatient to an outpatient setting. J Perinatol 2012;32(6):425.

48. Maalouf FI, Cooper WO, Slaughter JC, et al. Outpatient pharmacotherapy for neonatal abstinence syndrome. J Pediatr 2018;199:151–7.e1.

49. Loudin S, Werthammer J, Prunty L, et al. A management strategy that reduces NICU admissions and decreases charges from the front line of the neonatal abstinence syndrome epidemic. J Perinatol 2017;37(10):1108.

50. Kelly LE, Knoppert D, Roukema H, et al. Oral morphine weaning for neonatal abstinence syndrome at home compared with in-hospital: an observational cohort study. Paediatr Drugs 2015;17(2):151–7.

51. Smirk CL, Bowman E, Doyle LW, et al. Home-based detoxification for neonatal abstinence syndrome reduces length of hospital admission without prolonging treatment. Acta Paediatr 2014;103(6):601–4.

52. Grossman MR, Berkwitt AK, Osborn RR, et al. An initiative to improve the quality of care of infants with neonatal abstinence syndrome. Pediatrics 2017;139(6): e20163360.

53. Rodriguez CE, Klie KA. Pharmacological treatment of opioid use disorder in pregnancy. Semin Perinatol 2019;43(3):141–8.

54. Gomez-Pomar E, Finnegan LP. The epidemic of neonatal abstinence syndrome, historical references of its' origins, assessment, and management. Front Pediatr 2018;6(33). https://doi.org/10.3389/fped.2018.00033.

55. Patrick SW, Schiff DM. A public health response to opioid use in pregnancy. Pediatrics 2017;139(3):e20164070.

56. Whalen BL, Holmes AV, Blythe S. Models of care for neonatal abstinence syndrome: what works? Semin Fetal Neonatal Med 2019;24(2):121–32.

57. Mangat AK, Schmölzer GM, Kraft WK. Pharmacological and non-pharmacological treatments for the neonatal abstinence syndrome (NAS). Semin Fetal Neonatal Med 2019;24(2):133–41.

58. Wachman EM, Lahav A. The effects of noise on preterm infants in the NICU. Arch Dis Child Fetal Neonatal Ed 2011;96(4):F305–9.

59. World Health Organization (WHO). Baby-friendly hospital initiative: revised, updated and expanded for integrated care. 2009. Available at: https://www.ncbi.nlm.nih.gov/books/NBK153471/. Accessed September 18, 2019.
60. Abrahams RR, Kelly SA, Payne S, et al. Rooming-in compared with standard care for newborns of mothers using methadone or heroin. Can Fam Physician 2007;53(10):1722–30.
61. Saiki T, Lee S, Hannam S, et al. Neonatal abstinence syndrome—postnatal ward versus neonatal unit management. Eur J Pediatr 2010;169(1):95.
62. Hünseler C, Brückle M, Roth B, et al. Neonatal opiate withdrawal and rooming-in: a retrospective analysis of a single center experience. Klin Paediatr 2013; 225(05):247–51.
63. Holmes AV, Atwood EC, Whalen B, et al. Rooming-in to treat neonatal abstinence syndrome: improved family-centered care at lower cost. Pediatrics 2016;137(6): e20152929.
64. McKnight S, Coo H, Davies G, et al. Rooming-in for infants at risk of neonatal abstinence syndrome. Am J Perinatol 2016;33(05):495–501.
65. Cleveland LM, Gill SL. "Try not to judge": mothers of substance exposed infants. MCN Am J Matern Child Nurs 2013;38(4):200–5.
66. Short VL, Gannon M, Abatemarco DJ. The association between breastfeeding and length of hospital stay among infants diagnosed with neonatal abstinence syndrome: a population-based study of in-hospital births. Breastfeed Med 2016;11(7):343–9.
67. Tsai LC, Doan TJ. Breastfeeding among mothers on opioid maintenance treatment: a literature review 2016. p. 521–9. Los Angeles (CA).
68. Wachman EM, Byun J, Philipp BL. Breastfeeding rates among mothers of infants with neonatal abstinence syndrome. Breastfeed Med 2010;5(4):159–64.
69. Bogen DL, Whalen BL. Breastmilk feeding for mothers and infants with opioid exposure: what is best? Semin Fetal Neonatal Med 2019;24(2):95–104.
70. Demirci JR, Bogen DL, Klionsky Y. Breastfeeding and methadone therapy: the maternal experience. Subst Abuse 2015;36(2):203–8.
71. Favara M, David C, Jensen E, et al. Maternal breast milk feeding and length of treatment in infants with neonatal abstinence syndrome. J Perinatol 2019;39(6): 876–82.
72. Welle-Strand GK, Skurtveit S, Jansson LM, et al. Breastfeeding reduces the need for withdrawal treatment in opioid-exposed infants. Acta Paediatr 2013; 102(11):1060–6.
73. Tsai LC, Doan TJ. Breastfeeding among mothers on opioid maintenance treatment: a literature review. J Hum Lact 2016;32(3):521–9.
74. Pritham UA. Breastfeeding promotion for management of neonatal abstinence syndrome. J Obstet Gynecol Neonatal Nurs 2013;42(5):517–26.
75. Schiff DM, Grossman MR. Beyond the Finnegan scoring system: novel assessment and diagnostic techniques for the opioid-exposed infant. Semin Fetal Neonatal Med 2019;24(2):115–20.
76. Jones HE, Seashore C, Johnson E, et al. Psychometric assessment of the neonatal abstinence scoring system and the MOTHER NAS Scale. Am J Addict 2016;25(5):370–3.
77. Grossman MR, Lipshaw MJ, Osborn RR, et al. A novel approach to assessing infants with neonatal abstinence syndrome. Hosp Pediatr 2018;8(1):1–6.
78. Zimmermann-Baer U, Nötzli U, Rentsch K, et al. Finnegan neonatal abstinence scoring system: normal values for first 3 days and weeks 5–6 in non-addicted infants. Addiction 2010;105(3):524–8.

79. Wachman EM, Grossman M, Schiff DM, et al. Quality improvement initiative to improve inpatient outcomes for Neonatal Abstinence Syndrome. J Perinatol 2018;38(8):1114–22.

80. Rouse CL, Zaidel Y, DuPerry M, et al. Supporting newborn transition in perinatal areas by keeping at-risk babies with their mothers. J Obstet Gynecol Neonatal Nurs 2019;48(3):S67–8.

81. Patrick SW, Burke JF, Biel TJ, et al. Risk of hospital readmission among infants with neonatal abstinence syndrome. Hosp Pediatr 2015;5(10):513–9.

82. Uebel H, Wright IM, Burns L, et al. Reasons for rehospitalization in children who had neonatal abstinence syndrome. Pediatrics 2015;136(4):e811.

83. Liu G, Kong L, Leslie DL, et al. A longitudinal healthcare use profile of children with a history of neonatal abstinence syndrome. J Pediatr 2019;204:111–7.e1.

84. Bogen DL, Hanusa BH, Baker R, et al. Randomized clinical trial of standard- versus high-calorie formula for methadone-exposed infants: a feasibility study. Hosp Pediatr 2018;8(1):7.

85. Corr TE, Schaefer EW, Paul IM. Growth during the first year in infants affected by neonatal abstinence syndrome.(Report). BMC Pediatr 2018;18(1). https://doi.org/10.1186/s12887-018-1327-0.

86. Younger WJ, Chu FL, D'arcy TN, et al. Prescription opioid analgesics rapidly change the human brain. Pain 2011;152(8):1803–10.

87. Lin JC, Chu LF, Stringer EA, et al. One month of oral morphine decreases gray matter volume in the right amygdala of individuals with low back pain: confirmation of previously reported magnetic resonance imaging results. Pain Med 2016; 17(8):1497.

88. Ford DH, Rhines RK. Prenatal exposure to methadone HCL in relationship to body and brain growth in the rat. Acta Neurol Scand 1979;59(5):248–62.

89. Zagon IS, MacLaughlin PJ. Endogenous opioid systems regulate cell proliferation in the developing rat brain. Brain Res 1987;412(1):68–72.

90. Zagon IS, McLaughlin PJ. Comparative effects of postnatal undernutrition and methadone exposure on protein and nucleic acid contents of the brain and cerebellum in rats. Dev Neurosci 1982;5(5–6):385–93.

91. Robinson SE. Effect of prenatal opioid exposure on cholinergic development. J Biomed Sci 2000;7(3):253–7.

92. Willson N, Schneider J, Roizin L, et al. Effects of methadone hydrochloride on the growth of organotypic cerebellar cultures prepared from methadone-tolerant and control rats. J Pharmacol Exp Ther 1976;199(2):368–74.

93. Towers CV, Hyatt BW, Visconti KC, et al. Neonatal head circumference in newborns with neonatal abstinence syndrome. Pediatrics 2019;143(1). https://doi.org/10.1542/peds.2018-0541.

94. Visconti KC, Hennessy KC, Towers CV, et al. Chronic opiate use in pregnancy and newborn head circumference. Am J Perinatol 2015;32(01):027–32.

95. Yuan Q, Rubic M, Seah J, et al. Do maternal opioids reduce neonatal regional brain volumes? A pilot study. J Perinatol 2014;34(12). https://doi.org/10.1038/jp.2014.111.

96. Monnelly VJ, Anblagan D, Quigley A, et al. Prenatal methadone exposure is associated with altered neonatal brain development. Neuroimage Clin 2018; 18:9–14.

97. Walhovd KB, Watts R, Amlien I, et al. Neural tract development of infants born to methadone-maintained mothers. Pediatr Neurol 2012;47(1):1–6.

98. Walhovd KB, Moe V, Slinning K, et al. Volumetric cerebral characteristics of children exposed to opiates and other substances in utero. Neuroimage 2007; 36(4):1331–44.
99. Nygaard E, Slinning K, Moe V, et al. Neuroanatomical characteristics of youths with prenatal opioid and poly-drug exposure. Neurotoxicol Teratol 2018;68: 13–26.
100. Sirnes E, Oltedal L, Bartsch H, et al. Brain morphology in school-aged children with prenatal opioid exposure: a structural MRI study. Early Hum Dev 2017; 106:33–9.
101. Nygaard E, Moe V, Slinning K, et al. Longitudinal cognitive development of children born to mothers with opioid and polysubstance use. Pediatr Res 2015; 78(3):330.
102. Ornoy A, Daka L, Goldzweig G, et al. Neurodevelopmental and psychological assessment of adolescents born to drug-addicted parents: effects of SES and adoption. Child Abuse Negl 2010;34(5):354–68.
103. Fill M-MA, Miller AM, Wilkinson RH, et al. Educational disabilities among children born with neonatal abstinence syndrome. Pediatrics 2018;142(3):e20180562.
104. Oei JL, Melhuish E, Uebel H, et al. Neonatal abstinence syndrome and high school performance. Pediatrics 2017;139(2). https://doi.org/10.1542/peds. 2016-2651.
105. Maguire DJ, Taylor S, Armstrong K, et al. Long-term outcomes of infants with neonatal abstinence syndrome. Neonatal Netw 2016;35(5):277–86.
106. Beckwith AM, Burke SA. Identification of early developmental deficits in infants with prenatal heroin, methadone, and other opioid exposure. Clin Pediatr 2015; 54(4):328–35.
107. Konijnenberg C, Sarfi M, Melinder A. Mother-child interaction and cognitive development in children prenatally exposed to methadone or buprenorphine. Early Hum Dev 2016;101:91–7.
108. Sundelin Wahlsten V, Sarman I. Neurobehavioural development of preschool-age children born to addicted mothers given opiate maintenance treatment with buprenorphine during pregnancy. Acta Paediatr 2013;102(5):544–9.
109. Ornoy A, Segal J, Bar-Hamburger R, et al. Developmental outcome of school-age children born to mothers with heroin dependency: importance of environmental factors. Dev Med Child Neurol 2001;43(10):668–75.
110. Sirnes E, Griffiths ST, Aukland SM, et al. Functional MRI in prenatally opioid-exposed children during a working memory-selective attention task. Neurotoxicol Teratol 2018;66:46–54.
111. Hans SL. Developmental consequences of prenatal exposure to methadone. Ann N Y Acad Sci 1989;562(1):195–207.
112. Nygaard E, Slinning K, Moe V, et al. Behavior and attention problems in eight-year-old children with prenatal opiate and poly-substance exposure: a longitudinal study. PLoS One 2016;11(6):e0158054.
113. Konijnenberg C, Melinder A. Executive function in preschool children prenatally exposed to methadone or buprenorphine. Child Neuropsychol 2015;21(5): 570–85.
114. Ornoy A, Michailevskaya V, Lukashov I, et al. The developmental outcome of children born to heroin-dependent mothers, raised at home or adopted. Child Abuse Negl 1996;20(5):385–96.
115. Kaltenbach K, O'Grady KE, Heil SH, et al. Prenatal exposure to methadone or buprenorphine: early childhood developmental outcomes. Drug Alcohol depend 2018;185:40–9.

116. Peacock-Chambers E, Leyenaar J, Foss S, et al. Early intervention referral and enrollment among infants with neonatal abstinence syndrome. J Dev Behav Pediatr 2019;40(6):441–50.
117. Belcher MEH, Butz MA, Wallace HP, et al. Spectrum of early intervention services for children with intrauterine drug exposure. Infants Young Child 2005; 18(1):2–15.
118. Waite D, Greiner MV, Laris Z. Putting families first: how the opioid epidemic is affecting children and families, and the child welfare policy options to address it. J Appl Res Child 2018;9(1):4.

Pain, Opioids, and Pregnancy
Historical Context and Medical Management

Caitlin E. Martin, MD, MPH[a], Mishka Terplan, MD, MPH[b],*, Elizabeth E. Krans, MD, MSc[c]

KEYWORDS

- Addiction • Opioid use disorder • Pain • Trauma-informed care
- Gender differences • Substance use screening

KEY POINTS

- The biological and social pathways to substance use are different for women and men, including pain and trauma histories.
- A maternal substance use disorder should not be perceived as a disease of pregnancy but rather as a time when the reproductive health life course intersects with the addiction life course and when patients have the most access to preventative health care services.
- Although untreated opioid use disorder can have a profound effect on maternal and neonatal health outcomes, substance use disorders are chronic, relapsing, remitting disorders that continue to affect women well beyond the pregnancy episode.
- Pharmacotherapy remains central to care, and maternal engagement in prenatal care and addiction treatment is associated with birth outcomes that largely mirror that of a population of women without addiction.

INTRODUCTION

Opioid overdose deaths claim 130 Americans lives every day.[1] Although the opioid epidemic crosses all geographic, demographic, and social lines, this crisis has had a severe and arguably disproportionate impact on pregnant women and their children. Since 1999, opioid use disorder has increased 333% among pregnant women and in 2014, complicated approximately 1% of all births in the United States.[2] Opioid use now accounts for 50% of all drug treatment admissions during pregnancy[3] and is

The authors have nothing to disclose.
[a] Department of Obstetrics and Gynecology, Virginia Commonwealth University, 1250 East Marshall Street, Richmond, VA 23298-0268, USA; [b] Friends Research Institute, 1040 Park Ave, Suite 103, Baltimore MD 21202, USA; [c] Department of Obstetrics, Gynecology and Reproductive Sciences, University of Pittsburgh, Magee-Womens Research Institute, 300 Halket Street, Pittsburgh, PA 15213, USA
* Corresponding author.
E-mail address: Mishka.Terplan@vcuhealth.org

associated with a 4-fold increase in mortality during the delivery hospitalization.[4] Although opioid use disorder has had a profound effect on maternal and neonatal health outcomes, substance use disorders are chronic, relapsing, remitting disorders that continue to affect women well beyond the pregnancy episode. In fact, overdose death has become the leading cause of pregnancy-associated mortality in the United States with overdose rates most frequently occurring 7 to 12 months postpartum.[5–7] The purpose of review is to provide an evidence-based perspective on the historical relationships between gender, pain, and opioids and offer clinical management solutions for the treatment of opioid use disorder in pregnancy.

HISTORICAL CONTEXT

Although opioids have been part of human culture and medical practice for millennia, the adverse health effects of opioid use, misuse, and dependence have only recently emerged as a social and public health concern. At the turn of the twentieth century, the first opioid crisis occurred largely among white middle- and upper-class women whose addiction resulted from the prescribing practices of physicians for gynecologic pain such as dysmenorrhea.[8] Opioids were explicitly marketed to women as a "cure-all" medicine for a variety of ailments that resulted in gender disparities in the prevalence of addiction, as two-thirds of individuals addicted to opioids in the 1900s were women.[8] Over 100 years later, the social, health, and economic effects of the current US opioid crisis continues to disproportionally affect women and is far more complex. Opioid prescribing, the primary driver of the current epidemic, is more common for women who are more likely to use opioids chronically and at higher doses than men.[9] As a result, prescription opioid overdose events escalated among women.[10] In an evaluation of national demographic trends from 1993 to 2010, the rate of prescription opioid overdose hospitalizations among women increased from 2.4 to 15.9 per 100,000 US persons and exceeded the rate among men for all study years. A "triple wave epidemic," the first wave of opioid overdose deaths in the 1990s, largely involved prescription opioids but quickly transitioned to heroin in 2010 because it is cheaper and more readily available than prescription opioids.[11] From 2002 to 2013, reproductive-aged individuals experienced the largest increase (108.6%) in heroin use compared with other age groups, with a greater percentage of increase found among women (100%) compared with men (50%).[12] In 2013, synthetic opioids such as fentanyl replaced heroin as the leading cause of opioid overdose death.[13] Synthetic opioids are involved in 59.8% of all opioid-involved overdose deaths and have increased 850% in women between 1999 and 2015.[14]

WOMEN, PAIN, AND TRAUMA

The biological and social pathways to substance use are different for women and men.[15] Even though women typically start using substances at older ages, they progress to physical dependence more quickly than men, a phenomenon known as "telescoping."[16] They present to treatment with more impairments[17] and are at higher risk of opioid overdose than men, even when prescribed lower doses.[18] Predisposing factors associated with the risk of developing a substance use disorder differ for women compared with men. Higher rates of psychological distress,[19] comorbid psychiatric disorders such as depression,[20] and physical and emotional abuse increase the risk of substance use among women. More than half of women with a substance use disorder have experienced intimate partner violence, compared with less than 20% of non-substance use disorder women, and 55% to 99% report a history of trauma, with abuse commonly occurring in childhood.[21,22] As a result, women are more likely to report using substances to reduce negative mood states such as depression or cope with a history of trauma or violence including posttraumatic stress disorder.[17]

Chronic pain disorders are also more common among women,[23] who typically experience pain differently and at more body sites[24] compared with men. Not only are women more sensitive to painful stimuli[25] but they also experience higher levels of emotional distress and anxiety when faced with pain.[26] This negative emotional response to pain is thought to explain a large part of gender differences in reported pain severity[27] and disproportionate rates of opioid prescribing among women compared with men.[28] When caring for persons with opioid use disorder, comorbid pain conditions are more commonly encountered among women than men[29] and their management in this setting is complex.[30] Women with co-occurring substance use and chronic pain disorders also present to treatment with worse social functioning and a higher prevalence of medical, psychiatric, and traumatic comorbidities.[15,31] Thus, using a gender-informed, biopsychosocial approach to treatment, which includes therapies targeting emotional processes (eg, cognitive behavioral therapy), may be uniquely effective for supporting women in their recovery. Further, with women disproportionately represented in the current opioid crisis, a trauma-informed approach to care should be universally adopted across health care settings.[32]

SUBSTANCE USE AND SCREENING DURING PREGNANCY

Pregnancy is a "window of opportunity" for behavior change,[33,34] as most women who use substances, including tobacco, alcohol, and illicit drugs, either reduce or eliminate substance use during pregnancy. In an evaluation of substance use across pregnancy, 83% of women achieved abstinence to at least one substance and women were more likely to achieve abstinence from alcohol (hazard ratio [HR]: 7.24), marijuana (HR: 4.06), and cocaine (HR: 3.41). Similarly, opioid misuse is lower among pregnant than nonpregnant women.[35] According the National Survey of Drug Use and Health, from 2007 to 2014, 13.9% of nonpregnant women were in need of substance use disorder treatment compared with 7.6% of pregnant women with decreasing prevalence by trimester: 9.5% in the first to 7.7% in the second and 5.7% in the third trimester. In contrast, pregnant women who continue to use drugs during pregnancy likely have a substance use disorder[36] and providers have the responsibility to identify substance use and engage patients in treatment. Thus, a maternal substance use disorder should not be perceived as a disease of pregnancy. Instead, pregnancy should be perceived as a time when the reproductive health life course (getting pregnant, staying pregnant, and delivering) intersects with the addiction life course (use, misuse, addiction) (**Fig. 1**) and when patients have the most access to preventative health care services. **Fig. 1** illustrates opportunities for the assessment and management of substance use before pregnancy as well as the importance of the postpartum period.

Identification of pregnant women with an opioid use disorder rests on timely assessment. Universal screening for substance use is recommended by public health agencies and professional societies including American College of Obstetricians Gynecologists and American Academy of Pediatrics[37–40] and avoids the reproduction of stigma and stereotype inherent in risk-based screening.[41] Utilization of a validated instrument is ideal,[42] and positive screens should be followed by a proper diagnostic assessment, which details the diagnostic criteria for an opioid use disorder. Although point-of-care biological testing (eg, urine drug screen) is commonly used in health care settings, it is an insufficient and problematic substitute for screening and diagnosis using validated instruments and evidence-based methods (eg, SBIRT). Biological tests

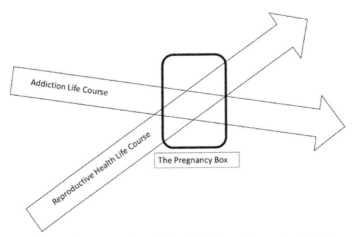

Fig. 1. Pregnancy is at the intersection of the addiction and reproductive life courses.

that capture drug metabolites vary by substance and assay used, have a short window of detection resulting in false-negative results, and false-positive results are often misinterpreted by nonlaboratory personnel[43] and can have legal consequences. Finally, biological tests capture nothing about maternal behavior, on which diagnosis rests, or an individual's parenting fitness.[44]

PRENATAL MANAGEMENT OF OPIOID USE DISORDER

Optimization of maternal health is a core principle of prenatal care.[45] Individuals with addiction need treatment to optimize maternal and neonatal health outcomes.[46] Since the 1970s, the provision of addiction treatment with prenatal care has demonstrated birth outcomes similar to that of a population of women without addiction,[47–49] an observation confirmed with recent data.[50] Pharmacotherapy with either methadone or buprenorphine, as part of a comprehensive addiction treatment program, is the standard of care for women with opioid use disorder.[51–53] Recent SAMHSA Clinical Guidance for Treating Pregnant Women with Opioid Use Disorder recommends either buprenorphine or methadone as the safest medications and advises against transitioning from one to the other during pregnancy.[54] Naltrexone, approved by Food and Drug Administration for the treatment of opioid use disorder, is not recommended in pregnancy due to a paucity of published data, although data do not indicate any evidence of harm.[55,56] Buprenorphine monotherapy has predominantly been used in pregnancy, but access to monotherapy is increasingly limited, diversion risks are higher, and, consequentially, many providers have switched to using the combination product (buprenorphine/naloxone).[57] Detoxification, or medically supervised withdrawal, is not recommended during pregnancy[54,58] due to its association with addiction recurrence.[59] A comparison of the different pharmacotherapies is in **Fig. 2**.

The principle of pharmacotherapy for opioid use disorder, initially, is control of withdrawal symptoms (which interrupts the negative reinforcing property of opioids), followed by opioid craving cessation and, finally, achievement of an "opioid blockade" (which interrupts the positive reinforcing property of opioids).[60] These clinical outcomes correlate with increasing dose, as they relate to medication binding to the mu-opioid receptor, the neurobiological target of the medications.[61] Physiologic changes of pregnancy alter both methadone and buprenorphine pharmacokinetics.[62,63] Therefore, some women may require split dosing or dose increases,

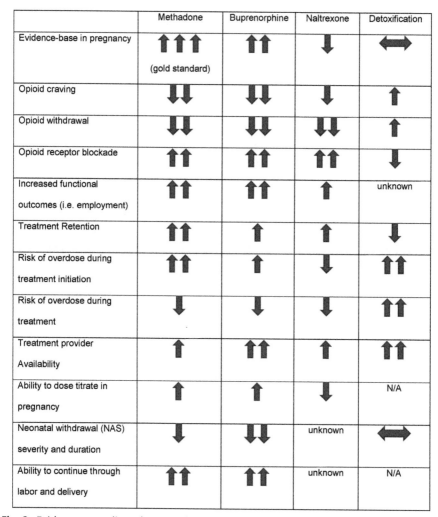

	Methadone	Buprenorphine	Naltrexone	Detoxification
Evidence-base in pregnancy	↑↑↑ (gold standard)	↑↑	↓	↔
Opioid craving	↓↓	↓↓	↓	↑
Opioid withdrawal	↓↓	↓↓	↓↓	↑
Opioid receptor blockade	↑↑	↑↑	↑↑	↓
Increased functional outcomes (i.e. employment)	↑↑	↑↑	↑	unknown
Treatment Retention	↑↑	↑	↑	↓
Risk of overdose during treatment initiation	↑↑	↑	↓	↑↑
Risk of overdose during treatment	↓	↓	↓	↑↑
Treatment provider Availability	↑	↑↑	↑	↑↑
Ability to dose titrate in pregnancy	↑	↑	↓	N/A
Neonatal withdrawal (NAS) severity and duration	↓	↓↓	unknown	↔
Ability to continue through labor and delivery	↑↑	↑↑	unknown	N/A

Fig. 2. Evidence regarding pharmacotherapy treatment options for opioid use disorder in pregnancy. Arrows represent strength of evidence in favor of treatment option, with 3 arrows being the max and a horizontal arrow meaning neutral.

especially as pregnancy progresses.[64,65] Medication dose, however, should be individualized, with attention to avoid underdosing, which is associated with treatment attrition and illicit drug use.[66,67]

Although opioid pharmacotherapy is the recommended, evidence-based treatment approach for opioid use disorder in pregnancy, comprehensive treatment of opioid use disorder extends beyond pharmacotherapy use.[54] Because of high prevalence rates, all pregnant women with opioid use disorder should be screened for infectious comorbidities associated with illicit drug use (eg, hepatitis C virus, human immunodeficiency virus,[68] co-occurring psychiatric disorders [eg, depression, anxiety],[69,70] intimate partner violence, and trauma).[71] Behavioral health interventions such as group or individual counseling and cognitive behavioral therapy can be also be effective adjuncts to pharmacotherapy especially among patients with prescription opioid dependence.[72] Because women with opioid use disorder often have multiple medical and psychosocial comorbidities that can negatively affect treatment engagement, a clinical checklist can help providers confirm that each component of care has been provided and that referral mechanisms are in place for women with positive screens. **Table 1** provides an example of clinical checklist for common medical and psychosocial comorbidities among women with opioid use disorder.

LABOR AND DELIVERY

Delivery is a painful event that all pregnant women anticipate and experience. However, effective analgesia can be achieved,[73] and methadone and buprenorphine should be continued, without dose change, throughout labor and delivery.[74] Multimodal therapies should be used, and regional anesthesia is recommended.[39] When opioids are given, their dosing should be individualized,[75,76] and there is no difference in perioperative opioid requirement between individuals receiving methadone versus those receiving buprenorphine.[77] Partial opioid agonists should be avoided (eg, nalbuphine, butorphanol) because they may precipitate withdrawal, and increasing the dose of methadone or buprenorphine will not improve pain control and should not be done.

Women with opioid use disorder may express concern regarding pain management during labor and delivery. Hence, providers should develop a pain management plan with patients prenatally, document such conversations,[74] and consult with OB anesthesia as needed. Most importantly, communication between these medical teams (eg, obstetric and addiction providers, anesthesia, labor and delivery nursing) should occur before the delivery admission to formulate and agree on a peripartum pain plan. Doing so will ensure consistency in management as the patient traverses through the outpatient and inpatient clinical settings. Again, involving the patient in the planning and execution of peripartum pain management plan in a transparent manner is crucial to optimize outcomes.

After delivery, routine opioid prescribing may not be indicated, especially following vaginal birth.[78,79] Following cesarean section, women with opioid use disorder may require higher than standard opioid doses,[75,76] and there is no evidence that opioid prescribing for acute pain leads to relapse.[80] In fact, poorly controlled pain may interfere with one's recovery progress serving as a risk factor for relapse.[81,82] Thus, opioid prescriptions should be individualized with the goal of providing adequate pain relief after discharge. Clear communication and close follow-up are key to optimize both effective analgesia and addiction recovery postpartum.

POSTPARTUM—THE FOURTH TRIMESTER

The postpartum period, or the "fourth trimester," is a time of increased vulnerabilities for women with opioid use disorder as pregnancy-related insurance eligibility lapses[83,84] and newborn care can be stressful and isolating. Breastfeeding carries a myriad of benefits for the mother-infant dyad in general. For infants exposed to medication-assisted treatment of opioid use disorder, breastfeeding carries additional benefits of decreasing severity of neonatal abstinence syndrome, and mothers should be counseled as such on this recommendation.[85] Having comorbid hepatitis C infection is not a contraindication to breastfeeding, and these mothers should also be encouraged to breastfeed their infants.[86]

The postpartum period is also characterized by poor sleep and mood changes, specifically postpartum depression, which is especially common among women with substance use disorders and behavioral health conditions.[87] Continuing health

Table 1
Clinical checklist for pregnant women with opioid use disorder

	Clinical Pathway	Tools
Initial prenatal visit/First trimester		
Opioid use disorder	Assess for opioid pharmacotherapy use (eg, methadone, buprenorphine) and engagement in behavioral health therapy Obtain appropriate consent to communicate with treatment provider Monitor dose and engagement with treatment provider Discuss with patient expectations regarding pharmacotherapy and OUD treatment during pregnancy and postpartum	DSM-5 diagnostic criteria SAMHSA patient handout: https://store.samhsa.gov/system/files/sma18-5071fs1.pdf
Overdose prevention	Provide naloxone prescriptions and instructions	Harm Reduction Coalition Manuals and Best Practice Documents: https://harmreduction.org/issues/overdose-prevention/tools-best-practices/manuals-best-practice/
Second/Third trimester		
Peripartum pain management	Continue pharmacotherapy through labor and delivery Consider OB anesthesia consultation visit Formulate and document peripartum pain management plan with anesthesia, labor, and delivery staff, obstetric and addiction provider Discuss pain management plan with patient	SAMHSA Clinical Guidance for Treating Pregnant and Parenting Women with Opioid Use Disorder
Neonatal withdrawal (NAS)	Discuss NAS expectations with family Consider prenatal consultation with pediatrics/neonatology	SAMHSA patient handout: https://store.samhsa.gov/system/files/sma18-5071fs3.pdf
Breastfeeding	Discuss benefits of breastfeeding with patient, including positive effects on NAS	SAMHSA patient handout: https://store.samhsa.gov/system/files/sma18-5071fs4.pdf
Family planning	Contraception counselling and postpartum method choice	Bedsider.org

(continued on next page)

Table 1
(continued)

	Clinical Pathway	Tools
Child welfare	Discuss with patient expectations regarding involvement of child protective services	SAMHSA patient handout: https://store.samhsa.gov/system/files/sma18-5071fs1.pdf
Postpartum		
Opioid use disorder	Coordinate early and frequent follow-up with both OB and addiction providers Continue pharmacotherapy at same dose	SAMHSA Clinical Guidance for Treating Pregnant and Parenting Women with Opioid Use Disorder
Ongoing assessment and management of comorbidities		
Tobacco use	Smoking cessation counselling Pharmacotherapy (eg, nicotine replacement) if indicated and desired	5 As (Ask, Advise, Assess, Assist, Arrange)
Psychiatric disorders	Screen for depression and other behavioral health conditions Referral to behavioral health provider or psychiatry	Edinburgh Postnatal Depression Scale (EPDS); Patient Health Questionnaire 9 (PHQ-9)
Infectious disease	Screen for HIV and HCV during the initial prenatal visit and third trimester if injection/intranasal drug use continues HCV-infected patients should be referred to hepatology and receive immunizations for hepatitis A and B HIV-infected patients should be referred to infectious disease	HCV and HIV antibody for initial screening If HCV antibody (+), HCV genotype, viral load, liver transaminases
Intimate partner violence (IPV)	Screen during the initial prenatal care visit and periodically as needed Referral to social work and/or case management	Abuse Assessment Screen (AAS) HITS Screening Assessment
Trauma	Screening during initial visit and periodically as needed	Trauma Assessment for Adults (TAA) Posttraumatic Stress Disorder (PTSD) Symptom Scale

Abbreviations: HCV, hepatitis C virus; HIV, human immunodeficiency virus; OB, obstetric; OUD, opioid use disorder.

care and treatment engagement beyond the 6 week postpartum period is critical to the long-term recovery process for women with opioid use disorder.[88] Although many women initiate substance use disorder treatment during pregnancy,[89] most experience gaps in care following delivery,[90] leading to relapse,[91] overdose, and overdose death.[5,7] Overdose is currently the leading cause of pregnancy-associated mortality in the United States with most of the overdose deaths occurring postpartum.[5,92]

Importantly, the postpartum is also an opportune time to address reproductive health care needs, including contraception, as unintended pregnancy is more common among women with opioid use disorder.[93] Although many women with substance use disorders want family planning services,[94] few receive effective reproductive health care. In an analysis of Pennsylvania Medicaid data, only 18% of postpartum women with opioid use disorder received an effective contraceptive method within 90 days of delivery.[95] Immediate postpartum contraception services may reduce barriers to contraception, especially for women who desire long-acting reversible contraception,[96] as most women with opioid use disorder fail to attend the postpartum visit.

SUMMARY

Five decades of published science attests to the safe and effective management of opioid use disorder during pregnancy. Pharmacotherapy remains central to care, and maternal engagement in prenatal care and addiction treatment is associated with birth outcomes that largely mirror that of a population of women without addiction. Despite the clear benefit of treatment engagement, most pregnant women with opioid use disorder fail to receive effective health care services. Even among women who receive care, addiction treatment is often disrupted in the postpartum period due to the loss of health insurance coverage and other structural conditions. Further, despite the clear benefit of treatment, the response to the opioid crisis among women has, arguably, trended toward the punitive.[97] Criminalization including the arrest, prosecution, and incarceration of pregnant women for drug use[98,99] far from benefits maternal and child health, conflicts with principles of reproductive autonomy, and overwhelmingly punishes poor and black women.[100] Instead, maternal management of opioid use disorder demands an evidence-based approach to care and an equitable public health response.

REFERENCES

1. Opioid Overdose. Understanding the epidemic. Center for Disease Control and Prevention. Available online at: https://www.cdc.gov/drugoverdose/epidemic/index.html. Accessed September 21, 2019.

2. Haight SC, Ko JY, Tong VT, et al. Opioid use disorder documented at delivery hospitalization - United States, 1999-2014. MMWR Morb Mortal Wkly Rep 2018;67(31):845–9.

3. Short VL, Hand DJ, MacAfee L, et al. Trends and disparities in receipt of pharmacotherapy among pregnant women in publically funded treatment programs for opioid use disorder in the United States. J Subst Abuse Treat 2018;89:67–74.

4. Whiteman VE, Salemi JL, Mogos MF, et al. Maternal opioid drug use during pregnancy and its impact on perinatal morbidity, mortality, and the costs of medical care in the United States. J Pregnancy 2014;2014:906723.

5. Metz TD, Rovner P, Hoffman MC, et al. Maternal deaths from Suicide and overdose in Colorado, 2004-2012. Obstet Gynecol 2016;128(6):1233–40.

6. Koch AR, Rosenberg D, Geller SE. Higher risk of homicide among pregnant and postpartum females aged 10-29 years in Illinois, 2002-2011. Obstet Gynecol 2016;128(3):440–6.

7. Schiff DM, Nielsen T, Terplan M, et al. Fatal and nonfatal overdose among pregnant and postpartum women in Massachusetts. Obstet Gynecol 2018;132(2):466–74.

8. Terplan M. Women and the opioid crisis: historical context and public health solutions. Fertil Steril 2017;108(2):195–9.

9. Campbell CI, Weisner C, Leresche L, et al. Age and gender trends in long-term opioid analgesic use for noncancer pain. Am J Public Health 2010;100(12):2541–7.

10. Unick GJ, Rosenblum D, Mars S, et al. Intertwined epidemics: national demographic trends in hospitalizations for heroin- and opioid-related overdoses, 1993-2009. PLoS One 2013;8(2):e54496.

11. Ciccarone D. Heroin in brown, black and white: structural factors and medical consequences in the US heroin market. Int J Drug Policy 2009;20(3):277–82.

12. Jones CM, Logan J, Gladden RM, et al. Vital signs: demographic and substance use trends among heroin users—United States, 2002–2013. MMWR Morb Mortal Wkly Rep 2015;64(26):719.

13. Ciccarone D. The triple wave epidemic: supply and demand drivers of the US opioid overdose crisis. Int J Drug Policy 2019. [Epub ahead of print].

14. Rudd RA, Aleshire N, Zibbell JE, et al. Increases in drug and opioid overdose deaths–United States, 2000-2014. MMWR Morb Mortal Wkly Rep 2016; 64(50–51):1378–82.

15. McHugh RK, Devito EE, Dodd D, et al. Gender differences in a clinical trial for prescription opioid dependence. J Subst Abuse Treat 2013;45(1):38–43.

16. Lewis B, Hoffman LA, Nixon SJ. Sex differences in drug use among polysubstance users. Drug Alcohol Depend 2014;145:127–33.

17. McHugh RK, Votaw VR, Sugarman DE, et al. Sex and gender differences in substance use disorders. Clin Psychol Rev 2018;66:12–23.

18. Liang Y, Goros MW, Turner BJ. Drug overdose: differing risk models for women and men among opioid users with non-cancer pain. Pain Med 2016;17(12):2268–79.

19. Green KM, Zebrak KA, Robertson JA, et al. Interrelationship of substance use and psychological distress over the life course among a cohort of urban African Americans. Drug Alcohol Depend 2012;123(1–3):239–48.

20. Wilkinson AL, Halpern CT, Herring AH, et al. Testing longitudinal relationships between binge drinking, marijuana use, and depressive symptoms and moderation by sex. J Adolesc Health 2016;59(6):681–7.

21. Engstrom M, El-Bassel N, Gilbert L. Childhood sexual abuse characteristics, intimate partner violence exposure, and psychological distress among women in methadone treatment. J Subst Abuse Treat 2012;43(3):366–76.

22. Greenfield SF, Back SE, Lawson K, et al. Substance abuse in women. Psychiatr Clin 2010;33(2):339–55.

23. Tsang A, Von Korff M, Lee S, et al. Common chronic pain conditions in developed and developing countries: gender and age differences and comorbidity with depression-anxiety disorders. J Pain 2008;9(10):883–91.

24. Andersson HI, Ejlertsson G, Leden I, et al. Chronic pain in a geographically defined general population: studies of differences in age, gender, social class, and pain localization. Clin J Pain 1993;9(3):174–82.

25. Fillingim RB, King CD, Ribeiro-Dasilva MC, et al. Sex, gender, and pain: a review of recent clinical and experimental findings. J Pain 2009;10(5):447–85.

26. Sullivan MJ, Tripp DA, Santor D. Gender differences in pain and pain behavior: the role of catastrophizing. Cognit Ther Res 2000;24(1):121–34.

27. Edwards RR, Haythornthwaite JA, Sullivan MJ, et al. Catastrophizing as a mediator of sex differences in pain: differential effects for daily pain versus laboratory-induced pain. Pain 2004;111(3):335–41.
28. Sharifzadeh Y, Kao MC, Sturgeon JA, et al. Pain catastrophizing moderates relationships between pain intensity and opioid prescription: nonlinear sex differences revealed using a learning health system. Anesthesiology 2017;127(1):136–46.
29. Hser YI, Mooney LJ, Saxon AJ, et al. Chronic pain among patients with opioid use disorder: results from electronic health records data. J Subst Abuse Treat 2017;77:26–30.
30. Chang YP, Compton P. Management of chronic pain with chronic opioid therapy in patients with substance use disorders. Addict Sci Clin Pract 2013;8:21.
31. Campbell ANC, Barbosa-Leiker C, Hatch-Maillette M, et al. Gender differences in demographic and clinical characteristics of patients with opioid use disorder entering a comparative effectiveness medication trial. Am J Addict 2018;27(6): 465–70.
32. Amaro H, Dai J, Arevalo S, et al. Effects of integrated trauma treatment on outcomes in a racially/ethnically diverse sample of women in urban community-based substance abuse treatment. Bull N Y Acad Med 2007;84(4):508–22.
33. Chisolm MS, Coleman-Cowger VH. Response: how to use a window of opportunity. Addict Sci Clin Pract 2011;6(1):71–2.
34. Olander EK, Darwin ZJ, Atkinson L, et al. Beyond the 'teachable moment' - a conceptual analysis of women's perinatal behaviour change. Women Birth 2016;29(3):e67–71.
35. Smith K, Lipari RN. Women of childbearing age and opioids. The CBHSQ Report: January 17, 2017. Rockville (MD): Center for Behavioral Health Statistics and Quality, Substance Abuse and Mental Health Services Administration. Available at: https://www.samhsa.gov/data/sites/default/files/report_2724/ShortReport-2724. html. Accessed September 21, 2019.
36. American Society of Addiction Medicine Public POlicy Statement on "women alcohol and other drugs and pregnancy". Available at: https://www.asam.org/advocacy/find-a-policy-statement/view-policy-statement/public-policy-statements/2011/12/15/women-alcohol-and-other-drugs-and-pregnancy. Accessed September 21, 2019.
37. Committee Opinion No. 711: opioid use and opioid use disorder in pregnancy. Obstet Gynecol 2017;130(2):e81–94.
38. Levy SJ, Williams JF. Substance use screening, brief intervention, and referral to treatment. Pediatrics 2016;138(1) [pii:e20161211].
39. Jones HE, Deppen K, Hudak ML, et al. Clinical care for opioid-using pregnant and postpartum women: the role of obstetric providers. Am J Obstet Gynecol 2014;210(4):302–10.
40. Chalmers B, Mangiaterra V, Porter R. WHO principles of perinatal care: the essential antenatal, perinatal, and postpartum care course. Birth 2001;28(3):202–7.
41. Terplan M, Minkoff H. Neonatal abstinence syndrome and ethical approaches to the identification of pregnant women who use drugs. Obstet Gynecol 2017; 129(1):164–7.
42. Wright TE, Terplan M, Ondersma SJ, et al. The role of screening, brief intervention, and referral to treatment in the perinatal period. Am J Obstet Gynecol 2016; 215(5):539–47.
43. Nichols JH, Christenson RH, Clarke W, et al. Executive summary. The National Academy of Clinical Biochemistry Laboratory Medicine Practice Guideline:

evidence-based practice for point-of-care testing. Clin Chim Acta 2007;
379(1–2):14–28 [discussion: 29–30].

44. Polak K, Kelpin S, Terplan M. Screening for substance use in pregnancy and the
newborn. Semin Fetal Neonatal Med 2019;24(2):90–4.

45. Organization WH. WHO recommendations on health promotion interventions for
maternal and newborn health 2015. World Health Organization; 2015.

46. Kampman K, Jarvis M. ASAM national practice guideline for the use of medications in the treatment of addiction involving opiod use. J Addict Med 2015;9(5):
358–67.

47. Strauss M, Andresko M, Stryker J, et al. Methadone maintenance during pregnancy: pregnancy, birth, and neonate characteristics. Am J Obstet Gynecol
1974;120(7):895–900.

48. Finnegan LP. Management of pregnant drug-dependent women. Ann N Y Acad
Sci 1978;311:135–46.

49. Stimmel B, Adamsons K. Narcotic dependency in pregnancy: methadone maintenance compared to use of street drugs. JAMA 1976;235(11):1121–4.

50. Kotelchuck M, Cheng ER, Belanoff C, et al. The prevalence and impact of substance use disorder and treatment on maternal obstetric experiences and birth
outcomes among singleton deliveries in Massachusetts. Matern Child Health J
2017;21(4):893–902.

51. Klaman SL, Isaacs K, Leopold A, et al. Treating women who are pregnant and
parenting for opioid use disorder and the concurrent care of their infants and
children: literature review to support national guidance. J Addict Med 2017;
11(3):178–90.

52. Reddy UM, Davis JM, Ren Z, et al. Opioid use in pregnancy, neonatal abstinence syndrome, and childhood outcomes: executive summary of a joint work-
shop by the Eunice Kennedy Shriver National Institute of Child Health and
Human Development, American College of Obstetricians and Gynecologists,
American Academy of Pediatrics, Society for Maternal-Fetal Medicine, Centers
for Disease Control and Prevention, and the March of Dimes Foundation. Obstet
Gynecol 2017;130(1):10–28.

53. Minozzi S, Amato L, Bellisario C, et al. Maintenance agonist treatments for opiate-
dependent pregnant women. Cochrane database Syst Rev 2013;(12):Cd006318.

54. Campus FH. Clinical guidance for treating pregnant and parenting women with
opioid use disorder and their infants 2018.

55. Jones CW, Terplan M. Pregnancy and naltrexone pharmacotherapy. Obstet Gynecol 2018;132(4):923–5.

56. Kelty E, Hulse G. A retrospective cohort study of birth outcomes in neonates
exposed to naltrexone in utero: a comparison with methadone-, buprenorphine-
and non-opioid-exposed neonates. Drugs 2017;77(11):1211–9.

57. Wiegand SL, Stringer EM, Stuebe AM, et al. Buprenorphine and naloxone
compared with methadone treatment in pregnancy. Obstet Gynecol 2015;
125(2):363–8.

58. World Health Organization (WHO). Guidelines for identification and management of substance use and substance use disorders in pregnancy. Geneva
(Switzerland): WHO; 2014. Available at: https://www.who.int/substance_abuse/
publications/pregnancy_guidelines/en/. Accessed September 21, 2019.

59. Terplan M, Laird HJ, Hand DJ, et al. Opioid detoxification during pregnancy: a
systematic review. Obstet Gynecol 2018;131(5):803–14.

60. Dole VP, Nyswander M. The treatment of heroin addiction. JAMA 1966;
195(11):972.

61. Greenwald MK, Comer SD, Fiellin DA. Buprenorphine maintenance and mu-opioid receptor availability in the treatment of opioid use disorder: implications for clinical use and policy. Drug Alcohol Depend 2014;144:1–11.
62. Shiu JR, Ensom MH. Dosing and monitoring of methadone in pregnancy: literature review. Can J Hosp Pharm 2012;65(5):380–6.
63. Caritis SN, Bastian JR, Zhang H, et al. An evidence-based recommendation to increase the dosing frequency of buprenorphine during pregnancy. Am J Obstet Gynecol 2017;217(4):459.e1-6.
64. Albright B, de la Torre L, Skipper B, et al. Changes in methadone maintenance therapy during and after pregnancy. J Subst Abuse Treat 2011;41(4):347–53.
65. Bastian JR, Chen H, Zhang H, et al. Dose-adjusted plasma concentrations of sublingual buprenorphine are lower during than after pregnancy. Am J Obstet Gynecol 2017;216(1):64.e1-7.
66. Wilder CM, Hosta D, Winhusen T. Association of methadone dose with substance use and treatment retention in pregnant and postpartum women with opioid use disorder. J Subst Abuse Treat 2017;80:33–6.
67. Lo-Ciganic WH, Donohue JM, Kim JY, et al. Adherence trajectories of buprenorphine therapy among pregnant women in a large state Medicaid program in the United States. Pharmacoepidemiol Drug Saf 2019;28(1):80–9.
68. Krans EE, Zickmund SL, Rustgi VK, et al. Screening and evaluation of hepatitis C virus infection in pregnant women on opioid maintenance therapy: a retrospective cohort study. Subst Abuse 2016;37(1):88–95.
69. Tuten M, Heil SH, O'Grady KE, et al. The impact of mood disorders on the delivery and neonatal outcomes of methadone-maintained pregnant patients. Am J Drug Alcohol Abuse 2009;35(5):358–63.
70. ACOG Committee Opinion No. 757: screening for perinatal depression. Obstet Gynecol 2018;132(5):e208–12.
71. McLafferty LP, Becker M, Dresner N, et al. Guidelines for the management of pregnant women with substance use disorders. Psychosomatics 2016;57(2): 115–30.
72. Carroll KM, Weiss RD. The role of behavioral interventions in buprenorphine maintenance treatment: a review. Am J Psychiatry 2017;174(8):738–47.
73. Jones HE, O'Grady K, Dahne J, et al. Management of acute postpartum pain in patients maintained on methadone or buprenorphine during pregnancy. Am J Drug Alcohol Abuse 2009;35(3):151–6.
74. SAMHSA. Clinical guidance for treating pregnant and parenting women with opioid use disorder and their infants. Rockville (MD): Substance Abuse and Mental Health Services Administration; 2018. HHS Publication No. (SMA) 18-5054.
75. Meyer M, Paranya G, Keefer Norris A, et al. Intrapartum and postpartum analgesia for women maintained on buprenorphine during pregnancy. Eur J Pain 2010;14(9):939–43.
76. Meyer M, Wagner K, Benvenuto A, et al. Intrapartum and postpartum analgesia for women maintained on methadone during pregnancy. Obstet Gynecol 2007; 110(2 Pt 1):261–6.
77. Vilkins AL, Bagley SM, Hahn KA, et al. Comparison of post-cesarean section opioid analgesic requirements in women with opioid use disorder treated with methadone or buprenorphine. J Addict Med 2017;11(5):397–401.
78. Jarlenski M, Bodnar LM, Kim JY, et al. Filled prescriptions for opioids after vaginal delivery. Obstet Gynecol 2017;129(3):431–7.

79. Mills JR, Huizinga MM, Robinson SB, et al. Draft opioid-prescribing guidelines for uncomplicated normal spontaneous vaginal birth. Obstet Gynecol 2019; 133(1):81–90.

80. Alford DP, Compton P, Samet JH. Acute pain management for patients receiving maintenance methadone or buprenorphine therapy. Ann Intern Med 2006; 144(2):127–34.

81. Arout CA, Waters AJ, MacLean RR, et al. Minocycline does not affect experimental pain or addiction-related outcomes in opioid maintained patients. Psychopharmacology (Berl) 2018. [Epub ahead of print].

82. Karasz A, Zallman L, Berg K, et al. The experience of chronic severe pain in patients undergoing methadone maintenance treatment. J Pain Symptom Manage 2004;28(5):517–25.

83. Tully KP, Stuebe AM, Verbiest SB. The fourth trimester: a critical transition period with unmet maternal health needs. Am J Obstet Gynecol 2017;217(1):37–41.

84. Daw JR, Hatfield LA, Swartz K, et al. Women in the United States experience high rates of coverage 'churn' in months before and after childbirth. Health Aff (Millwood) 2017;36(4):598–606.

85. Mangat AK, Schmolzer GM, Kraft WK. Pharmacological and non-pharmacological treatments for the Neonatal Abstinence Syndrome (NAS). Semin Fetal Neonatal Med 2019;24(2):133–41.

86. Cottrell EB, Chou R, Wasson N, et al. Reducing risk for mother-to-infant transmission of hepatitis C virus: a systematic review for the U.S. Preventive Services Task Force. Ann Intern Med 2013;158(2):109–13.

87. Cox EQ, Sowa NA, Meltzer-Brody SE, et al. The perinatal depression treatment cascade: baby steps toward improving outcomes. J Clin Psychiatry 2016;77(9): 1189–200.

88. Krans EE, Cochran G, Bogen DL. Caring for opioid-dependent pregnant women: prenatal and postpartum care considerations. Clin Obstet Gynecol 2015;58(2):370–9.

89. Terplan M, Garrett J, Hartmann K. Gestational age at enrollment and continued substance use among pregnant women in drug treatment. J Addict Dis 2009; 28(2):103–12.

90. Wilder C, Lewis D, Winhusen T. Medication assisted treatment discontinuation in pregnant and postpartum women with opioid use disorder. Drug Alcohol Depend 2015;149:225–31.

91. Ebrahim SH, Gfroerer J. Pregnancy-related substance use in the United States during 1996-1998. Obstet Gynecol 2003;101(2):374–9.

92. Koch AR, Geller SE. Addressing maternal deaths due to violence: the Illinois experience. Am J Obstet Gynecol 2017;217(5):556.e1-6.

93. Heil SH, Jones HE, Arria A, et al. Unintended pregnancy in opioid-abusing women. J Subst Abuse Treat 2011;40(2):199–202.

94. Robinowitz N, Muqueeth S, Scheibler J, et al. Family planning in substance use disorder treatment centers: opportunities and challenges. Substance Use Misuse 2016;51(11):1477–83.

95. Krans EE, Kim JY, James AE 3rd, et al. Postpartum contraceptive use and interpregnancy interval among women with opioid use disorder. Drug Alcohol Depend 2018;185:207–13.

96. Kotha A, Chen BA, Lewis L, et al. Prenatal intent and postpartum receipt of long-acting reversible contraception among women receiving medication-assisted treatment for opioid use disorder. Contraception 2019;99(1):36–41.

97. Terplan M, Kennedy-Hendricks A, Chisolm MS. Prenatal substance use: exploring assumptions of maternal unfitness. Subst Abuse 2015;9(Suppl 2):1–4.
98. Paltrow LM, Flavin J. Arrests of and forced interventions on pregnant women in the United States, 1973-2005: implications for women's legal status and public health. J Health Polit Policy Law 2013;38(2):299–343.
99. Angelotta C, Appelbaum PS. Criminal charges for child harm from substance use in pregnancy. J Am Acad Psychiatry L 2017;45(2):193–203.
100. Goodwin M. How the criminalization of pregnancy robs women of reproductive autonomy. Hastings Cent Rep 2017;47(Suppl 3):S19–27.

UNITED STATES POSTAL SERVICE®

Statement of Ownership, Management, and Circulation
(All Periodicals Publications Except Requester Publications)

1. Publication Title	2. Publication Number	3. Filing Date
CLINICS IN PERINATOLOGY	001 - 744	9/18/2019

4. Issue Frequency	5. Number of Issues Published Annually	6. Annual Subscription Price
MAR, JUN, SEP, DEC	4	$309.00

7. Complete Mailing Address of Known Office of Publication (Not printer) (Street, city, county, state, and ZIP+4®)

ELSEVIER INC.
230 Park Avenue, Suite 800
New York, NY 10169

Contact Person
STEPHEN R. BUSHING

Telephone (Include area code)
215-239-3688

8. Complete Mailing Address of Headquarters or General Business Office of Publisher (Not printer)

ELSEVIER INC.
230 Park Avenue, Suite 800
New York, NY 10169

9. Full Names and Complete Mailing Addresses of Publisher, Editor, and Managing Editor (Do not leave blank)

Publisher (Name and complete mailing address)

TAYLOR BALL, ELSEVIER INC.
1600 JOHN F KENNEDY BLVD. SUITE 1800
PHILADELPHIA, PA 19103-2899

Editor (Name and complete mailing address)

KERRY HOLLAND, ELSEVIER INC.
1600 JOHN F KENNEDY BLVD. SUITE 1800
PHILADELPHIA, PA 19103-2899

Managing Editor (Name and complete mailing address)

PATRICK MANLEY, ELSEVIER INC.
1600 JOHN F KENNEDY BLVD. SUITE 1800
PHILADELPHIA, PA 19103-2899

10. Owner (Do not leave blank. If the publication is owned by a corporation, give the name and address of the corporation immediately followed by the names and addresses of all stockholders owning or holding 1 percent or more of the total amount of stock. If not owned by a corporation, give the names and addresses of the individual owners. If owned by a partnership or other unincorporated firm, give its name and address as well as those of each individual owner. If the publication is published by a nonprofit organization, give its name and address.)

Full Name	Complete Mailing Address
WHOLLY OWNED SUBSIDIARY OF REED/ELSEVIER, US HOLDINGS	1600 JOHN F KENNEDY BLVD. SUITE 1800 PHILADELPHIA, PA 19103-2899

11. Known Bondholders, Mortgagees, and Other Security Holders Owning or Holding 1 Percent or More of Total Amount of Bonds, Mortgages, or Other Securities. If none, check box ▶ ☐ None

Full Name	Complete Mailing Address
N/A	

12. Tax Status (For completion by nonprofit organizations authorized to mail at nonprofit rates) (Check one)
The purpose, function, and nonprofit status of this organization and the exempt status for federal income tax purposes:
☒ Has Not Changed During Preceding 12 Months
☐ Has Changed During Preceding 12 Months (Publisher must submit explanation of change with this statement)

PS Form **3526**, July 2014 [Page 1 of 4 (see instructions page 4)] PSN: 7530-01-000-9931   PRIVACY NOTICE: See our privacy policy on www.usps.com.

13. Publication Title	14. Issue Date for Circulation Data Below
CLINICS IN PERINATOLOGY	JUNE 2019

15. Extent and Nature of Circulation			Average No. Copies Each Issue During Preceding 12 Months	No. Copies of Single Issue Published Nearest to Filing Date
a. Total Number of Copies (Net press run)			536	588
b. Paid Circulation (By Mail and Outside the Mail)	(1)	Mailed Outside-County Paid Subscriptions Stated on PS Form 3541 (Include paid distribution above nominal rate, advertiser's proof copies, and exchange copies)	391	446
	(2)	Mailed In-County Paid Subscriptions Stated on PS Form 3541 (Include paid distribution above nominal rate, advertiser's proof copies, and exchange copies)	0	0
	(3)	Paid Distribution Outside the Mails Including Sales Through Dealers and Carriers, Street Vendors, Counter Sales, and Other Paid Distribution Outside USPS®	96	111
	(4)	Paid Distribution by Other Classes of Mail Through the USPS (e.g., First-Class Mail®)	0	0
c. Total Paid Distribution (Sum of 15b (1), (2), (3), and (4))			487	557
d. Free or Nominal Rate Distribution (By Mail and Outside the Mail)	(1)	Free or Nominal Rate Outside-County Copies included on PS Form 3541	36	14
	(2)	Free or Nominal Rate In-County Copies Included on PS Form 3541	0	0
	(3)	Free or Nominal Rate Copies Mailed at Other Classes Through the USPS (e.g., First-Class Mail)	0	0
	(4)	Free or Nominal Rate Distribution Outside the Mail (Carriers or other means)	0	0
e. Total Free or Nominal Rate Distribution (Sum of 15d (1), (2), (3) and (4))			36	14
f. Total Distribution (Sum of 15c and 15e)			523	571
g. Copies not Distributed (See Instructions to Publishers #4 (page #3))			13	17
h. Total (Sum of 15f and g)			536	588
i. Percent Paid (15c divided by 15f times 100)			93.12%	97.55%

* If you are claiming electronic copies, go to line 16 on page 3. If you are not claiming electronic copies, skip to line 17 on page 3.

PS Form **3526**, July 2014 (Page 2 of 4)

16. Electronic Copy Circulation	Average No. Copies Each Issue During Preceding 12 Months	No. Copies of Single Issue Published Nearest to Filing Date
a. Paid Electronic Copies ▶		
b. Total Paid Print Copies (Line 15c) + Paid Electronic Copies (Line 16a) ▶		
c. Total Print Distribution (Line 15f) + Paid Electronic Copies (Line 16a) ▶		
d. Percent Paid (Both Print & Electronic Copies) (16b divided by 16c × 100) ▶		

☒ I certify that 50% of all my distributed copies (electronic and print) are paid above a nominal price.

17. Publication of Statement of Ownership

☒ If the publication is a general publication, publication of this statement is required. Will be printed ☐ Publication not required.
in the DECEMBER 2019 issue of this publication.

18. Signature and Title of Editor, Publisher, Business Manager, or Owner

[signature] Stephen R. Bushing   Date 9/18/2019

STEPHEN R. BUSHING - INVENTORY DISTRIBUTION CONTROL MANAGER

I certify that all information furnished on this form is true and complete. I understand that anyone who furnishes false or misleading information on this form or who omits material or information requested on the form may be subject to criminal sanctions (including fines and imprisonment) and/or civil sanctions (including civil penalties).

PS Form **3526**, July 2014 (Page 3 of 4)   PRIVACY NOTICE: See our privacy policy on www.usps.com

Moving?

Make sure your subscription moves with you!

To notify us of your new address, find your **Clinics Account Number** (located on your mailing label above your name), and contact customer service at:

Email: journalscustomerservice-usa@elsevier.com

800-654-2452 (subscribers in the U.S. & Canada)
314-447-8871 (subscribers outside of the U.S. & Canada)

Fax number: 314-447-8029

Elsevier Health Sciences Division
Subscription Customer Service
3251 Riverport Lane
Maryland Heights, MO 63043

*To ensure uninterrupted delivery of your subscription, please notify us at least 4 weeks in advance of move.

Printed and bound by CPI Group (UK) Ltd, Croydon, CR0 4YY

03/10/2024

01040405-0002